Managing the Critically Ill Child

A Guide for Anaesthetists and Emergency Physicians

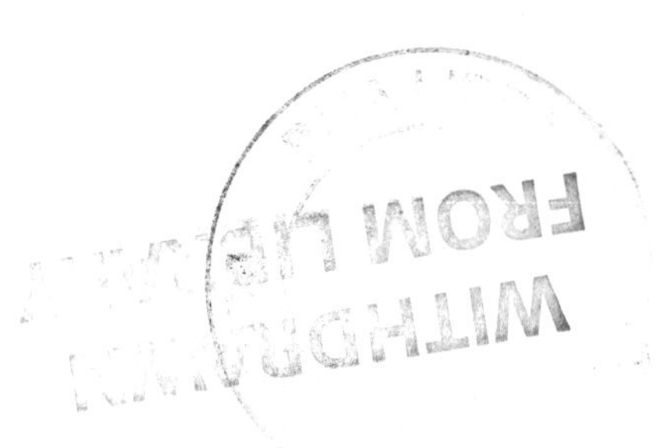

Managing the Critically Ill Child

A Guide for Anaesthetists and Emergency Physicians

Edited by

Richard Skone
Specialist Registrar, Paediatric Intensive Care Medicine and Anaesthetics, Birmingham Children's Hospital, Birmingham, UK

Fiona Reynolds
Paediatric Intensivist, Paediatric Intensive Care Unit, Birmingham Children's Hospital, Birmingham, UK

Steven Cray
Consultant Paediatric Anaesthetist, Birmingham Children's Hospital, Birmingham, UK

Oliver Bagshaw
Consultant in Anaesthesia and Intensive Care, Birmingham Children's Hospital, Birmingham, UK

Kathleen Berry
Consultant in Paediatric Emergency Medicine, Birmingham Children's Hospital, Birmingham, UK

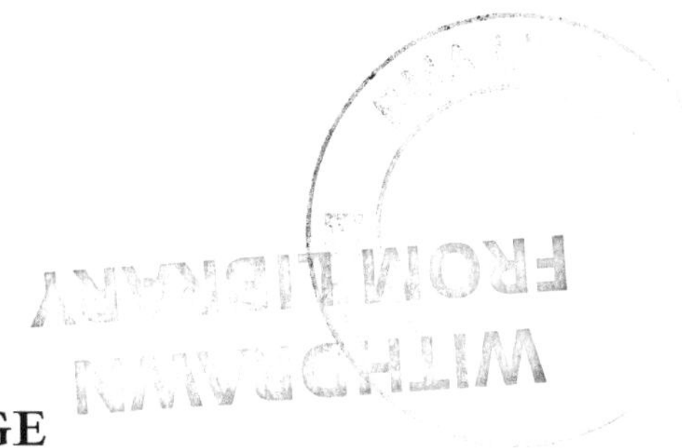

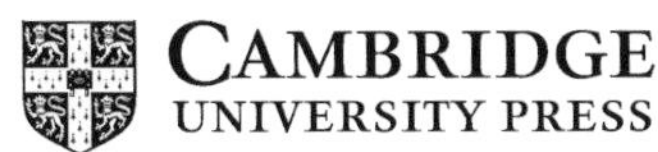
CAMBRIDGE
UNIVERSITY PRESS

CAMBRIDGE UNIVERSITY PRESS
Cambridge, New York, Melbourne, Madrid, Cape Town,
Singapore, São Paulo, Delhi, Mexico City

Cambridge University Press
The Edinburgh Building, Cambridge CB2 8RU, UK

Published in the United States of America by
Cambridge University Press, New York

www.cambridge.org
Information on this title: www.cambridge.org/9781107652323

First published 2013

A catalogue record for this publication is available from the British Library

Library of Congress Cataloguing in Publication data

Managing the critically ill child : a guide for anaesthetists and emergency physicians / edited by Richard Skone ... [et al.].
p. cm.
Includes index.
ISBN 978-1-107-65232-3 (Paperback)
1. Pediatric emergencies. 2. Critically ill children–Medical care.
I. Skone, Richard
RJ370.M34 2013
618.92′0025–dc23

2012028035

ISBN 978-1-107-65232-3 Paperback

Contents

List of contributors

Suren Arul
Consultant Paediatric Surgeon, Birmingham Children's Hospital, Birmingham, UK

Oliver Bagshaw
Consultant in Anaesthesia and Intensive Care, Birmingham Children's Hospital, Birmingham, UK

Paul Baines
Consultant in Paediatric Intensive Care, Alder Hey Children's NHS Foundation Trust; Wellcome Trust Biomedical Ethics Research Fellow, Department of Professional Ethics, Keele University, Staffordshire, UK

Andrew J. Baldock
Specialist Registrar in Anaesthesia, Southampton University Hospital, Southampton, UK

Helga Becker
Consultant Anaesthetist, Dudley Group NHS Foundation Trust, West Midlands, UK

Julian Berlet
Consultant Anaesthetist, Worcester Royal Hospital, Worcester, UK

Kathleen Berry
Consultant in Paediatric Emergency Medicine, Birmingham Children's Hospital, Birmingham, UK

Ed Carver
Consultant Paediatric Anaesthetist, Birmingham Children's Hospital, Birmingham, UK

Matthew D. Christopherson
Specialist Registrar in Paediatric Intensive Care, Alder Hey Children's NHS Foundation Trust, Liverpool, UK

Alistair Cranston
Consultant Anaesthetist, Birmingham Children's Hospital, Birmingham, UK

Steven Cray
Consultant Paediatric Anaesthetist, Birmingham Children's Hospital, Birmingham, UK

Tim Day-Thompson
Specialist Registrar in Anaesthesia, Birmingham School of Anaesthesia, Birmingham, UK

Geoff Debelle
Consultant Paediatrician, Birmingham Children's Hospital, Birmingham, UK

Ursula Dickson
Consultant in Paediatric Anaesthesia, Birmingham Children's Hospital, Birmingham, UK

Stuart Hartshorn
Consultant in Paediatric Emergency Medicine, Birmingham Children's Hospital, Birmingham, UK

Marius Holmes
Specialist Registrar in Emergency Medicine, West Midlands Deanery, UK

Phil Hyde
Consultant Paediatric Intensivist, Paediatric Intensive Care Unit, Southampton General Hospital, Southampton, UK

Rhian Isaac
Paediatric Pharmacist, Birmingham Children's Hospital, Birmingham, UK

Kasyap Jamalapuram
Specialist Registrar, Paediatric Emergency Medicine, West Midlands Deanery, UK

Ian Jenkins
Consultant in Paediatric Anaesthesia and Intensive Care, Royal Hospital for Children, Bristol, UK

Adrian P. Jennings
Specialist Registrar in Paediatric Anaesthesia, Birmingham Children's Hospital, Birmingham, UK

Gareth D. Jones
Consultant in Anaesthesia and Paediatric Intensive Care, University Hospital Southampton NHS Trust, Southampton, UK

Mazyar Kanani
Fellow in Congenital Cardiothoracic Surgery, Great Ormond Street Hospital, London, UK

Josephine Langton
Specialist Registrar in Paediatric Emergency Medicine, Birmingham Children's Hospital, Birmingham, UK

Mark D. Lyttle
Consultant in Paediatric Emergency Medicine, Bristol Royal Hospital for Children, Bristol, UK

Oliver Masters
Specialist Registrar in Anaesthesia, Birmingham Children's Hospital, Birmingham, UK

Richard Pierson
Specialist Registrar in Anaesthetics, West Midlands Deanery, UK

Adrian Plunkett
Consultant Paediatric Intensivist, Birmingham Children's Hospital, Birmingham, UK

J. Nick Pratap
Assistant Professor in Anaesthesia and Paediatrics, Cincinnati Children's Hospital and University of Cincinnati, Cincinnati, OH, USA

Fiona Reynolds
Paediatric Intensivist, Paediatric Intensive Care Unit, Birmingham Children's Hospital, Birmingham, UK

Saikat Santra
Consultant in Paediatric Inherited Metabolic Disorders, Birmingham Children's Hospital, Birmingham, UK

Nick Sargant
Consultant in Paediatric Emergency Medicine, Bristol Royal Hospital for Children, Bristol, UK

Barney Scholefield
Clinical Research Fellow, Paediatric Intensive Care Unit, Birmingham Children's Hospital, Birmingham, UK

Brian Shields
Specialist Registrar in General Paediatrics, University Hospitals Coventry and Warwickshire NHS Trust, Coventry, UK

Kate Skone
Specialist Registrar in Paediatric Neurodisability, Birmingham Children's Hospital, Birmingham, UK

Richard Skone
Specialist Registrar, Paediatric Intensive Care Medicine and Anaesthetics, Birmingham Children's Hospital, Birmingham, UK

John Smith
Consultant Paediatric Cardiothoracic Anaesthetist, Paediatric Intensive Care Unit, Freeman Hospital, Newcastle upon Tyne, UK

Benjamin Stanhope
Clinical Lead, Emergency Department, Birmingham Children's Hospital, Birmingham, UK

Manu Sundaram
Specialist Registrar in Paediatric Emergency Medicine, Birmingham Children's Hospital, Birmingham, UK

Andy Tatman
Consultant Anaesthetist, Birmingham Children's Hospital, Birmingham, UK

Karl Thies
Consultant in Paediatric Anaesthesia, Birmingham Children's Hospital, Birmingham, UK

Sapna Verma
Consultant in Paediatric Emergency Medicine, Birmingham Children's Hospital, Birmingham, UK

Ian Wacogne
Consultant Paediatrician, Birmingham Children's Hospital, Birmingham, UK

Katie Z. Wright
Specialist Registrar in Paediatric and Adult Emergency Medicine, Birmingham Children's Hospital, Birmingham, UK

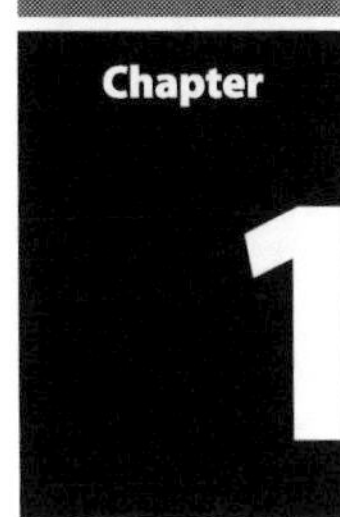

Chapter 1

Setting up a department for managing a sick child

Adrian P. Jennings and Julian Berlet

Introduction

In 2009 nearly 5000 UK children were admitted to 28 paediatric intensive care units (PICUs) from outlying hospitals, accounting for 64% of their unplanned workload. A designated retrieval team performed the transfer to PICU in 80% of cases with a median time of arrival at the patient's bedside of 2 hours.

Life-saving interventions required during the first few hours of stabilization remain the responsibility of the referring district general hospital (DGH) and cannot be deferred until the arrival of the retrieval team. Figure 1.1 demonstrates the frequency with which referring teams perform interventions. Any hospital that potentially manages sick children should have a series of systems in place that anticipate and ease the process of managing a critically ill child.

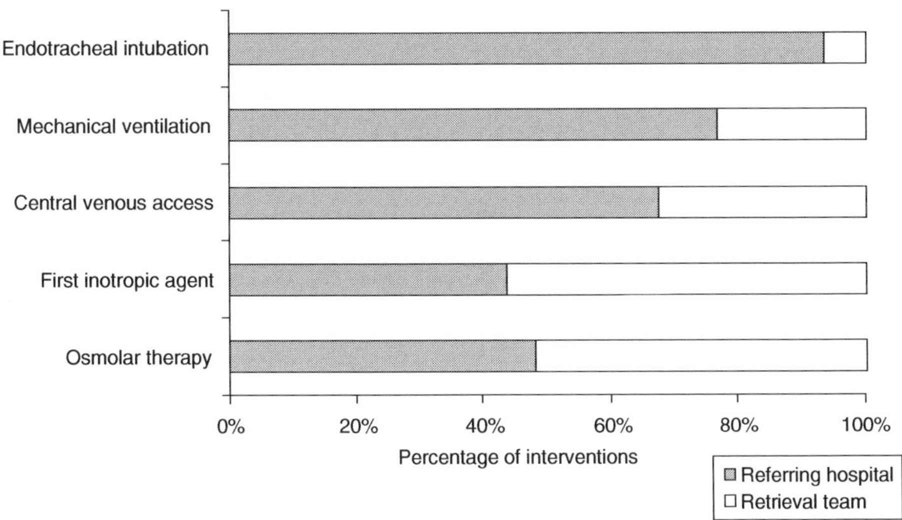

Figure 1.1. Proportion of interventions performed by referring hospitals and intensive care retrieval teams during stabilization of critically ill children. (Reproduced from S Lampariello, M Clement, AP Aralihond, *et al.* Stabilization of critically ill children at the district general hospital prior to intensive care retrieval: a snapshot of current practice. *Arch Dis Child* 2010;95:681–685, with permission from BMJ Publishing Group Ltd.)

Managing the Critically Ill Child, ed. Richard Skone *et al.* Published by Cambridge University Press.

Changing practice in district general hospitals (DGH)

Decreasing experience

Many UK hospitals have withdrawn surgical services for children younger than 2 years of age. This leaves many non-specialist anaesthetists with a duty of care to manage sick children out of normal working hours. Nevertheless, public expectation of standards of care has increased and DGH emergency departments (EDs) have maintained open access for all children.

The Tanner report

In 2006 the Department of Health published a report entitled 'The acutely or critically sick or injured child in the district general hospital – a team response'. The working group established that concerns about deskilling in the management of critically ill children were shared by many specialties, including paediatrics and ED medicine.

The report recommended that services for the critically ill child should be planned within a network, with the local tertiary hospital acting as a source of advice and support while stabilization is performed in the local DGHs. It suggested six generic skills which can be expected of all personnel involved in the care of critically sick or injured children in the DGH:

- to recognize the critically sick or injured child
- to initiate appropriate immediate treatment
- to work as part of a team
- to maintain and enhance skills
- to be aware of issues around safeguarding children
- to communicate effectively with children and carers.

There was also emphasis on the importance of considering the whole patient pathway.

Pre-hospital

The report commented that paramedic crews should transport sick children to the most appropriate paediatric facility, and make a clinical judgement to 'drive-by' a local DGH if the hospital does not have a team capable of stabilizing the critically ill child.

Resuscitation/stabilization

The report encouraged a team approach with shared responsibility. It emphasized that 'following the initial stages of resuscitation of a critically ill /collapsed child, stabilization and further management should not be left solely to the anaesthetist'.

Transfer

The sickest children require transfer to the local tertiary paediatric centre and this transfer should be performed by a designated paediatric retrieval team. However, in certain cases, it may be necessary for the DGH team to facilitate transfer (see Chapter 24).

Organizing a DGH to manage a critically ill child

Preparation

Relative to adult practice, the resuscitation and stabilization of critically ill children is a rare event. This increases the need for clear planning in order to ensure a smooth pathway for each patient. As a minimum each hospital should aim to have in place:

- clear communication pathways within and between departments
- easily available hospital protocols and guidelines for the management of common paediatric emergencies
- appropriate range of drugs and equipment
- adequate, ongoing training of staff in paediatric emergencies.

Location

Critically ill children usually present to the ED; however, they may also deteriorate in theatre, wards or other clinical areas. It is not practical to equip all clinical areas to stabilize a sick child. Local guidelines should be in place stating where resuscitation and stabilization should occur until the child's condition improves or the retrieval team arrives.

Designated areas should have appropriate neonatal and paediatric resuscitation equipment (see Table 1.1).

Children should ideally not be managed directly alongside adults and the need to support the family should be remembered. Parents and, where possible, children should be consulted when designing areas of care.

Equipment

Studies show that DGHs continue to perform the vast majority of key stabilization procedures on critically ill children (Figure 1.1). Therefore it is essential that paediatric and neonatal emergency equipment be readily available, well maintained and organized in a systematic fashion. Staff should undergo regular updates on its use, especially if used infrequently. A robust system should be in place to ensure that every area has rapid access to this equipment in the event of a paediatric emergency. Formal checks of drugs and equipment should be performed daily.

When equipment is procured in the DGH, it is useful to ensure suitability for use with both adult and paediatric patients as this will allow adult practitioners to use equipment with which they are familiar, and minimize cost.

The emergency equipment should be arranged in a structured manner so that staff using it infrequently can find the necessary items quickly and easily. This can be achieved in different ways:

- system-based
  - airway equipment of all sizes in one drawer, circulation in another
- weight-based
  - one tray containing all the equipment for a child of a given weight.

Team composition

Stabilization of a critically ill child requires a team of competent individuals. As a minimum this should include:

- a paediatrician or ED consultant
- an anaesthetist or intensivist
- a paediatric trained nurse.

Clinicians from other services such as surgery or radiology may also need to be involved. All staff should be trained in the specific needs of children and their families, including child protection and consent.

It may sometimes be necessary for staff within the DGH to undertake transfer to the regional PICU if the condition is time-critical (see Chapter 24) or if the retrieval team is unavailable. Suitably trained staff to facilitate the transfer must be available at all times.

Support services

Services such as haematology, chemical pathology, radiology and blood transfusion should meet the requirements of children. Pharmacy staff with specialist paediatric knowledge should be available to ensure safe and effective drug management.

Hospitals with no acute paediatric units

Where a DGH with no on-site inpatient paediatric facilities offers children unrestricted access via the ED, the challenges of being able to manage the critically ill child are even greater. 'Drive-by' policies agreed with the ambulance service and close links to other hospitals with paediatric facilities are crucial.

Table 1.1. Minimum set of equipment for paediatric emergency trolley. Further equipment should be kept easily accessible if needed, e.g. ventilators.

System	Suggested equipment needed
Airway and breathing	Oxygen mask with reservoir bag Self-inflating ventilation bag Oropharyngeal airway (size 00 to 4) Nasopharyngeal airway Face mask (all sizes) Endotracheal tubes Uncuffed (from size 2.5 up) Cuffed (from size 3.5 up) Laryngoscope Spare batteries Range of blades (straight and curved) Bougie (size 5 and 10 Fr) End-tidal CO_2 monitor Laryngeal mask airway (all sizes) Stethoscope Yankeuer sucker Magill's forceps Nebulizer mask Tracheostomy tubes
Circulation	Intravenous cannulas (24G upwards) Intraosseous needles Wide range of syringes Selection of needles Arterial blood gas syringe/capillary blood gas tubes IV administration/blood giving set Dressings Three-way taps and bungs Defibrillator with size appropriate pads
Drugs	Locally agreed emergency drugs should be kept on the trolley, e.g. adrenaline
Other	Blood glucose monitor Lubricating gel Scissors Nasogastric tubes Tape Blood sampling bottles Monitoring equipment, including ECG electrodes etc. Stopwatch Resuscitation chart Algorithms, protocols and guidelines

Teamwork and training

A team approach is essential in order to utilize the skill-mix of different practitioners.

Local policies should define the members of the paediatric resuscitation team, the team leader (for example, emergency medicine consultant or paediatrician) and the roles expected to be performed by each member of the team.

Front-line medical staff should be trained in paediatric resuscitation and receive annual updates. The departments should aim to support staff as they improve their knowledge and skills through:

- practising skills such as intraosseous needle insertion on purpose-built equipment
- completion of an accredited paediatric life-support course
- repeated attendance at these courses for the purpose of recertification/revalidation
- secondment to a local paediatric centre
- locally organized training (involving all departments)
- regular audit
- interdepartmental morbidity/mortality meetings
- tutorials and e-learning modules.

Practice scenarios are a good opportunity to test equipment and review or develop local guidelines. Audit and morbidity/mortality meetings are an essential opportunity for the team to reflect on how actual cases are managed and identify areas of improvement.

Table 1.2. Factors to be taken into consideration when planning paediatric emergency management.

Factors	Actions needed in preparing for a sick child
Staff	Regular scenario training Audit Multidisciplinary morbidity and mortality meetings Adequate clinical governance Paediatric life-support training Trained in using/setting up appropriate equipment
Equipment	Age-appropriate Laid out systematically Familiar to practitioners, i.e. same as adult if appropriate Appropriate drug availability Immediate availability of life-saving equipment Central store of more specialized equipment
Environment	Prompts, e.g. wall chart with age-appropriate GCS Clear guidelines and protocols Child-friendly Support for family
Procedural	Age-specific early warning scores to identify sick inpatients Rapid escalation policy Paediatric trained 'emergency response' team Good communication with support services Clear lines of communication with tertiary centre Policies for transferring patient – staff availability, training, etc.

Relationship with the tertiary centre

A good relationship between a DGH and the local tertiary paediatric centre is essential if care of the acutely ill or injured child is to be well organized and effective. Links and coordination need to exist on several different levels.

Networks

The creation of paediatric service networks has helped improve communication over the last decade. In many regions, paediatricians, surgeons and paediatric anaesthetists have formed groups that create regional guidelines, conduct peer reviews of services and organize study days. There is no substitute for face-to-face meetings between clinicians as a way of developing closer links between local and tertiary centres. Outreach education and feedback sessions in local units help to foster the feeling of partnerships between DGHs and regional PICUs.

Retrieval services

In the UK, the development of regional retrieval teams has greatly improved links with DGHs. They provide facilities such as:

- single point of access to PICU
- rapid response
- advice throughout the process of managing a child
- web-based drug calculators
- feedback sessions (two-way)
- teaching days
- attendance at morbidity and mortality meetings.

Much of the responsibility for achieving a good relationship with the tertiary centre still lies with staff in the DGH. Liaising with specialist clinicians regarding equipment purchases, agreeing joint protocols and discussing individual patients is an effective way of forging links. Visiting the tertiary centre to observe or participate in a clinical attachment often helps to create strong links.

Summary

The burden of stabilizing critically ill children falls to all members of the ED, anaesthetic and paediatric team within a DGH. It is important that plans are put in place to help make the situation as straightforward and safe as possible.

Golden rules

- Preparation is key to managing a sick child
- Have appropriate equipment available and easy to access
- Develop clear guidelines that are easy to access
- In-hospital, scenario-based training can improve teamwork and highlight potential problems

Further reading

Guidance on the provision of Paediatric Anaesthesia Services. Royal College of Anaesthetists, 2010. www.rcoa.ac.uk/docs/GPAS-Paeds.pdf.

Lunn JN. Implications of the national confidential enquiry into perioperative deaths for paediatric anaesthesia. *Paediatric Anaesthesia* 1992;**2**:69–72.

Standards for Children and Young People in Emergency Care Settings 2012: Developed by the Intercollegiate Committee for Standards for Children and Young People in Emergency Care Settings. www.rcpch.ac.uk/emergencycare.

The acutely or critically sick or injured child in the District General Hospital: A team response. Department of Health, 2006. http://www.dh.gov.uk/Consultations/ClosedConsultations/ClosedConsultationsArticle/fs/en?CONTENT_ID=4124412&chk=lIVmJg.

Tomlinson A. Anaesthetists and care of the critically ill child. *Anaesthesia* 2003;**58**:309–311.

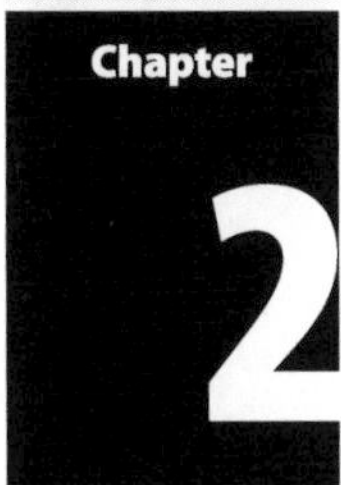

Team approach and organization

Richard Skone

Introduction

A critically ill/injured child, depending on where they present, will be looked after by many of the following professionals:

- paediatrician
- ED physician
- ED nurse
- paediatric nurse
- anaesthetist
- intensivist
- surgeon
- operating department practitioner (ODP).

Within this team there are often two specific groups: those who have a paediatric background but who do not frequently manage critically ill patients and those who are used to managing critically ill adults but have little paediatric experience. A good team will use the skills and experience of both groups and allow them to work freely and calmly.

The following chapter aims to cover the factors that make the team looking after a critically ill child function well.

Differences in paediatric emergencies

The major difference in the team composition compared to most other medical emergencies is the presence of paediatric doctors and nurses.

Some paediatricians will have spent a considerable amount of time on neonatal units as part of their training. They will have acquired a lot of skills such as intubation and insertion of arterial lines in babies. This can alleviate some of the pressure on anaesthetists who might otherwise feel that the burden of stabilizing small children lies with them.

It should be remembered, however, that neonatal emergencies seen in ED may not be similar to those in a maternity unit. The major difference in ED is that the children are less well 'controlled' in their presentation. A child may present at any point during their illness (rather than after birth or on a neonatal intensive care unit (NICU)). In this respect the ED doctor or anaesthetist will be more familiar with time-critical emergencies such as fulminant sepsis or trauma.

Managing the Critically Ill Child, ed. Richard Skone *et al.* Published by Cambridge University Press.

Organizing the team

Approaches to team management

Vertical management

In the past much has been made of vertical management systems when dealing with medical emergencies (Figure 2.1). In this structure all information is relayed to the team leader, and then disseminated to the team. The team leader is responsible for all decision-making and tells the team members what to do at each stage.

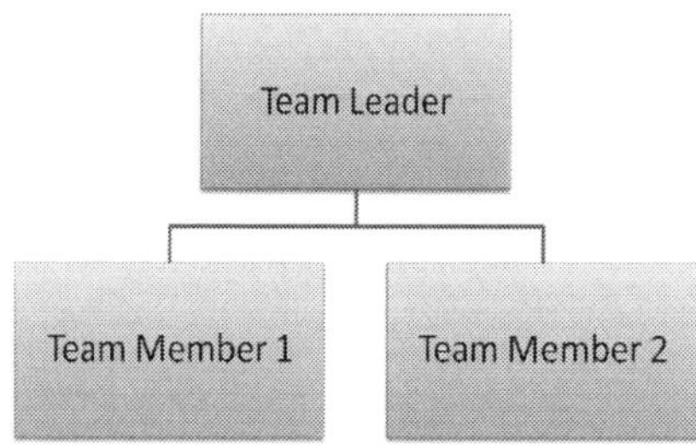

Figure 2.1. Vertical management.

Vertical management has its place. In particular, it is useful when managing an inexperienced team, or when a child has a single life-threatening problem that needs immediate attention.

Horizontal management

When compared to vertical management, horizontal management has greater responsibility and involvement for all members (Figure 2.2). Team members make decisions, carry out tasks and communicate with each other and the team leader in a controlled, calm fashion.

The advantage of the horizontal structure is that it recognizes that people within a team have their own skills and abilities. It also recognizes that it is very rare for the management of medical emergencies to occur in a stepwise fashion. The key to this management structure is communication.

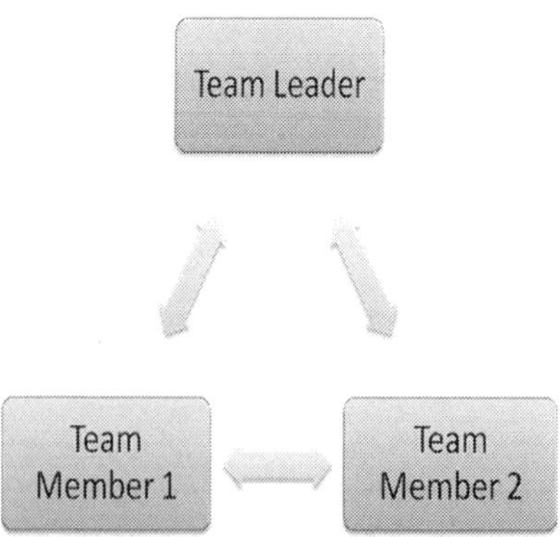

Figure 2.2. Horizontal management.

Team leader

The team leader for a paediatric emergency should not be chosen purely on the basis of seniority. Experience either within the required specialty or of managing emergency teams should determine the best person to manage the situation.

This experience is essential as the team leader's role will involve core skills such as:

- keeping an overview of the situation
- integrating information as it feeds back
- prioritizing treatments
- keeping everyone aware of their tasks and overall plan.

Team member

As well as having roles, team members have responsibilities. It is up to each member to:

- work within their competencies
- take appropriate decisions
- listen
- communicate clearly in a timely manner.

When a team member feels that they have a piece of information that needs to be raised urgently, they need to remember that they are working within a team. Other members may also have similarly urgent problems. Hence timely and concise relaying of information is essential.

If at any point in the emergency someone has been allocated a role which has no pressing problem, they should mention this at an opportune moment so that they can be reassigned further tasks within the resuscitation.

Why mistakes happen

As mentioned in Chapter 1, preparation and practice are the best way to try to improve team interaction. Errors occur for various reasons. Systems should be put in place to minimize the potential for errors. However, human factors will still contribute to problems if not addressed.

Technical skills

Technical procedures performed on small children are difficult especially if not done often. Simulation and practical experience are important in order to stop fear of performing procedures impacting on other aspects of the team interactions. Time-critical skills should be performed by the most skilled person. The team leader also has a role in keeping the emergency room calm, as anxiety will worsen performance.

Knowledge

Like technical skills, it is up to individual doctors to make sure that their knowledge is up to date. Hospitals should facilitate relevant CPD in paediatric practice for appropriate staff members.

Team dynamic

Communication is a two-way process. Each team member needs to feel comfortable raising concerns with the team leader, while remaining clear and concise when reporting facts.

Mistakes happen within hierarchical teams when 'junior' members feel unable to raise concerns. This can be due to lack of confidence in their clinical ability or due to intimidation from the team leader.

When reporting a problem the team member needs to:

- be clear and concise about what needs to be done
- emphasize importance of corrective action
- escalate the issue calmly if they feel that the point has not been addressed.

At all points group responsibility needs to be emphasized by the team member so as not to seem confrontational. An example of raising a concern would therefore be:

> 'We need to intubate this child urgently because the saturations are low and I'm not able to ventilate her with a mask'

Differences of opinion

Differences of opinion between specialists are difficult to manage. Should a disagreement arise the involvement of the most experienced physicians should be sought. Many PICUs have a consultant on call or a retrieval team that could provide advice. At no point should the situation be allowed to degenerate into an argument.

Before the child arrives

If the child is being brought in as an emergency it is likely that the emergency team will assemble before the patient arrives. In this instance the time should be used to:

- introduce each member of the team (name and background)
- allocate roles appropriately
- brief the team about any information given by the paramedics
- give initial instructions and plan (the team leader)
- check equipment.

The time available to perform these tasks may vary and in cases of urgency it should be kept brief but thorough.

If the child is already present

Assembling a team

A pre-hospital emergency call from an ambulance crew enables swift team assembly. It is often harder to assemble a team promptly for a patient who is already in hospital. If a child deteriorates in ED, on a ward or in theatre there needs to be a clear policy within the hospital on how to escalate the situation to have the relevant people present quickly. The escalation policy needs to make certain that rapid escalation does not have to pass through a chain of seniority. Instead, if a senior member is needed, they should be contacted as a first line.

A paediatric inpatient who is deteriorating rapidly needs the same level of attention as the child brought in by ambulance. Each hospital needs to make sure that there is an appropriate senior doctor available 24 hours a day who can make themselves available at short notice.

Integrating the team

The health professional who put out the call to assemble an emergency team for an inpatient should assume the role of the team leader initially. They will need to:

- organize people as they arrive
- give a brief overview of the child
- describe what has happened since admission
- explain the plan for ongoing management
- hand over the team leader responsibility if appropriate.

Summary

The stress of infrequent paediatric emergencies can lead to teams underperforming. It is important that all hospitals rehearse paediatric emergency scenarios, both illness and injury, and have protocols and guidelines in place to ensure optimal management of sick and injured children.

Chapter 3

Equipment

Fiona Reynolds

Introduction

Having the correct equipment available in an emergency can make the management of a sick child much more straightforward. This chapter does not aim to tell people which particular pieces or brand of equipment to use. Instead it aims to highlight common problems in using medical equipment in children. It also offers a guide to which sizes to use in smaller children.

Airway and ventilation equipment

Airway

Endotracheal (ET) tubes

There are a number of formulae for the appropriate size of ET tube in children. The most commonly used in children in the UK is:

Size of ET tube (mm) = Age (yrs)/4 + 4

This, however, may either over- or underestimate the tube size so the size above and below should be immediately available. A common mistake is not to upsize a tube which is too small and has too great a leak.

Cuffed tubes have traditionally been used after puberty although more modern cuffed tubes have proved safe in children as small as term babies. These smaller cuffed tubes tend only to be available in children's hospitals as there is little need for them in an emergency situation.

Children suffering from serious burns should have a cuffed ET tube inserted, if the appropriate size is available locally, as changing the tube will be difficult once facial swelling has occurred. An uncut tube should also be used in this situation whether or not a cuffed tube is used.

Suction catheters for ET tube suctioning

Suction catheters should be available for ET tube suctioning. The appropriate size of suction catheter can be calculated using the formula:

Suction catheter size (Fr) = ET tube size (mm) × 2
(maximum size 14 Fr for an adolescent)

Managing the Critically Ill Child, ed. Richard Skone *et al.* Published by Cambridge University Press.

Suction systems

Wall or portable suction may be used in children. For endotracheal suction a pressure of 60–80 mmHg (8–10 kPa) is appropriate for neonates and up to 120 mmHg (< 16 kPa) for older children. It should be used for the minimum period of time.

Tracheostomy

The care-givers of children with a tracheostomy are usually expert in the management of the tracheostomy. Emergency supplies of a change of tracheostomy tube, including a smaller tube and suctioning equipment, usually accompany the child wherever they go. Most children with tracheostomies will have uncuffed tubes although occasionally a child may have a cuffed tube. Fenestrated tubes are rare before adolescence.

The care of the child with a tracheostomy mirrors that of an adult, with the understanding that the smaller tubes are more likely to block with secretions.

Ventilation

Mechanical ventilators

Most ICU ventilators used to ventilate adult-sized patients are capable of ventilating even the smallest of patients when used appropriately. An adult ventilator may be used with pressure control mode of ventilation, titrating the pressure to the measured tidal volume achieved or to the degree of chest movement and blood gases. Alternatively a volume control mode may be used provided the software allows a small enough tidal volume to be delivered (6–10 ml/kg).

The sedated, muscle-relaxed patient can be placed on a controlled mode of ventilation and the mechanics of triggering and synchronization are less important. Weaning from ventilation usually requires synchronization and triggering with the ventilator. Pressure triggering in children is usually not successful. Flow triggering commonly used in adult ICU is also used in paediatric practice (see Chapter 31).

Breathing circuits for ventilators

Breathing circuits come in two main sizes: 15 mm and 22 mm diameter tubing. The smaller tubing is used in children less than 20 kg.

The compression volume lost in the 15 mm ventilator tubing is smaller, i.e. the volume change of the circuit with each breath. However, some ventilators are able to compensate for any lost compression volume. In this case the size of the tubing is less of an issue.

The larger tubing often requires a catheter mount to connect from the 'Y' piece of the breathing circuit to the ET tube. The volume of the catheter mount contributes to dead space. For a child over 20 kg on mandatory ventilation this is usually not significant as the ventilator rate can be set to compensate. During the ventilator weaning phase when the patient is improving the dead space from the catheter mount can be an impediment to successful weaning.

The smaller 15 mm breathing circuits tend to have a single elbow connector. This connects directly to the ET tube without the need for a catheter mount and the attendant concerns about dead space.

Continuous positive airway pressure devices

Continuous positive airway pressure (CPAP) devices are commonly used for infants with moderate respiratory distress who do not require urgent intubation. The most common scenario is the neonate or infant with bronchiolitis. These babies may present with apnoea or moderate respiratory distress, which often improves with CPAP.

A variety of devices are used for this purpose and for the most part the paediatricians are usually familiar with the set-up in their own hospital. Anaesthetists and emergency department physicians should also make themselves familiar with the device used locally.

Most devices rely on an oxygen blender to titrate the percentage of inspired oxygen between 21% and 100%. The blender supplies a constant flow of gas maintained at a near constant pressure by an adjustable pressure valve. Alternatively the gas flow can be bubbled through an adjustable head of water (bubble CPAP). CPAP devices for infants typically use up to 15 l/min of gas and can generate pressures of up to 10 cmH_2O.

Non-invasive ventilation

Non-invasive ventilation is used in children for the same indications as used in adults. The same ventilators are used in children over 10 kg as are used in adult practice. Children require smaller interfaces such as nasal, full face or face shield masks. It may be difficult to move a child requiring non-invasive ventilation between hospitals without intubation.

Humidification

Active humidification is generally achieved by a warmed water bath evaporator/humidifier. The principles and temperatures used are identical to those used in adults. In general humidification aims at 100% relative humidity at body temperature for patients with an ET tube *in situ*. The humidifier dead space and resistance are not relevant in a fully ventilated patient or in the situation where a flow trigger is in use.

Passive humidification is achieved using a heat–moisture exchanger (HME). Care should be taken to use an appropriately sized HME. This is usually indicated on the device itself, giving a range of suggested tidal volumes where the device is suitable for use. An HME provides a lower level of humidity than is available using active humidification.

Chest drains

Insertion of a chest drain follows the same principles as in adult practice. Smaller sizes are used for draining a pneumothorax, with larger sizes used for draining fluid or blood (see Table 3.1). Underwater seals used for adults are identical to those used for children. Current guidance supports the use of ultrasound to guide the drainage of fluid.

Table 3.1. Guide to size of chest drain to use in a child.

Age	Chest drain size (French)
Newborn	8–12 Fr
Infant	12–16 Fr
Child	16–24 Fr
Adolescent	20–32 Fr

Arterial and venous access

Intravenous access

Peripheral lines

Peripheral lines start at 26G, which is primarily used for premature neonates under 1 kg. 24G cannulae are commonly used for term neonates although it is usually possible to insert a 22G cannula in the long saphenous vein at term.

The veins in the feet are commonly used in paediatric practice. Scalp veins are sometimes used in babies, making sure the temporal artery is not cannulated. In an emergency, the external jugular vein may be useful to gain intravenous access.

Intraosseous access

If intravenous access cannot be obtained in a timely manner, intraosseous access should be secured. The most common site used is the proximal tibia, although the distal femur and proximal humerus may also be used. The hand-held needles are being replaced by battery-powered devices such as the EZ-IO® as these are associated with a higher success rate. More experienced clinicians are more likely to choose to use an intraosseous needle at an earlier stage in a patient's treatment.

Central lines

The main sites of central venous line insertion are the internal jugular and femoral veins. Both should be accessed under ultrasound guidance using strict aseptic technique. The subclavian route is rarely used in paediatric practice. In the neonate the jugular vein usually measures up to three times the diameter of the femoral vein, but tends only to be used by expert practitioners. Complications of femoral vein puncture are much rarer. Unlike adult data there are no paediatric data to suggest a higher infection rate in femoral central lines.

The most commonly used central lines in children from 3 to 25 kg are 4.5 or 5 Fr triple-lumen central lines, which are available from 5 to 12.5 cm in length. The 5–8 cm length can be used for most situations where central venous access is required in an emergency. Above a weight of 25 kg, a 7 Fr adult line is commonly used.

Arterial access

Arterial lines

Specific cannulae designed for use as arterial lines for adults may be used in children above 25 kg. Under 25 kg these lines may be too large in relation to the child's artery.

In smaller children, it is common practice to use cannulae intended for intravenous insertion. Lines must be clearly marked to indicate the arterial nature of the line and any side port used for injection must be occluded by covering over with a dressing to prevent its use.

A 24G cannula is commonly used from 3 to 10 kg and a 22G above 10 kg. The radial artery and posterior tibial arteries are commonly used, with the femoral artery being used when more peripheral insertion sites prove impossible. The brachial and axillary arteries can be used. However, their use should be avoided in preterm babies due to the lack of collateral arterial flow.

Blood gas sampling devices

Arterial blood samples are taken in the same way as in adults. In-line sampling devices used for adults may be used in children. It is common practice to return the dead-space sample through either the inline sampling device or a syringe if an in-line sampling device is not used.

The minimum volume of blood should be taken; most modern blood gas machines need less than 1 ml per sample.

Monitoring and defibrillators

Monitoring

Minor modifications of the interfaces for physiological monitoring are necessary depending on the size of the patient. These modifications are smaller ECG stickers, pulse oximeter probes, blood pressure cuffs and temperature probes.

Invasive monitoring may rely on the insertion of smaller arterial and central lines but the transducers used in paediatric practice are the same as used in adult practice. In children less than 10 kg, many PICUs will use a flush of 1 ml per hour connected to a syringe driver by a 'Y' connector rather than the pressure transducer's default 3 ml/h flush. In the emergency situation the default 3 ml/h flush is entirely appropriate for a term baby or older child.

Defibrillators

Manual defibrillators have a range of energy levels that are suitable for even the smallest neonate. The energy required is dependent on the rhythm to be treated and is calculated from the weight of the child.

Two sizes of hands-free stick-on pads are available: small for children less than 10 kg and adult size for use in adults and children greater than 10 kg. The small pads are applied in the same position used in adults. If the only pads available are adult pads, they may be used in an emergency on the anterior and posterior chest wall using the same energy calculated according to the weight of the child and rhythm to be treated.

External pacing

Many external defibrillators have an external pacing mode which may be used for bradyarrhythmias. External pacing uses the same principles as in adults. The capture current is relatively lower and the paced rate should be higher according to the normal heart rate for the age of child.

Other equipment

Nasogastric tubes

Nasogastric tube length is measured from the nose to ear then to the stomach. Insertion in a child is usually simpler than in an adult. The site of placement must be confirmed by pH testing or X-ray. The size of nasogastric tube is usually:

- 6–8 Fr in a neonate
- 10–12 Fr in a toddler
- 14–16 Fr in an adolescent.

A nasogastric tube may be used to deflate the stomach when ventilating a child using a face mask and may be crucial to the ease of bagging in an emergency. For this reason, a nasogastric tube should always be available when intubating a paediatric patient.

Cervical hard collars

A properly sized hard collar can be used for cervical spine immobilization along with blocks and tapes for children over the age of 3 years. Single-piece hard collars used by the ambulance service and EDs do not fit most children under the age of 3 years.

There are hard two-piece collars designed for this younger age group, e.g. Miami Jr® from Ossur, but these tend to only be available in children's hospitals. In the absence of an appropriately sized hard collar, manual in-line immobilization should be maintained. If a small enough hard collar is not available for a toddler, after intubation and ventilation the sedated and muscle-relaxed patient may be immobilized using blocks and tapes pending admission to PICU. Care must be taken to minimize flexion and extension of the neck.

Summary

It is important that the right equipment is available to team members as they strive to stabilize a child. Delays in finding the right equipment can make an already fraught situation more stressful. As always, preparation and planning can make the process of stabilizing a sick patient more efficient.

Golden rules

- Most equipment used in adult practice is suitable for use with appropriate adjustments for size
- Equipment should be stored in a systematic way so that it is immediately available
- Advice on equipment can be obtained from the local PICU

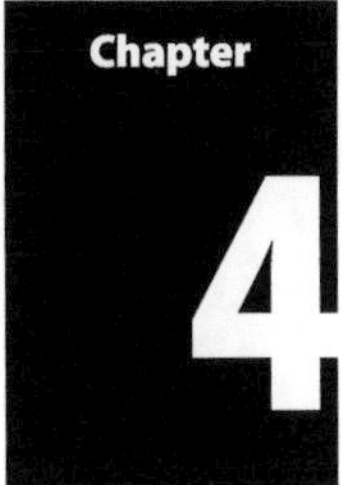

Chapter 4

Stabilization of the critically ill child: the initial approach

Richard Skone

Introduction

Most acutely critically ill children present first to their local DGH. However, they still remain a rare occurrence outside paediatric intensive care. The chances are slim therefore of a child presenting to a team with regular experience of resuscitating critically ill children.

There is plenty of knowledge, expertise and experience available amongst the team members outside specialized centres that can be applied to managing the critically ill child. This chapter aims to help to overcome some of the most common hurdles that adult physicians face, and address the most common fears.

All doctors in a specialty that may manage sick children should already be familiar with the treatment algorithms provided by resuscitation groups. This chapter will focus on the emergency care provided by DGH ED physicians and anaesthetists.

Differences between children and adults

When sitting exams from medical school to postgraduate training the list of differences between adults and children is usually learnt as in Table 4.1. In reality these differences make little difference if you:

- stick meticulously to the same gold standard principles of care delivered to adults, i.e. optimize oxygen delivery, fluid balance, electrolytes and temperature
- refer to reliable reference sources to remind you of normal values and drug doses
- ask for help from regional PICU retrieval teams early.

Managing the Critically Ill Child, ed. Richard Skone *et al.* Published by Cambridge University Press.

Table 4.1. Classic list of differences between adults and children.

Common issues	Consequences	How do I sort it out?
Anatomy and physiology		
Relatively large head	Trauma to head more common, greater forces on neck Airway positioning more challenging	Be aware of potential for isolated head injuries and position the head as carefully as possible Make sure that the head is supported at all times
Large body surface area for weight/volume	Temperature more difficult to maintain	Use active warming when needed Give warmed fluids
Relatively deep subcutaneous tissues/ small vessels	Cannulation technically difficult	Ask for help from paediatricians Use sensible sizes of cannulas Low threshold for IO needle
High metabolic rate Small glycogen stores	Rapid use of reserves Hypoglycaemia	Check blood sugars regularly Dextrose should be included in the maintenance fluid
Age-dependent normal values	Impossible to remember	Have correct values printed and attached to all areas that children might be managed in
Congenital disease, e.g. heart disease Rare syndromes and other diseases	Lack of familiarity with anatomy/ physiology/treatment	Seek advice from the PICU team
Airway and breathing		
Upper airway anatomy	Obstruction Difficult laryngoscopic view	Have an experienced anaesthetist on all paediatric emergency teams
Smaller airways	Resistance high – increased work of breathing Effect of secretions or oedema significant	Be aware that children tire quickly Have a low threshold for CPAP or intubation
Fewer alveoli	Reduced surface area for gas exchange Increased work of breathing	As above
High O_2 consumption	Rapid use of reserves Reduced time for intervention	Prepare and be thorough before intubation Do not persevere with laryngoscopy if you cannot intubate (Bag and mask)
Compliant chest wall Immature intercostal and diaphragm musculature	Energy wasted Increased work of breathing	Have a low threshold for CPAP and intubation

Table 4.1. *(cont.)*

Common issues	Consequences	How do I sort it out?
Cardiovascular		
Left ventricle less compliant	Less responsive stroke volume Tachycardia in an attempt to increase cardiac output	Pay close attention to response to fluid challenges Optimize electrolytes (especially calcium in neonates)
Myocardial failure/ vasoconstriction in response to sepsis	Blood pressure not useful to predict cardiac output Vasodilatory agents precipitate significant hypotension	Same as in adults
Relatively high circulating blood volume Small total blood volume	Small losses have significant cardiovascular effect	Fluid challenges form the mainstay of assessing fluid balance Be aware of significance of small volume losses
Emotional		
Parents	History has to be obtained from care-givers Care-giver emotional upset affects team	Paediatricians on team will be useful
Emotional impact of resuscitating sick child	Team performance may be affected by fear and upset	Regular debriefing sessions

By focussing on the differences between adults and children, many teams forget that they have the skills at hand to manage children well. Working calmly and in an organized fashion can compensate, to a degree, for a lack of familiarity. This is best achieved as described in Table 4.2.

Table 4.2. Broad outline of approach to a sick child.

The essence of care for children is:

Don't make it more complicated than it has to be
• Be systematic
• Use basic principles
• Use/listen to the parents/carers
• Access help/expertise from your team and PICU
• Acknowledge fear and upset – in yourself and others – then put it aside
• Concentrate on making the team work – remember human factors have a huge impact on ability to perform
• Prepare for eventualities (see Chapters 1 and 2)
  o Display visible normal values charts
  o Display charts for ET tube size/length and other parameters
  o Advanced paediatric resuscitation course – staff up-to-date
  o Debrief each significant episode with learning points – not just those with poor outcomes!

Assessing the critically ill child – when to intervene

Approach to the child

How you approach a sick child will depend on the severity of their illness. If the child arrives in cardiac arrest then a team approach where each member assesses, reports and acts on their designated role should be used. It is always worth taking 5 seconds when the patient arrives for the team leader to make a quick assessment, even if it is to confirm a lack of cardiac output.

If a child comes in seriously unwell, but awake, a single person examining the child may be appropriate in order to not upset the child. The team may arrive in a staggered fashion and the approach can quickly fragment. It is worth the team leader periodically repeating the management plan and allocation of roles in order to maintain order.

Airway assessment

The narrow airway of a child makes obstruction more likely when conditions such as inflammation and oedema of the trachea occur. If any of the signs seen in Table 4.3 occur then it is important to find out whether it is normal for that child. If it is not then the anaesthetist should be prepared to intubate the child (see Chapter 15).

Table 4.3. Signs of potential airway obstruction.

- Stridor – biphasic (inspiration and expiration) stridor being more serious
- Stertor/snoring
- Position of child – the child may sit in a 'tripod' position (leaning forward) to maintain optimum airway position
- Accessory muscle use in the presence of other upper airway signs
- Tracheal tug – indrawing of skin above sternal notch – especially if stridor present

Indications for intubation

There are many indications for intubation in a child. Most are the same as in adults, but some differ. Typical indications for intubation are detailed in Table 4.4.

Table 4.4. Indications for ventilation.

- Respiratory failure
- Cardiovascular instability – fluid resuscitation greater than 40 ml/kg with no response should prompt consideration
- Active significant bleeding
- An unconscious child (GCS < 9)
- Head injury with a need for control of CO_2/neuroprotection, etc.
- Airway burns
- Cardiac/respiratory arrest
- Significant invasive procedures

It is usually necessary to intubate and ventilate small children if you are performing invasive procedures, such as a jugular central line or chest drain insertion, as these are tolerated less well. The threshold for ventilation usually favours earlier intubation.

Breathing assessment

Children have a very compliant chest wall, and respiratory muscles that fatigue quickly. Their work of breathing, even at rest, is high compared to adults. The cartilaginous component of the ribs in children means that there is less opposition to the chest wall elastance. This results in a high closing capacity and a tendency towards airway collapse and atelectasis.

However, children are also very good at maintaining 'normal values', such as saturations and $PaCO_2$. They may not always look as if they're about to decompensate. This might go some way to explaining why paediatricians seem to have a low threshold for requesting intubation and ventilation in their patients.

By the time children do look as if they are in need of support, their ability to continue to maintain 'normal values' including any semblance of cardiovascular stability may be significantly compromised. Clinical signs that would make you worry about a child's respiratory effort include those seen in Table 4.5.

Intercostal recession is a common finding in many children with chest infections. On its own it may not point towards respiratory compromise. However, when present with some of the other signs from Table 4.5 it may become significant.

Table 4.5. Clinical signs of significant respiratory pathology.

- Respiratory rate – tachypnoea is one of the most sensitive signs
- Grunting – an effort to generate positive end-expiratory pressure (PEEP)
- Intercostal and subcostal recession
- Appearing drowsy or tired
- Apnoeas – especially in babies

A slowing of the respiratory rate and bradycardia are potentially preterminal events.

Capillary gases can be used in the same way as arterial blood gases (ABG) when deciding on management plans. The $PaCO_2$ will equate to that of an ABG. See below for further information about capillary gases.

When making a decision about intervening, waiting for a child to become 'sick enough to need intubation' can turn a straightforward procedure into a highly pressured risky event.

Cardiovascular assessment

The circulating volume of small children is large relative to their size. However, the absolute volume is easy to overestimate. Fluid losses (GI, skin, respiratory, urine, third-spacing) have a significant impact. For example, a baby with a circulating volume of 80 ml/kg who weighs 4 kg will have a circulating volume of 320 ml. A loss of 80 ml equates to 25% of their circulating volume.

Blood pressure is well maintained despite significant illness in children. It should always be measured but never relied on as a single parameter to guide therapy. Capillary refill time

(CRT) is commonly used in paediatric practice to aid assessment of cardiovascular status. As a single parameter it is not useful either – however, CRT can be used along with other parameters such as:

- heart rate
- pulse quality
- blood pressure
- lactic acidosis
- response to therapies (e.g. volume bolus)
- urine output.

Children have a huge capacity for vasoconstriction in the face of a low cardiac output. When examining a child in shock, feel along the arms and legs. There is often a cut-off point at which the limb becomes cool. The higher up the level, the more the child is compensating for a poor cardiac output.

The 'cold shock' response to sepsis seen in smaller children differs from the more usual adult model of 'high output' shock as it can occur very early in the disease process. Myocardial failure and intense vasoconstriction is a difficult situation to manage. It needs early recognition and aggressive management (see below and Chapter 5).

Table 4.6. Signs of a child with cardiovascular compromise.

- Tachycardia – a child may look well, but have an elevated heart rate (the cause of the tachycardia needs to be treated)
- Weak pulses
- Cool peripheries – the level at which a limb becomes cool may extend proximally as the child becomes sicker
- Mottling – assuming the child is not cold
- Hepatomegaly – this is a sign of heart failure, e.g. congenital heart disease or severe sepsis
- Decreased conscious level

Electrolytes and temperature

Electrolytes and blood sugar

The advent of blood gas machines that measure electrolytes and blood sugars in addition to the usual parameters has made their management very straightforward. A separate blood sugar measurement should be performed immediately on arrival for any sick child. It should then be noted on every blood gas from there on, at regular intervals.

Temperature

Core temperature should also be measured on arrival and, as with blood sugars, should be monitored at regular intervals. Again, management is straightforward; it is forgetting to measure that forms the main stumbling block.

As well as hypothermia in sick children, pyrexia can cause significant problems. Pyrexia can make children appear disproportionately unwell with lethargy and tachycardia. Pyrexia can also worsen outcome in head injuries. It should be treated by:

- removing the child's clothes
- giving antipyretics such as paracetamol
- keeping the environment cool
- placing icepacks (head, axillae and over femoral arteries).

Carrying out the interventions – what to do when you *are* the specialist help

As mentioned above, anxiety can seriously affect performance. It is better to acknowledge fear and to deal with it than to drown under the pressure of expectation. If you have been called to manage a child, it is because you have the necessary skills that others in the team do not.

The major advantage of paediatric emergencies is that they attract a large team of people who are desperate to help. Use your team. Take a deep breath and manage the situation with the same calm reasoning as you would an adult.

Airway

As children get older the airway becomes more and more familiar to those working in adult medicine. By the time they reach the age of 1–2 years, the larynx is not as anterior, the tongue relatively smaller and the FRC greater. For children closer to the neonatal age paediatricians may become more helpful for practical procedures. Some will be very familiar with intubating and siting arterial lines on neonates.

Bag-mask ventilation

When bagging small children, the biggest problem by far is the anxiety-driven airway grip. Pressing on the soft tissue under the mandible easily obstructs the airways of children. Managing the airway in babies should be done by fingertip pressure on bony prominences, with the head in a neutral position.

The second biggest problem is gastric distension and is caused by even experienced paediatric anaesthetists. Air forced into the stomach during bagging can compromise ventilation. An early NG tube can make the situation much better. In fact it is commonplace to put in an NG tube for induction of anaesthesia in critically ill children.

Intubation

In small children, the occiput forms the biggest problem. The right size of roll underneath/between the shoulder blades can make a huge difference. If your intubation has failed, stop early, bag the patient and reposition (as you would in adults). Always intubate orally first. The retrieval team can make a decision on nasal intubation for transfer. Important things to consider when intubating critically ill children are mentioned in Table 4.7.

There are situations where a gas induction in theatre should be the method of choice for induction. These are discussed in Chapters 15 and 16. Endotracheal intubation is covered in Chapter 37.

Table 4.7. Tips for intubating a sick child.

- If possible place a tube for gastric decompression prior to induction – expect gastric distension and high risk of aspiration
- Have access secured (peripheral or IO under local anaesthetic)
- Have volume already given and/or available to give during induction
- Have inotrope attached and/or running (depending on cardiovascular status)
- Consider carefully the choice of induction agents (ketamine 1–2 mg/kg is the default choice for most retrieval teams)
- Use a cuffed ET tube for burns, and if high airway pressures are anticipated, e.g. asthma
- Be ready to abandon laryngoscopy and attempts to intubate at any stage and sooner than expected – have a timekeeper and agree time allowed for each attempt (usually 30 seconds)
- Do not cut the length of an ET tube until its position has been checked on a CXR

Breathing

It has already been mentioned that smaller patients have to work harder to maintain a 'normal state'. They also fatigue more quickly. The relatively immature chest wall of small children means that they have a high closing capacity and a tendency towards airway collapse and atelectasis.

Pressure-control ventilation

Once intubated the settings for the ventilator need to be set. In general, pressure-control ventilation will compensate for leaks around the ET tube. The pressures should be the same as in adults. Because the tidal volume measurements become less reliable as children become smaller, always look at the movement of the child's chest, to check that it is sufficient (but not too much).

Positive end-expiratory pressure (PEEP)

The tendency towards airway collapse means that PEEP is essential when setting a ventilator. Start off with the same pressure as you would in adults (about 5 cmH_2O) and titrate as needed. The biggest problem in small children is that as the PEEP increases, the venous return becomes compromised. If this occurs, first give a fluid bolus then back off the pressure (back to 5 cmH_2O).

Difficulty ventilating

If you are having difficulty in ventilating a child, the commonest problems are:

- the ET tube is not in the trachea – use end-tidal CO_2 monitoring
- the ET tube is too far in (very common) – clinical examination and a CXR will confirm this
- the ET tube is blocked – pass a suction catheter
- the ET tube is too small and there is a large leak
- the child has significant lung pathology or fluid overload
- there is a pneumothorax
- the child has pulmonary hypertension.

Table 4.8. Setting a ventilator for a child.

- Always use end-tidal CO_2
- Use lowest FiO_2 necessary to achieve adequate oxygenation (check what is normal for the child)
- Use lung protective strategies, aiming for tidal volumes of 6–10 ml/kg
- Start inspiratory pressures at 15–20 cmH_2O then titrate to tidal volume
- Use the same inspiratory pressure limits as used in adults
- Use PEEP
- If PEEP causes hypotension, give fluid before backing off
- Inspiratory times may need to be long – start with a minimum of 0.6 seconds for a neonate. Use up to 1.0 s for older patients or young patients with difficult oxygenation
- Permissive hypercapnoea should be used for lung protection where necessary with pH of 7.25 being acceptable (caution in pulmonary hypertension and neuroprotective strategies)
- Perform a CXR
- Use adequate sedation/analgesia and muscle relaxation to keep ET tube *in situ* and promote best ventilation

As in adults, there are conditions where different ventilator strategies are applied. These include asthma (Chapter 8) and bronchiolitis (Chapter 7). Ventilation strategies in children with congenital heart disease are also covered (Chapter 6). However, even in these conditions, the settings mentioned in Table 4.8 will be adequate as an initial set-up to be titrated.

Cardiovascular

It is regularly taught that small children cannot increase their stroke volume to compensate for a low systemic vascular resistance (SVR). However, small babies who are unwell will present with relative volume depletion. Therefore their stroke volume will increase as normovolaemia returns. There will be a decrease in heart rate, and evidence of improved cardiac output.

Hypovolaemia should be treated aggressively, with boluses of 20 ml/kg given as quickly as possible whilst maintaining very close observation of response (with the exception of resuscitation in trauma – 10 ml/kg). A good response to a fluid bolus should include:

- a reduction in heart rate
- improvement in quality of pulses and pulse pressure
- improved capillary refill time
- improved lactic acidosis
- increased urine output.

How much fluid?

Many adult physicians struggle with changing measurement values when giving fluid, i.e. using ml/kg rather than absolute volume. When working out whether you have given a lot of fluid or not, there are two easy methods:

- compare it to the circulating volume – 40 ml/kg is already half of the circulating volume
- multiply it by 70 to work out the equivalent volume in an 'average' adult – 40 ml/kg would be 2.8 litres.

For children who are likely to receive a lot of fluid, e.g. severe sepsis, take a cross-match sample early and request blood products as soon as possible. It is likely that you will need blood products once you have reached 60–80 ml/kg of fluid resuscitation (see Chapter 21 for giving blood products).

Sepsis and fluids

For sepsis, the evidence points strongly to early rapid fluid resuscitation being associated with the largest reduction in mortality (accompanied with early antibiotic administration). By the time the patient gets to PICU the timeliness of early fluid administration has disappeared. If a child is septic, resuscitate quickly using crystalloid first (see Chapter 5 for further choice of fluids). Although it is not the norm, volumes in excess of 150 ml/kg of fluid are sometimes given in severe sepsis.

Vascular access and IO needles

No one would argue that vascular access in children can be difficult. Intraosseous (IO) access should not be seen as a failure. Instead it should be seen as a pressure-relieving fallback that takes the stress out of gaining IV access. It is no coincidence that the more senior the paediatric ED or PICU doctor, the quicker they resort to IO access.

Central lines and arterial lines are rarely 'life-saving' procedures in children. The time is often better spent concentrating on the management of the child. If you are planning to place a central line, speak to the retrieval team first to help weigh up the pros and cons.

Remember that all drugs, including inotropes, can be given through an IO needle.

Table 4.9. Gaining vascular access.

- Remove people whose presence is unhelpful
- Have a timekeeper accurately record time spent attempting access
- Use intraosseous access early – one for vasoactive agents, one for everything else
- Formalize access once the patient is more stable (volume resuscitated, vasoactive agents in progress, intubated and ventilated) if there is time

Vasoactive agents

Inotropes and vasoactive drugs are chosen along the same principles as in adults. Adrenaline is usually the first-line inotrope. Dopamine, noradrenaline and dobutamine are used to achieve the same response as in adults. Adrenaline can be given peripherally if used in a suitable dilution (see Chapter 36).

Other agents may be suggested by the PICU retrieval team, but should not be started as a first line.

Sedation and muscle relaxants

Sedation for ventilated children is usually achieved with a morphine infusion 20–40 μg/kg/h. Midazolam 2–4 μg/kg/min is used from 3 months old (see Chapter 36 for how to make up these infusions). Propofol is not routinely used in children due to the risk of propofol infusion syndrome in critically ill children.

Insufficient sedation will confuse interpretation of haemodynamic parameters (such as heart rate). If in doubt bolus the equivalent of an hour's worth of both agents, i.e. if your morphine is running at 2 ml/h, give a 2 ml bolus. Be careful with midazolam, as it can lead to quite profound myocardial depression and hypotension.

For most paediatric emergencies a muscle-relaxant infusion is used. As well as aiding ventilation, it helps to ensure safety of the ET tube, which can otherwise be easily coughed out.

Glucose

The blood sugar should be checked on arrival of a patient, and at regular intervals thereafter (including with each blood gas). Many of the infusions, e.g. sedatives and inotropes, are made up in dextrose. This alone can supply enough dextrose to maintain the blood sugar in most cases. If not, then maintenance fluid (often 0.45% saline with 5% dextrose or 0.9% saline with 5% dextrose) can be run alongside the fluid boluses that are given.

Hypoglycaemia

If the blood sugar is below 3.0 mmol/l give 2 ml/kg of 10% dextrose and increase the amount given as an infusion, either by volume or by concentration of dextrose (up to 12.5% dextrose can be given peripherally through a good cannula). A single bolus will only raise the blood sugar level temporarily.

If the blood sugar remains low despite the increased maintenance consider whether it can be attributable to:

- severe sepsis
- inherited metabolic disease
- acute liver failure.

These should be discussed with the PICU retrieval consultant. It is worth calculating how much dextrose the child is receiving before considering these diagnoses. Greater than 10 mg/kg/min would prompt concern.

Temperature

Aim for normothermia in any critically ill child and remember that small patients lose heat quickly. Active rewarming should be easily available for all children who require it. As mentioned above, treat pyrexia aggressively, and contact the PICU retrieval team to discuss therapeutic hypothermia in cardiac arrest (see Chapter 23).

Care-givers

Parents are usually good sources of information, and may be able to remain nearby without compromising resuscitation. They tend to respond well to information, however inadequate and indefinite that information may be. Although an area of debate, there is some evidence that parents cope better with bad outcomes if they are present at the resuscitation. Where possible, a member of staff should be allocated to looking after parents.

Summary

Management of sick children needs a calm and structured approach. This chapter covers many of the details that need to be covered when managing a sick child. Oxygen therapy and fluid resuscitation form the mainstay of treatment along with attention to detail to electrolytes and temperature. Figure 4.1 shows a brief summary of the commonly asked management questions during resuscitation.

Golden rules

- Do not wait for a child to get 'too sick' before intubation
- Have a low threshold for IO needle insertion
- Do not be afraid of giving fluid boluses quickly, as long as the child is responding
- Check and correct electrolytes and glucose
- Pay close attention to temperature – especially if you are performing procedures on a small child

Question	Consideration
Do I need to intubate this child?	• Are any of the indications in Table 4.4 present? • Does the child appear to be tiring? • Are the blood /capillary gases worsening (increasing $PaCO_2$ or hypoxia refractory to oxygen therapy)? • Would I intubate an adult in this situation? IF THE ANSWER IS YES TO ANY OF THE ABOVE POINTS THEN CALL FOR HELP AND PREPARE TO INTUBATE
Do I need to go to theatre for a gas induction?	• Is there any sign of a narrowed airway? See Table 4.3 • Is the child likely to be a difficult intubation, i.e. is there a syndrome that might indicate one (ask the paediatrician and see Chapter 16)? • Is there time to move the child; are they well enough to transfer to theatre? IF THE ANSWER IS YES TO ANY OF THE ABOVE POINTS THEN CALL FOR HELP AND CALL THEATRES TO PREPARE EQUIPMENT
Do I need to use an IO needle?	• Have you had more than two attempts? • Have you taken longer than 2 minutes? • Does the child need immediate access for fluids or drugs e.g. adrenaline? • Have you ruled out contraindications e.g. fracture of bone to be accessed, overlying infection? IF THE ANSWER IS YES TO ALL OF THE ABOVE POINTS THEN INSERT AN IO NEEDLE
How much fluid should I give?	• Give up to 40 ml/kg then cross-match (if not done already) • After 60–80 ml/kg start giving blood products (FFP and packed red cells) • Keep giving fluid as long as you get a response (improved heart rate, blood pressure, etc.) • When the patient stops responding to fluid, start inotropes

Which inotropes should I use?	• If the child is in extremis and the diagnosis uncertain – start peripheral strength adrenaline (Chapter 36) or normal strength through an IO needle
	• If you have IO or CVC access:
	    • Is the child warm with bounding pulses? – noradrenaline
	    • Is it primarily a cardiac problem? – consider dobutamine
	    • Is there sepsis and myocardial dysfunction? – dopamine/dobutamine + noradrenaline, or adrenaline

Figure 4.1. Timeline for commonly asked questions during resuscitation.

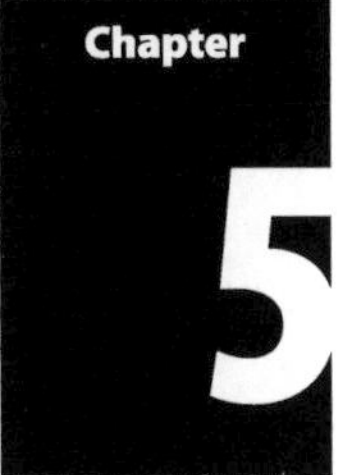

The child with sepsis

Matthew D. Christopherson and Paul Baines

Introduction

Infections in children are common. Around 1 in 14 of all infants will be hospitalized with an infectious disease. The majority of infections are mild and managed with careful observation, antibiotics and fluid management before discharge. Severe sepsis is uncommon, with about 0.6 cases per 1000 children in the USA and causing about 5% of UK PICU admissions. Sepsis affects the whole paediatric age range, peaking in the second month of life. Infections have a peak incidence over the winter months.

Sepsis in children

Severe sepsis is defined as systemic inflammatory response syndrome (SIRS) in the presence of or as a result of suspected or proven infection. The definition of paediatric SIRS reflects the normal age-dependent physiological parameters (Table 5.1).

Table 5.1. Criteria for SIRS in children.

Temperature (rectal)	< 36°C or > 38°C	
Heart rate (beats per minute)	Neonates (< 4 weeks)	< 100 or > 180
	Infants (1 month–1 year)	< 90 or > 180
	Children 1–5 years	> 140
	Children 6–12 years	> 130
	Children 13–18 years	> 110
Respiratory rate (breaths per minute)	Neonates (< 4 weeks)	> 50
	Infants (1 month–1 year)	> 34
	Children 1–5 years	> 22
	Children 6–12 years	> 18
	Children 13–18 years	> 14
White blood cell count	$< 4 \times 10^9$/l or $> 12 \times 10^9$/l	

Modified from Goldstein B, Giroir B, Randolph A, *et al.* International pediatric sepsis consensus conference: Definitions for sepsis and organ dysfunction in pediatrics. *Pediatr Crit Care Med* 2005;6:2–8.

Managing the Critically Ill Child, ed. Richard Skone *et al.* Published by Cambridge University Press.

The pathophysiological process of sepsis in children is broadly similar to that of adults. The complex interaction between pathogen and host provokes the release of pro- and anti-inflammatory mediators. These mediators have broad-ranging effects on myocardial function, vascular tone, permeability and coagulation, leading to hypotension, capillary leak and coagulopathy.

The pathogen causing sepsis varies with age. In neonates the main pathogens include:

- group B *Streptococci*
- *Escherichia coli*
- herpes simplex
- enterovirus.

In older children the main causes of sepsis are likely to be:

- *Neisseria meningitides*
- *Haemophilus influenzae*
- *Staphylococcus* sp.
- *Streptococcus* sp.

Fungal sepsis and other viruses such as adenovirus may present in the immunocompromised child. The general principles of managing severe sepsis in children are the same regardless of pathogen, with antibiotic therapy directed at the commonest causative organisms in the age group of the affected child. Care should be taken with chronically unwell children who may be colonized with *Pseudomonas* or *Klebsiella* species.

Around 10% of deaths in children younger than 4 years are as a result of infection and approximately 20% of the children admitted to UK PICUs with severe sepsis die. Higher mortality is associated with multi-organ dysfunction. Four or more affected organ systems increase the reported mortality to 50%; however, total mortality is declining.

Differences between paediatric sepsis and adult sepsis

Susceptibility to infection

Children are more susceptible to infection than adults for a wide variety of reasons. At birth, the skin and mucous membranes provide less effective passive protection because colonization with commensal flora is incomplete.

Neonates possess all the components of the immune system to mount an immune response; however, they are pathogen-naive. At birth, there is an absolute IgA and IgM deficiency, with levels rising over the first 6 months. Passive immunity is afforded by transplacentally acquired maternal IgG. This IgG declines rapidly over the first few weeks of life. To coincide with lasting antibody formation, the childhood immunization schedule commences at 2 months of age, with only high-risk infants being immunized against tuberculosis and hepatitis B prior to this.

Children's immune function matures as they grow. Some children remain at risk. These include:

- infants born prematurely
- infants with chronic lung disease (respiratory tract infections)
- children with short gut syndrome (parenteral nutrition through an indwelling vascular access device and may lead to line sepsis)
- children with hydrocephalus (infected ventriculo-peritoneal shunts)
- congenital or acquired immunodeficiency e.g. DiGeorge syndrome
- children with sickle cell disease (*Salmonella* and *Streptococcus*).

In older children, it is those with neurological disorders or those receiving immunosuppressive therapy who have an increased risk of sepsis.

Presentation

The presentation of sepsis is variable and remarkably non-specific. The child may be unsettled with muscle aches, listlessness or a reluctance to be separated from the main care-giver. Frequently, children refuse to eat or drink or may be vomiting, leading to dehydration and decreased urine output or number of wet nappies. Examination of the fontanelle may show it to be sunken in dehydration or bulging in meningitis. Despite presentation with mild symptoms, all children are at risk of rapidly deteriorating to complete collapse within a short period of time.

Variation in presentation

Pyrexia is one of the first clues to infection in children but neonates and infants may be hypothermic, especially in severe sepsis. Tachypnoea may be present as the child attempts to compensate for metabolic acidosis, but neonates and infants often suffer from apnoeas.

Hypoglycaemia is a reasonably frequent finding in infants with sepsis. Maintenance fluid with an adequate dextrose concentration should be commenced until enteral feeds start. Some septic children become hyperglycaemic, which may be due to relative insulin deficiency. Very high glucose levels are associated with increased mortality.

Clinical presentation of sick children can be misleading because:

- they compensate well until they suddenly collapse
- blood pressure measurements can be unreliable and hypotension is a late sign of impending collapse
- tachycardia is a useful indicator of illness but the heart rate may also be high in children who are not sick if they are pyrexial or distressed.

Blood tests

A full blood count can show either raised white cell counts (WCC $> 12 \times 10^9$/l) or low white cell counts ($< 4 \times 10^9$/l). Raised white cell counts are more likely in children who mount a normal response to infection. Very high white cell, especially lymphocyte, counts ($> 50 \times 10^9$/l) suggest infection with *Bordetella pertussis* though the first presentation of leukaemia should be borne in mind.

Infants under 3 months have reduced neutrophil stores and tend to drop their white cell count when septic. Bone marrow suppression may be found as part of a multiorgan dysfunction syndrome with anaemia, leucopenia and thrombocytopenia on investigation. Other markers of inflammation including C-reactive protein, erythrocyte sedimentation rate, procalcitonin and IL-6 can indicate sepsis; however, investigations are unreliable and may be normal, especially early on in overwhelming disease.

Cold shock

In septic adults cardiac output is usually maintained despite myocardial dysfunction because of reduced systemic vascular resistance. There is a decreased ejection fraction but maintenance of cardiac output via ventricular dilatation and an increased heart rate. Hyperdynamic–low systemic vascular resistance sepsis or 'warm shock' is frequently encountered in adults. Septic children, however, most frequently present with a low cardiac output–high systemic vascular resistance or 'cold shock' picture.

Children do not develop the ventricular dilatation seen in adults that maintains cardiac output and, whilst tachycardia contributes to compensatory mechanisms, the proportional increase in heart rate seen in adults is not sustainable in children. Septic children with low cardiac output have greater mortality than those with a cardiac index between 3.3 and 6.0 $l/min/m^2$. Because vasomotor regulatory mechanisms usually remain intact, the mainstay of treatment is aggressive fluid resuscitation and positive inotropes.

Monitoring degree of vasoconstriction

It is possible to observe the changing vascular tone by feeling the core–peripheral temperature gap and monitoring the progression from distal to proximal sites, e.g. from the feet upwards. Increased core–peripheral temperature gap is a marker of poor peripheral perfusion and one can use this clinical assessment alongside heart rate, capillary refill time and blood pressure to guide fluid resuscitation whilst invasive monitoring is established.

Continual assessment is required as the progression of sepsis evolves. Response to interventions can be variable and the symptoms may switch between those of cold and warm shock.

What are the warning signs that a child is really sick?

The presentation of sepsis can be misleading. Despite signs of hypotension and delayed capillary refill time, the child may remain alert. Children who lie still and passively endure interventions give cause for concern and children who seem to be 'good' or 'cooperative' may just be very ill.

Temperature

Infants who present with hypothermia often represent the more severe end of the spectrum of disease and present a challenge in the resuscitation room as vascular access can be difficult in a cold shut-down child. Whilst it is essential to remove clothes to allow examination of the whole child for signs of rash and the placement of lines, it is imperative that the child is kept warm in a ward room or by using a radiant heater.

Respiratory signs

Respiratory distress may be present in severely ill children. Tachypnoea may be respiratory compensation for metabolic acidosis. As exhaustion ensues, the child may start grunting. Apnoeas, if present, require intervention, as they suggest impending collapse.

Cardiovascular signs

Persistent tachycardia is a useful indicator of impending cardiovascular collapse in sick children. The pulse rate can be used to monitor the response to fluid resuscitation with the rate falling as adequate filling has been reached.

Neurological signs

If there is decreased conscious level or intractable seizures, intubation is necessary to protect the airway and facilitate transfer for neuroimaging. Signs of meningitis or raised intracranial pressure require intubation for neuroprotective management strategies (see Chapter 19).

Specific conditions

Meningitis

The presentation of meningitis in neonates and infants can be non-specific. A bulging, tense fontanelle or focal neurological signs may be present on examination; however, apnoeas and bradycardias may be the only feature. Children older than 1 year may appear generally unwell, with headache, neck stiffness, vomiting and photophobia. In all children, signs of raised intracranial pressure are features that require prompt intervention.

Diagnosis is made clinically with microbiological confirmation of cerebrospinal fluid (CSF) cultures. The decision to perform a lumbar puncture must balance the benefits of making a diagnosis, identifying the organism and obtaining antibiotic sensitivities against the risks of coning, bleeding and introducing infection. Lumbar puncture should not be performed in children who:

- are cardiovascularly unstable
- have decreased conscious level
- show focal neurological signs
- demonstrate a coagulopathy.

The responsible organism can be identified by blood cultures or polymerase chain reaction (PCR), or CSF PCR and CSF cell counts obtained when the child has improved.

Antibiotic therapy is initially broad-spectrum, guided by the age of the child and rationalized when the organism is identified. As a general rule, the organisms that cause meningitis may also cause sepsis. Here supportive management should be directed to maintaining normal parameters with neuroprotection (see Chapter 19).

Neonates with meningitis should receive antibiotics according to local policy, e.g. amoxicillin and cefotaxime. Aciclovir should also be considered. Infants and older children with meningitis should receive cefotaxime or ceftriaxone.

Dexamethasone 0.15 mg/kg (maximum dose 10 mg) 6 hourly in children over 3 months of age reduces the incidence of neurological sequelae.

Group B streptococcus

Group B streptococcus (GBS) is a normal commensal bacterium found in the rectum and vagina of around one-quarter of pregnant women. Approximately 1 in 2000 neonates develop invasive GBS, which presents either early (within the first week of life) or late (1 week to 90 days of age).

Early-onset GBS carries a risk of mortality of 5–15% in term infants and causes either meningitis or sepsis. The incidence of late-onset GBS has not reduced with intrapartum antibiotics. Presentation is similar to early-onset disease but with a mortality of less than 3%.

E. coli

Escherichia coli meningitis and sepsis can be particularly severe in neonates.

Listeria

Listeria monocytogenes is a rare cause of neonatal meningitis and sepsis. The organism is able to cross the placenta, infecting the fetus. Mortality is 80%; however, *Listeria* is sensitive to amoxicillin and prompt treatment may modify the disease course.

Pneumococcal meningitis

Pneumococcal meningitis is associated with significant neurological morbidity and mortality. Carriage of *Streptococcus pneumoniae* occurs in around half of all pre-school children. The organism reaches the meninges by haematological spread or direct transmission through a communication in sinusitis or otitis media.

Haemophilus influenzae type B

Haemophilus influenzae type B (Hib) meningitis is uncommon due to the inclusion of the conjugate vaccine in the immunization schedule. Mortality from this disease is around 5%; however, around 30% have neurological sequelae.

Meningoencephalitis

A number of other organisms may cause a meningoencephalitis-type picture (combined picture of meningitis and encephalitis). Bacterial infection with *Mycoplasma pneumoniae* is amongst the differential diagnoses and a macrolide antibiotic should be introduced if the history is not typical of one of the more common causes. Viruses including enterovirus and herpes simplex are uncommon causes of meningoencephalitis. Herpes simplex should be considered if there is recent contact with the virus or in the presence of herpetic lesions, and treatment with aciclovir commenced.

Meningococcal disease

Neisseria meningitides or the meningococcus is the organism most frequently associated with meningitis. Carriage occurs throughout the adult population; however, invasive disease mainly affects children. Recent influenza A infection, exposure to tobacco smoke and close-quarter living are known risk factors. Progression of the disease is rapid and, with sepsis, death can occur within hours. There is frequently a prodromal period with non-specific symptoms. Muscle aches and pains may be an early indicator. Invasive disease may present with a blanching pink macular rash or the more characteristic purpura; however, absence of a rash does not exclude meningococcal infection. Some children present with just signs of meningitis or sepsis but in the main it is a mixed picture. Children who have sepsis without evidence of meningitis carry a poor prognosis.

Table 5.2. Poor prognostic signs in meningococcal sepsis.

Low white cell count
Thrombocytopenia
Deranged clotting
Persisting shock
Rapidly progressing purpura
Decreased conscious level
No evidence of meningitis

Management is with antibiotic treatment and supportive measures. Electrolyte disturbance is common, with hypokalaemia, hypocalcaemia and hypomagnesaemia all potentially correctable. Myocardial dysfunction in meningococcal disease is common and high doses of inotropes may be necessary to support the circulation. Despite intensive care, the outcome may remain poor, with up to 5% dying. Immunization against serotype C has reduced the UK incidence and serotype B is now the dominant strain. Nasal carriage persists with cefotaxime therapy and carriage should be eliminated with ciprofloxacin or ceftriaxone.

Toxic shock syndrome

Infections with *Streptococcus* sp. and *Staphylococcus* sp. can cause SIRS secondary to toxin production. Streptococcal infections are usually mild, with pneumonia, impetigo and pharyngitis being common. Group A streptococcus can have serious effects when it becomes invasive (iGAS). Risk factors for iGAS are recent chicken pox (varicella zoster) or ibuprofen use.

Staphylococcus aureus may cause sepsis from chest or urinary tract infections or toxic shock syndrome, with a widespread fine erythematous rash, particularly on the soles of the hands and feet. Treatment is with flucloxacillin or cefuroxime with clindamycin.

Less commonly, children may present with methicillin-resistant *Staphylococcus aureus* (MRSA) or coagulase-negative *Staphylococcus* sepsis. Usually, these children have indwelling catheters or a history of prolonged hospital admissions. Intravenous immunoglobulin G is thought to reduce sepsis-related organ dysfunction and mortality in toxic shock syndrome and its use is recommended in this situation.

Neutropenic sepsis

Children with neutropenia develop sepsis from not only the common childhood causes but also a number of more unusual organisms. *Pseudomonas*, *Streptococcus viridans*, adenovirus and fungal infections can cause overwhelming sepsis in these patients. Cultures must be taken before the administration of antibiotics as isolation of pathogens dictates treatment. Oncology departments in conjunction with infectious disease specialists have often written a febrile neutropenia policy that guides treatment based on local infection patterns and antibiotic susceptibility. In the absence of a local policy, dual therapy with gentamicin and piperacillin/tazobactam (Tazocin®) is indicated and aciclovir added for herpes or varicella infection.

Targeted treatments

When faced with a septic child, it is important to place particular emphasis on assessing the child and making appropriate interventions quickly prior to collapse. Failure to apply the correct normal range to physiological observations is a recognized failure of care that continues to contribute to morbidity and mortality.

Figure 5.1 shows a timeline of specific interventions for sepsis in children. The first few minutes are critical once a child is recognized as being critically ill. When cannulating a child blood samples should be sent for:

- glucose
- full blood count
- clotting screen
- biochemistry
- blood cultures and PCR
- cross-match.

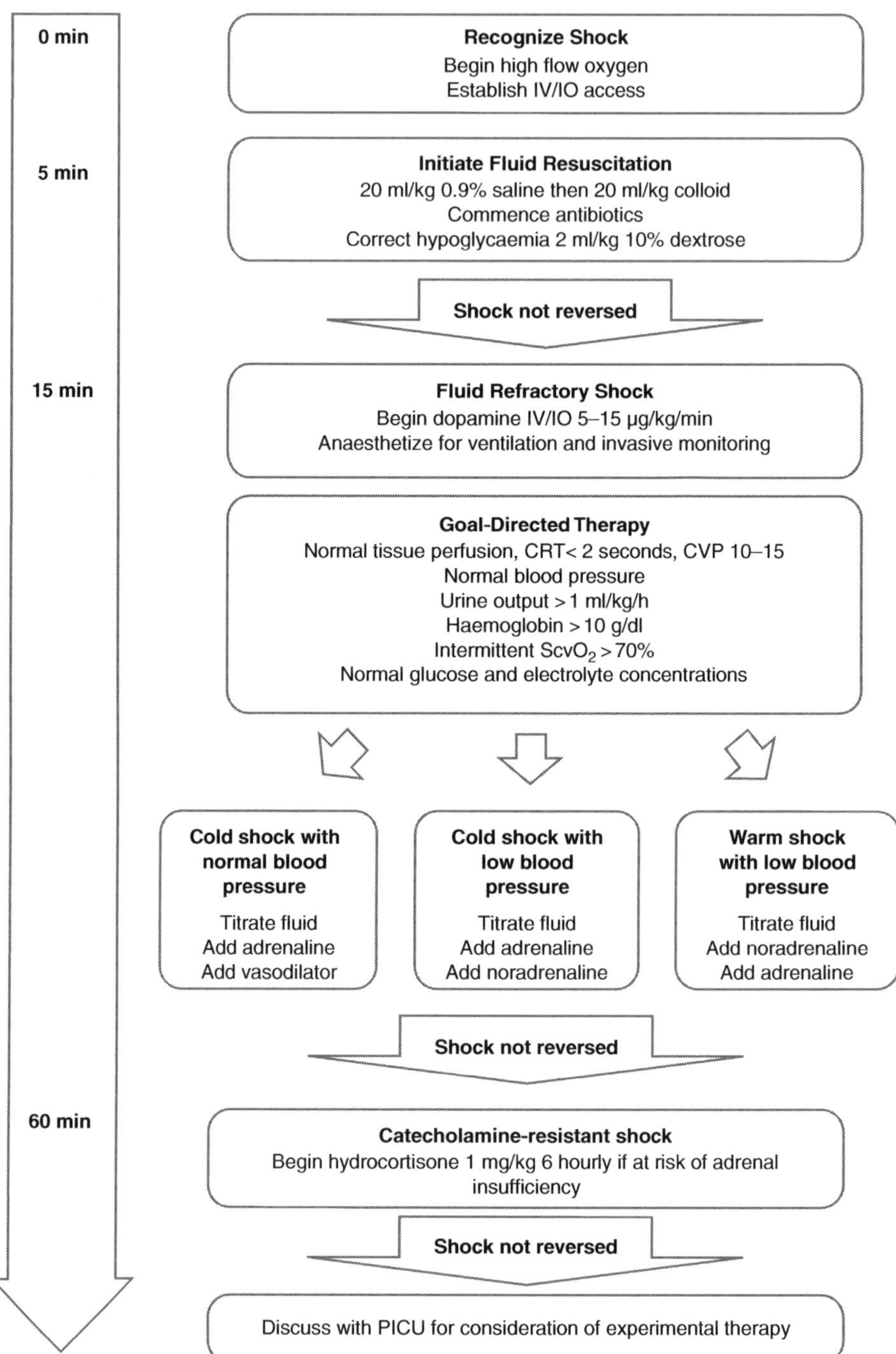

Figure 5.1. Goal-directed therapy in paediatric sepsis – the first hour.

Goal-directed therapy

Reductions in mortality are associated with early aggressive fluid resuscitation in children. Goal-directed therapy has reduced mortality from sepsis in adults.

Just as in adults, the aim of treatment is to restore tissue perfusion and improve oxygen delivery. Treatment is directed at normalizing:

- tissue perfusion
- pulse rate (which may remain high indicating severe disease)
- blood pressure
- urine output ($>$ 1 ml/kg/h in children)
- central venous oxygen saturations ($ScvO_2 > 70\%$)
- haemoglobin concentration ($>$ 100 g/l).

$ScvO_2$ is used as an assessment of oxygen delivery and consumption, with low results reflecting increased tissue oxygen extraction through an inadequate cardiac output. Improving cardiac output and optimizing oxygen delivery by increasing haemoglobin concentrations can increase the $ScvO_2$. Resuscitation targeting improved $ScvO_2$ has been associated with improved survival.

Raised serum lactate concentrations can also reflect poor tissue perfusion. High levels may take longer to fall in improving children, compared to adults, due to physiological differences in hepatic lactate metabolism.

Fluid resuscitation

Principles of fluid therapy in severe sepsis in children

- Severe sepsis needs rapid fluid resuscitation
- Each hour passing without reversal of shock doubles the risk of death
- 20 ml/kg aliquots should be infused over 5 min and the child reassessed for signs of improvement in perfusion or fluid overload
- Resuscitation fluid volumes of 60 ml/kg administered within the first hour improve outcome with no increased risk of ARDS or pulmonary oedema
- Fluid overload in this situation is uncommon
- Have blood products ready (see below)

Pulmonary oedema occurring early in children with septic shock is likely to be due to capillary leak and should be treated with ventilation with high positive end-expiratory pressure (PEEP). Over the first 24 hours, it is not uncommon for severely ill, septic children to receive between 150 and 200 ml/kg or more of fluid in addition to their maintenance requirement.

During the initial management give 20 ml/kg crystalloid followed by 20 ml/kg aliquots of 4.5% human albumin solution (HAS) for all subsequent boluses; however, resuscitation should not be delayed if HAS is unavailable (continue with crystalloid or other colloids). Central venous pressure (CVP) can be monitored to guide fluid therapy with a target range of 10–15 mmHg.

Blood products

Resuscitation with large volumes of crystalloids will reduce the haematocrit. Current guidance suggests maintaining the haemoglobin concentration above 10 g/dl to improve oxygen delivery to tissues. Coagulopathies are to be anticipated not only as part of the consumptive pathology but secondary to haemodilution. Infusions of cryoprecipitate and fresh frozen plasma are used to treat the clotting abnormalities and should be infused even with no active bleeding.

Platelets should be given to all children with a count of less than 10×10^9/l, or 10–40 $\times 10^9$/l and a risk factor for bleeding. Platelet levels should be maintained at more than 50×10^9/l for invasive procedures (see Chapter 21). It is unusual for the platelet count to fall in the early hours of sepsis and it may be an indicator of an additional underlying disease process. Blood products may also act as colloid within the fluid resuscitation process; however, fluid administration should not be delayed until these products become available.

Vasoactive drugs

The majority of septic children respond well to fluid; however, some need cardiovascular support. The aim is to counteract the myocardial dysfunction present in septic children.

If the cause of the collapse is uncertain adrenaline should be considered first-line inotropic therapy.

Dopamine infusion at 5–10 μg/kg/min to a maximum of 15 μg/kg/min is the first-line agent for both cold and warm shock in paediatric sepsis (see Chapter 35 for infusion strength). The positive inotropic and chronotropic effects increase cardiac output in both scenarios. Paediatric studies do not support the inferiority of dopamine when compared to noradrenaline and, as such, it remains the first-line inotrope in paediatric sepsis.

In warm shock, noradrenaline plays a similar role to that in adult practice and can be used as single-agent vasopressor therapy where central access is immediately available. The safety and efficacy of vasopressin infusion in paediatric sepsis is currently under investigation and its routine use is not currently recommended.

For dopamine/dobutamine-resistant cold shock, adrenaline (0.1–1 μg/kg/min) is the next inotrope to start (Figure 5.1). Dobutamine may cause vasodilatation, with further fluids required to prevent hypotension.

Type III phosphodiesterase inhibitors, e.g. milrinone, provide a theoretical advantage in cold shock, adding inotropic effects to vasodilatation independently of the catecholamine pathway. In reality, the steady state may take several hours to achieve so these agents may only have a place in the ongoing intensive care environment.

Endotracheal intubation and mechanical ventilation

The decision to intubate and ventilate needs to be made early in the resuscitation process. Indications for ventilation include:

- decreased conscious level
- respiratory failure or apnoeas
- persisting shock despite 40 ml/kg fluid resuscitation over a short period of time should also act as a trigger to prepare for intubation.

In reality, if further fluid resuscitation is required, central venous access is necessary to monitor CVP, measure $ScvO_2$ and reliably deliver vasoactive drugs. Such procedures are painful, require a cooperative child and therefore are most safely achieved under anaesthesia.

Mechanical ventilation has additional benefits in sepsis. Ventilation will relieve the work of breathing, which may be higher in septic shock. Children with low cardiac output and high systemic vascular resistance may receive benefit from the improved left ventricular function associated with with increased intrathoracic pressure. Pulmonary oedema may develop and can be treated with high PEEP.

Steroids

The role of steroids in paediatric sepsis is controversial. Some septic children have low steroid concentrations and those children are more likely to die. Current guidelines suggest the administration of hydrocortisone to children with sepsis and catecholamine-resistant shock, who are at risk of absolute adrenal insufficiency or adrenal pituitary axis failure, for example those with purpura fulminans, congenital adrenal hyperplasia or recent steroid use.

In reality, the practicalities of demonstrating cortisol deficiency prevent formal investigations in the acute situation and as such, if the child is deteriorating or on escalating catecholamines, give hydrocortisone at 1 mg/kg 6 hourly. A random cortisol can be requested on a sample taken before steroids were commenced.

What do I need to do pre/post intubation?

Intubation

When preparing to intubate a septic child, consideration should be given to the potential pitfalls. Pulmonary oedema bubbling up the trachea following induction may obscure the laryngeal inlet. An appropriately sized bougie can be useful to place through the cords to guide intubation. If there is pulmonary oedema use a high PEEP and consider asking PICU to prepare for high-frequency oscillatory ventilation. Hand ventilation in the presence of significant pulmonary oedema may also be difficult due to the inability to maintain a constant PEEP. Placing the child on a ventilator may improve the situation.

A rapid-sequence induction is usually required; however, giving thiopentone to shut-down and effectively hypovolaemic children can lead to loss of cardiac output. Ketamine (1–2 mg/kg) theoretically provides more cardiovascular stability but hypotension is not unknown. The change in physiology from negative to positive intrathoracic pressure on invasive positive-pressure ventilation exacerbates the fall in cardiac output. Continuous infusion of volume along with an inotrope infusion running may prevent arrest on induction.

Post intubation

Post intubation, arterial and central venous access should be placed, thus facilitating further stabilization. Insert a urinary catheter to monitor urine output and obtain a sample of urine to send for microbiological testing. If not done already, site a nasogastric tube to deflate the stomach and empty any contents.

At this point the child should be reassessed with particular attention paid to:

- correction of blood glucose and electrolytes
- continued fluid resuscitation
- regular temperature monitoring.

Parents are frequently asked to wait in the parents' room during the initial stabilization and intubation process. When invasive procedures are complete the parents should be informed of what has happened since they left their child and invited to return to their child's side. Appropriate support needs to be provided to explain their child's status and appearance. A further more detailed history can often be taken at this point.

What do I need to have done/organized before transfer?

Prior to transfer to PICU, a number of routine tasks should be completed whilst continuing to deliver intensive care (Figure 5.2). The checklist for transfer in Chapter 24 can be used to guide preparation of the child for transfer in order to speed up the process.

Airway

- Nasal endotracheal tube – caution in coagulopathy, may cause epistaxis
- Endotracheal tube secured appropriately for transfer
- Nasogastric tube placed to decompress the stomach
- Chest X-ray demonstrating position of endotracheal tube and nasogastric tube
- Inclusion of a heat moisture exchanger within the circuit

Breathing

- Placed on ventilator with clear settings and blood gas monitoring
- Positive end-expiratory pressure (PEEP) maintained as appropriate
    - High PEEP in pulmonary oedema

Circulation

- At least one good peripheral venous cannula
- Multi-lumen central venous catheter (CVC) sited and secured
    - Position confirmed on X-ray if internal jugular line
- Measurement of the central venous pressure (CVP)
- Arterial line sited, secured and transduced
    - If placing in the groin, preferably the same side as the CVC to keep the other side free for renal support catheter
- Inotrope infusions running via the CVC
- Urinary catheter

Investigations

- Blood cultures
- Full blood count, coagulation studies
- Urea and electrolytes, calcium, magnesium, lactate, C-reactive protein
- Blood glucose
- Arterial blood gas and intermittent $ScvO_2$
- Urine dipstick and cultures

Drugs

- Antibiotics prescribed with times administered
- Consider steroids if meningitis or escalating inotrope requirement
    - Request random cortisol
- Maintenance infusion containing dextrose to maintain normal blood glucose levels

Communication

- Parents
    - Outline diagnosis, management and prognosis
- With the transfer team
    - Copies of notes, X-rays, drug charts, management pre transfer
- Receiving PICU
    - History, current management, requests for specialist equipment (e.g. HFOV)

Figure 5.2. Beyond the first hour until transfer.

History

A detailed account of the history, initial examination, anaesthetic difficulties and interventions should be written. In particular, the timing of administration of antimicrobials, fluids, paracetamol and steroids should be recorded. Treatment can then safely be continued on PICU. A list of microbiological specimens sent and copies of radiological and blood investigations need to accompany the child upon transfer.

Blood products

Blood products are strictly regulated and the transfer of products between hospitals requires organization. With sepsis, coagulopathies can be expected due to the large fluid volumes administered during resuscitation along with the consumptive processes. Intensive care continues during ambulance transfers and the infusion of either blood or clotting products may become necessary.

Notification of disease

There is a statutory requirement to notify many causes of paediatric sepsis, including bacterial and viral meningitis, invasive group A streptococcus infection and haemolytic uraemic syndrome, to the local public health team. They arrange contact-tracing and chemoprophylaxis for those at high risk of infection. In meningococcal disease, chemoprophylaxis should be provided to household contacts and those exposed to a large amount of droplets from the respiratory tract around the time of admission.

What are the pitfalls in this kind of child?

Common pitfalls in managing paediatric sepsis

- Failing to appreciate severity of illness
- Not using age-appropriate values (see Chapter 35)
- Not exposing a child to see rashes
- Not giving fluids early – use an IO needle if necessary
- Not giving enough fluids
- Not intubating early enough
- Not preparing for unstable intubation
- Not cross-matching blood products early enough
- Allowing the child to become hypothermic with procedures

Summary

During the time following initial stabilization until the child is transferred to PICU it is imperative that the optimal management guidelines are followed. Advice for ongoing treatment can be obtained from the transport service or receiving PICU. Persisting shock on arrival at the PICU is associated with an increased risk of mortality. It has been shown that these children frequently do not receive the fluid and inotrope therapy they require. Continual assessment and early intervention thus maintaining our treatment goals should improve the outcome for this critical group of children in the future.

Further reading

Brierley J, Carcillo JA, Choong K, *et al.* Clinical practice parameters for haemodynamic support of pediatric and neonatal septic shock: 2007 update from the American College of Critical Care Medicine. *Crit Care Med* 2009;**37**:666–688.

Goldstein B, Giroir B, Randolph A, *et al.* International pediatric sepsis consensus conference: definitions for sepsis and organ dysfunction in pediatrics. *Pediatr Crit Care Med* 2005;**6**:2–8.

Meningitis Research Foundation website. http://www.meningitis.org/health-professionals.

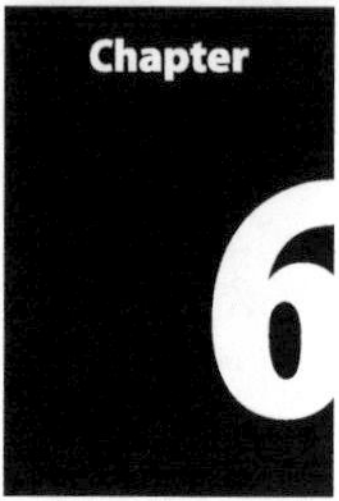

The child with cardiac disease

John Smith, with illustrations by Mazyar Kanani

Introduction

Abnormalities in the development of the heart and great vessels are the commonest congenital abnormalities, with a frequency of 5.2/1000 live births. Whilst many are not life-threatening and may require only conservative therapy there are a number that present in the newborn period or early infancy that require stabilization and urgent treatment.

In this chapter two different scenarios will be covered. The first is the collapsed neonate admitted to ED with possible congenital heart disease. The second is the child with known congenital heart disease (CHD).

Neonatal presentation of cardiac disease

The final switch from a fetal to an adult circulation by closure of the ductus arteriosus (DA) can unmask CHD. It is the most likely situation for an anaesthetist/ED doctor to encounter in the context of a baby with CHD returning to ED in extremis within 2 to 3 weeks of birth as the DA closes.

Suspecting CHD

The collapsed neonate presenting to ED is unlikely to have an obvious diagnosis of CHD. It is more likely that the child will present with an unknown cause of their illness where CHD may or may not be the underlying cause. For this reason CHD should always be kept in the differential diagnosis of a collapsed baby.

It would be reasonable to expect that the presentation of the sick child would depend on the anatomy of the cardiac lesion, i.e. low saturations in conditions with poor lung blood supply or systemic hypoperfusion/weak pulses in those with aortic outflow obstruction. However, in reality, a child brought back in to a DGH after duct closure is likely to present with a mixture of signs:

- low saturations that are refractory to oxygen therapy
- poor peripheral perfusion

Managing the Critically Ill Child, ed. Richard Skone *et al.* Published by Cambridge University Press.

- weak pulses (especially if normal upper limb but poor lower limb)
- high lactate
- cardiogenic shock.

Other potential diagnoses need to be considered. Most children are treated empirically with broad-spectrum antibiotics to cover sepsis.

Confirming CHD as a cause of collapse

Peripheral pulses

Peripheral and central pulses usually provide the first sign of CHD. Poor peripheral pulses and capillary refill would suggest that a bolus of fluid (20 ml of crystalloid) should be administered and the response assessed. However, if the femoral pulse is impalpable in the face of a good right brachial pulse then some form of left heart obstruction is likely. Palpable femoral and foot pulses are reassuring.

Saturations

A difference in saturation between the right arm and lower limbs suggests CHD (although not the exact lesion). The reason for the difference is that the DA joins the aorta close to the origin of the left subclavian artery (see Figure 6.1).

If there is a complete obstruction to flow from the left ventricle, any blood flowing in the aorta will be both anterograde and retrograde from the DA and pulmonary artery. It will therefore be deoxygenated equally as measured by the saturations in the hand and foot.

This diagnostic sign is not without its problems, as a shocked child coming into the ED may not have enough peripheral perfusion to give readable saturations.

Hepatomegaly

As with adults, right heart failure leads to increased inferior vena cava pressure. The liver can then become distended and easily palpable. It is possible to get false positives if a child has been given large volumes of resuscitation fluid or if they are ventilated with high airway pressures.

Chest X-ray

Pulmonary oedema has the same characteristics on X-rays to that of adults. Cardiomegaly should also raise the suspicion of CHD. Again, false positives from fluid resuscitation are possible.

Echocardiography

Some hospitals may have the facility to perform a cardiac ultrasound scan. This may help define whether there is a one- or two-ventricle pattern to the heart, whether there is a ventricular septal defect (VSD) or a duct present. However, complex lesions cannot always be excluded, especially if the practitioner in question is used to adult scans, or the correct scanner is not available.

The ductus arteriosus (DA)

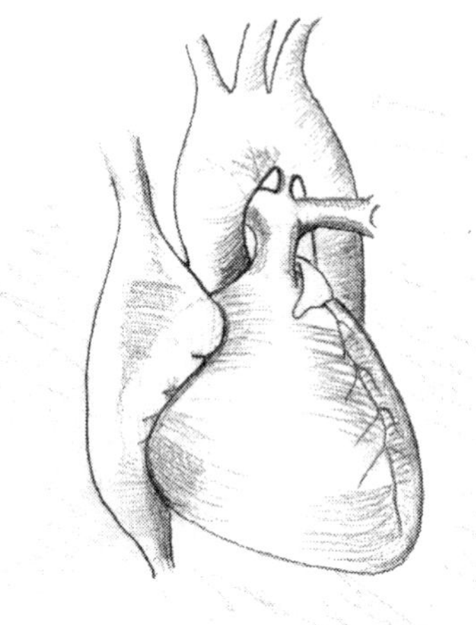

Figure 6.1. Ductus arteriosus. Note the DA arising from the bifurcation of the pulmonary artery and passing onto the inferior aspect of the aortic arch, opposite the left subclavian artery.

The DA is one of the two links in the fetal circulation that allow blood to bypass the high-resistance pulmonary circulation (the other is the foramen ovale). Once the lungs inflate and pulmonary vascular resistance drops the DA ceases to have a function in healthy babies. After birth the duct usually closes in two stages. First, it undergoes functional closure at about 15 hours, by smooth muscle contraction. This is triggered by a rise in blood oxygen levels, and a drop in maternal prostaglandins. The second stage is true anatomical closure, which can take a couple of weeks.

Persistence of the DA causes long-term problems such as pulmonary hypertension or heart failure. This is because the DA directly connects the high-pressure aorta with the pulmonary arteries.

The initial management of CHD relies on the fact that the duct can be re-opened temporarily (after functional closure) by the use of prostaglandin E1 or E2 (PgE). After true anatomical closure PgE will not be effective. However, CHD which is 'duct-dependent' may prolong the amount of time that the DA remains open, and therefore allow the DA to re-open in response to PgE infusion up to 3–4 weeks after birth.

Prior to its closure the DA can mask the presence of CHD in one of three ways:

- supplying blood to the lungs from the aorta if there is an interruption to the pulmonary artery, e.g. pulmonary atresia (left to right shunt across the DA)
- supplying blood to the systemic circulation from the pulmonary artery if there is an interruption or obstruction to the outflow of the left heart, e.g. severe coarctation (right to left shunt across the DA)
- providing a 'mixing point' where oxygenated blood can get from the pulmonary to the systemic side, e.g. transposition of the great vessels.

Specific conditions affecting neonates

Conditions with duct-dependent pulmonary blood flow

Critical pulmonary stenosis/pulmonary atresia/tricuspid atresia

The primary problem is a restriction to blood flow out of the right ventricle into the pulmonary artery (PA) (Figure 6.2). The DA, from the aorta, then becomes the main blood supply to the PA. Without reasonable blood flow through the DA these children will have very low saturations. Most conditions will have a second mixing point (atrial septal defect (ASP) or VSD) to allow blood to pass from the pulmonary to the systemic side, which will allow for a cardiac output to be maintained. This is essential as it would not be possible to maintain a circulation in conditions such as pulmonary atresia.

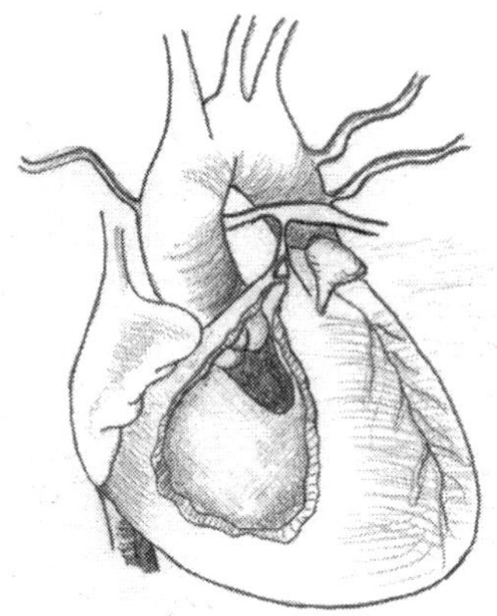

Figure 6.2. Pulmonary atresia. Note the very small (atretic) pulmonary artery (PA) and branch Pas. The VSD allows blood to escape from the right ventricle into the left ventricle. This diagram shows MAPCAs, which are anomalous blood vessels which supply the lungs directly from the aorta, under high pressure.

Conditions with duct-dependent systemic blood flow

Coarctation of the aorta

The classic presentation is of an infant who presents with feeding difficulties, breathlessness or collapse within the first week of birth. The contraction of ductal tissue within the distal aortic arch narrows the lumen of the aorta (see Figure 6.1 for point of insertion of DA on the aorta) and makes the lower half of the body dependent upon the flow of desaturated blood from pulmonary artery, via the DA. The closure of the duct then precipitates the presentation. Physical examination will reveal weak or absent femoral pulses as blood fails to travel past the narrowing (coarctation) in the aorta, while managing to supply the upper part of the body.

Once the diagnosis is suspected, treatment should include appropriate resuscitation, PgE1/PgE2 (which may or may not be effective depending on the age at presentation) and assessment for surgical repair.

Hypoplastic left heart syndrome (HLHS)

This condition used to be lethal in the neonatal period. The clinical presentation is similar to that of coarctation of the aorta. Mitral atresia (failure of development of the mitral valve)

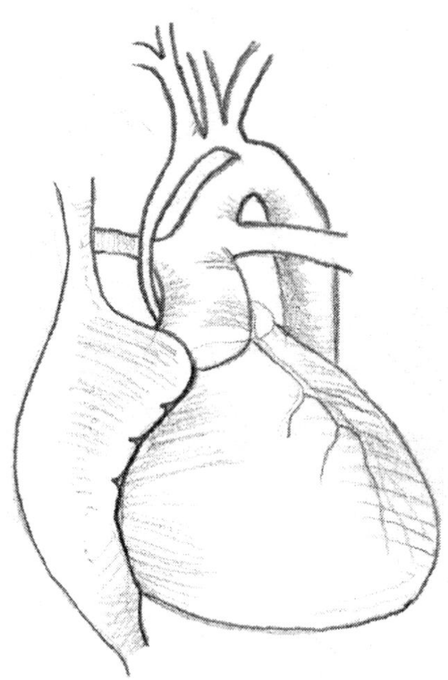

Figure 6.3. Hypoplastic left heart syndrome. Note the very small aorta passing around the pulmonary artery. The aorta enlarges at the point of insertion of the DA. This diagram does not show the small left ventricle or the fact that the coronary arteries arise from the small aorta.

leads to a condition where the left ventricle and first part of the aorta fail to develop properly (see Figure 6.3). As a result, blood supply to the systemic circulation is dependent on the DA.

Blood passing out of the right ventricle and into the PA can flow either along the branch pulmonary arteries to the lungs, or down the DA to the systemic circulation. *The direction of flow will be decided by the balance between pulmonary and systemic vascular resistance.*

Aiming for high systemic arterial oxygen Saturation (SaO_2) in these children may result in a low cardiac output or cardiac arrest.

A high PaO_2 will reduce pulmonary vascular resistance (by abolishing hypoxic pulmonary vasoconstriction). Blood will then flow along the path of least resistance, into the lungs, leaving very little flow to the systemic circulation, compromising blood flow down the coronary arteries, and may cause cardiac arrest.

The key to adequate resuscitation is to ensure that the aims are conservative, i.e. SaO_2 of 75% with a normal or slightly high $PaCO_2$ so that the pulmonary vascular resistance is not reduced. Heart rate and cardiac function need to be optimized with volume boluses and inotropes if oxygen delivery is compromised. Once stabilized and appropriately assessed these children undergo early surgery.

Conditions with duct-dependent mixing of pulmonary and systemic blood

Transposition of the great arteries (TGA)

In this condition the systemic and pulmonary circulations exist as two parallel circuits and cyanosis is present from birth (Figure 6.4). Blood mixes between the two otherwise independent circuits by passing across a patent arterial duct or across the foramen ovale. A VSD, if present, is another point at which mixing can occur. The amount of mixing will depend on the patency of the DA (or septal defects) and the relative pressures in the pulmonary and systemic circulations.

A single mixing point, such as an ASD, may not be enough to sustain a child with a TGA. PgE2 should be started in these children. If it does not lead to an increase in the arterial saturations then the usual strategies of assessing and treating cardiovascular filling, the administration of inotropes and controlling ventilation should be instituted before emergency balloon atrial septostomy (BAS) to improve mixing.

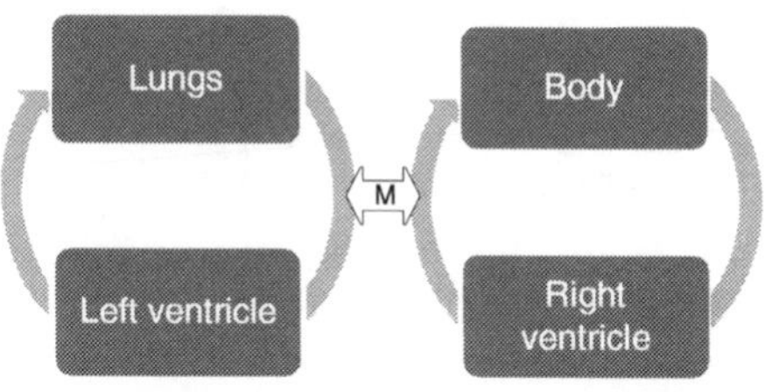

Figure 6.4. Transposition of the great arteries (with connecting DA).

Duct-independent condition causing cyanosis

Total anomalous pulmonary venous connection (TAPVC)

The pulmonary veins drain, either partially or fully, into the systemic veins, e.g. inferior vena cava. There is an absence or much reduced pulmonary venous connection to the left atrium. The consequences are reduced blood flow to the left heart with a subsequent increase in pulmonary blood flow. This results in pulmonary hypertension, breathing difficulties secondary to the volume of blood in the pulmonary circulation and right heart failure. If the pulmonary venous drainage is 'obstructed' the condition is a true surgical emergency. This is because there is very little flow to the left atrium and the lungs become very oedematous secondary to pulmonary venous hypertension. This in turn leads to compensatory pulmonary arterial hypertension. Despite the need for urgent surgery proper resuscitation prior to urgent transfer to theatre is needed.

Conditions presenting with signs of poor cardiac function in infants and older children

Congenital heart disease may present when the child is no longer a neonate. The presenting symptom is more likely to be breathlessness on a background of poor feeding and faltering growth. Fluid overload of the right ventricle, e.g. from a VSD, will lead to pulmonary hypertension and right heart failure. Obstructive conditions such as tetralogy of Fallot or subclinical coarctation of the aorta will cause right and left ventricular hypertrophy respectively.

Heart failure

An infant or older child who presents with fluid retention, breathlessness and signs of a low cardiac output may well be suffering from cardiac failure. Causes of heart failure in children include:

- large left to right shunts, e.g. VSD or persistent DA
- chronic arrhythmias, e.g. supravertricular tachycardias (SVTs) from channelopathies
- primary cardiomyopathy, e.g. dilated cardiomyopathy
- outflow tract obstruction, e.g. undiagnosed coarctation of the aorta

- cyanotic CHD, e.g. truncus arteriosus (although this is rarely undiagnosed)
- myocarditis.

A very brief history of breathlessness with symptoms and signs of heart failure, but without a very enlarged heart on chest X-ray, should raise concerns about fulminant myocarditis. Although, as mentioned above, classic presentations may not occur in CHD.

Left to right shunts

An infant who presents with breathlessness, signs of fluid retention and a murmur is likely to have a lesion with a large left to right shunt, e.g. VSD, complete atriovertricular septal defect (AVSD) or truncus arteriosus. These children do not present when the DA closes but present some weeks after birth when the pulmonary vascular resistance (PVR) falls (it does not achieve adult levels until approximately 6 months of age).

When the PVR drops, blood flows freely across the VSD and back into the pulmonary circulation. This increases pulmonary blood flow and lung water while the relative under-filling of the systemic circulation causes fluid retention. This results in an increase in the work of breathing and heart failure.

Tetralogy of Fallot (ToF)

The main problem in the tetralogy of Fallot (ToF) is obstruction to the right ventricular outflow tract (RVOT) as it passes into the pulmonary artery (see Figure 6.5). It is the main reason that the right ventricle hypertrophies. The obstruction to the RVOT is dynamic in that it worsens when the infundibulum at the base of the pulmonary artery goes into spasm. With increased resistance to blood passing out of the right ventricle, it passes instead through a VSD into the left ventricle. This can cause profound cyanosis. Giving oxygen may not correct the hypoxia, as this is a true shunt. Giving oxygen is important though as it will optimize oxygenation of the blood that does pass through the lungs. Severe desaturations associated

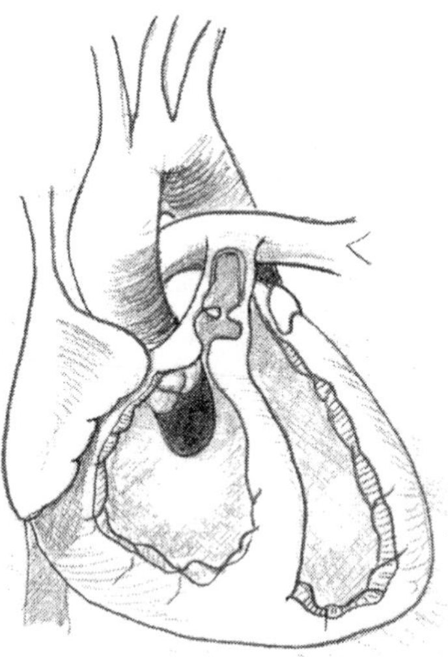

Figure 6.5. Tetralogy of Fallot. Note the VSD (with the root of the aorta shown overriding the VSD). There is also pulmonary stenosis and a hypertrophied right ventricle.

with right ventricular outflow tract obstruction are known as 'spells'. The steps in managing a child who is spelling are detailed in Figure 6.7.

Hypertrophic ventricles

As mentioned previously ToF leads to right ventricular hypertrophy whereas coarctation of the aorta causes the left ventricle to hypertrophy. Children with hypertrophic ventricles have a similar problem to adults. The decreased compliance means that a greater pressure is required to achieve the same ventricular filling. Also, the myocardial oxygen requirement can outstrip the coronary blood supply. The principle of aiming for a low normal heart rate with adequate coronary perfusion is the same.

Arrhythmias

An arrhythmia is usually well tolerated in children. However, they may be associated with collapse or dyspnoea. It is often not easy to distinguish between a physiological tachycardia and a pathological rhythm. A good-quality ECG and a long rhythm strip are essential for diagnosis.

The arrhythmias can be caused by:

- electrolyte abnormalities
- channelopathies
- conduction pathway abnormalities, e.g. re-entrant tachycardias
- structural abnormalities, e.g. hypertrophic ventricle
- postoperative, e.g. AVSD repair causing complete heart block.

The principles of treatment of arrhythmias in children are the same as in adults and are detailed below under 'Problems with known/treated/palliated CHD'. Advice can be sought from the local cardiac centre.

Child with known CHD (post surgery)

As paediatric cardiac surgery becomes more successful, the prevalence of children with CHD increases. It is not uncommon for children with known cardiac disease to present to a local emergency department with any of the common intercurrent infections or other diseases of childhood. They may also be suffering from an acute deterioration of their cardiac problem. The management of these conditions is described below under 'Problems with known/treated/palliated CHD'.

Managing the neonate with CHD

The collapsed neonate with CHD

The question in neonates is often not 'what type of CHD does the child have?' but 'does this child have CHD?' The initial assessment may not reveal the diagnosis and therefore a structured approach is essential. First manage the collapsed child as the initial approach recommends in Chapter 4 and in Table 6.1.

Once a diagnosis of CHD is suspected, it is important to continue to stabilize the patient rather than spend time attempting to diagnose the type of CHD. A child with an acyanotic heart condition will be cyanotic if they are sick enough.

Table 6.1. Initial management of a neonate with suspected cardiac disease.

Phase of management	Assessment	Action
Initial phase On presentation of the child (see Chapter 4 for initial management)	Assess need for intubation or CPR	Give oxygen • Ventilate by hand if needed Gain IV access • IO if more than three IV attempts Give fluid bolus • 20 ml/kg of crystalloid Take blood including ABG, clotting and cross-match Treat for other pathologies if uncertain of cause, e.g. give antibiotics
After initial assessment Once imminently life-threatening risks have been addressed and CHD is suspected	Consider CHD and look for confirmation • Pulses, peripheral and central • Differential saturations pre- and post-ductal • Poor peripheral perfusion • Organomegaly Reassess after starting PgE2	Start PgE2 Airway • Consider intubation if PgE2 dose rising Breathing • Do not aim too high with SaO_2 (> 75% is often adequate) Circulation • Continue with fluid boluses • Consider inotropes
Further stabilization Not immediately lifesaving procedures	Continue to reassess clinical condition and blood results Definitive plan (transfer vs. operate) Decide on further monitoring	Contact tertiary centre for advice, e.g. via regional retrieval team Arterial line (preferably right radial artery) especially when: • Starting inotropes • Repeated blood gases required CVC if: • More definitive access needed • Starting inotropes • Giving high-concentration drugs Correct coagulopathy

Prostaglandin E

Prostaglandins are rapidly metabolized and therefore given by IV infusion. PgE2 is made up as a solution with a concentration of 1 μg/ml and given at a dose of 5–20 ng/kg/min. When given to a child with CHD the response is rapid, within minutes. SaO_2 and clinical signs of cardiac function should be assessed regularly once treatment has begun in order to measure the response.

Side effects of prostaglandin E treatment include hypotension, apnoea, fever, tachycardia, bradycardia and hypoglycaemia. An increasing dose of prostaglandin is an indication for intubation in otherwise stable babies with CHD, as apnoeas may become significant with higher doses.

Once the question has been raised of potential CHD in a sick child, the default position should be to start PgE2 treatment (and monitor response). Table 6.2 gives a broad outline of when to start PgE.

Table 6.2. Should I start PgE?

Findings that would prompt a trial of prostaglandin therapy in a neonate
Weak femoral pulses (especially if brachial pulse good)
Low saturations (< 90%) on maximal oxygen therapy
Pre-ductal (right arm) saturations higher than post-ductal (lower limb)

Inotropes

The need for fluid resuscitation in excess of 40 ml/kg, on the basis of poor pulses or capillary refill, or a metabolic acidosis should prompt ventilation and inotrope therapy. Inotropes should be started early if CHD is suspected. The choice of inotrope follows a similar rationale to that in adults. In the case of conditions where inotropy and reduced SVR are ideal, e.g. heart failure or conditions with excessive left to right shunts, dobutamine and milrinone can be considered. However, for a sick child who presents in a state of shock, adrenaline is also a reasonable choice as a first-line inotrope. Remember that inotropes may be administered through an IO needle if necessary.

A regional PICU retrieval team should have been contacted both for advice and to initiate the transfer of the child by this point.

Invasive monitoring

Once the child is ventilated, an arterial line can be placed, preferably in the right arm (radial rather than brachial) or a femoral artery and a blood gas and lactate obtained. This should be monitored continuously for blood pressure with regular intermittent blood gases.

A central line is desirable, but, as with other children, should only really be attempted if the practitioner is confident of their skill in the procedure in small children.

Aims of management of neonatal CHD

The aim of managing neonates with CHD is to have:

- adequate cardiac output
- adequate blood flow to the pulmonary and systemic circulations
- adequate oxygen saturations to meet demand.

When deciding on oxygen delivery remember that neonates will usually have a higher haemoglobin concentration than adults (if not, early transfusion is indicated).

Cardiac output

Achieving a good cardiac output involves the basics discussed in Chapter 4, i.e. adequate oxygenation and fluid resuscitation. Inotropes can be used as discussed above.

'Balancing' circulations – directing blood flow to the correct side of the circulation

The DA provides an unregulated, low-resistance path for blood to flow between the systemic and pulmonary circulations. As a result, the direction of blood flow will depend on the balance between SVR PVR. A similar situation can occur in conditions such as truncus arteriosus (TA) when both main arteries effectively come from a common outlet, i.e. blood will flow via the path of least resistance.

Managing SVR is familiar to most adult physicians. Managing PVR on the other hand may be a bit less familiar. Once intubated, managing the PVR of a child is straightforward. Factors that will increase PVR include:

- raised $PaCO_2$ – allowing the CO_2 to rise will increase PVR
- hypoxia – hypoxia increases PVR, by means of hypoxic pulmonary vasoconstriction
- acidosis – acidosis will increase PVR.

On the other hand PVR can be reduced by:

- low CO_2 – hyperventilation will reduce the PVR
- high FiO_2 – hyperoxia will reduce PVR
- nitric oxide – inhaled nitric oxide will reduce PVR
- drugs – nitrates, beta-agonists and phosphodiesterase inhibitors will lower PVR.

In a situation where too much of the cardiac output is being diverted to the pulmonary circulation and poor peripheral perfusion exists, relative hypoventilation with an FiO_2 titrated to keep SaO_2 at 75–80% maximum may help 'balance' the blood flow towards an improved systemic output (by raising PVR).

Oxygen saturations

If a child has a true right to left shunt then no amount of oxygen will improve their SaO_2. Adaptations in utero, such as fetal haemoglobin, allow SaO_2 of 70–80% to be tolerated in neonates with cyanotic heart disease. If the oxygen delivery does not match the baby's needs then markers of anaerobic metabolism such as lactate will increase.

The stable neonate with CHD

If a neonate with CHD is assessed and found to be stable it is reasonable not to 'chase the saturations'. There is no need to ventilate to improve the SaO_2 alone; SaO_2 above 70% can be tolerated in these circumstances until diagnosis. The SaO_2 should be measured in the right arm (pre-ductal) as well as in the legs (post-ductal). A difference between the two readings (lower SaO_2 in the lower limbs) suggests a significant shunt but not a precise diagnosis.

Managing the older child with CHD

Infants or young children with cardiac conditions can present with breathlessness, drowsiness, oedema or nausea. Cardiac diseases can also mimic gastrointestinal problems (abdominal pain and poor feeding in infants and children). Other signs of heart failure are similar to those seen in adults, e.g. added heart sounds and distended veins. Although cardiac problems are a rare cause of breathlessness in the general paediatric population, shortness of breath is a common presentation for heart failure.

The initial management of sick children with CHD follows the pattern set out in Chapter 4.

Initial management of the older child with CHD

It should come as no surprise that, even though the causes are different, the management of cardiac disease in children is very similar to that in adults. It follows the same principles:

- give oxygen, aiming for $SaO_2 > 90\%$, unless the child is known to 'normally' have lower SaO_2 saturations
- check for arrhythmias
- induce a diuresis, e.g. with furosemide 0.5–1 mg/kg
- vasodilate and offload the heart.

The examination may reveal signs such as bilateral fine crackles, distended neck veins, a gallop rhythm and an enlarged liver. An ECG and chest X-ray should be performed at the earliest possible opportunity. The chest X-ray may confirm the size of the heart and the presence or absence of any pleural effusions.

Further interventions such as intubation or inotropes will be required if:

- inappropriate cyanosis persists in the face of high flow oxygen
- there are poor peripheral pulses
- tachycardia persists
- a metabolic acidosis persists.

Inotropes

Often on PICU dobutamine or milrinone is used as a first-line therapy for heart failure. However, given that many children will present to ED *in extremis* it is reasonable to use adrenaline as a first-line inotrope. The choice of agent will need to be decided based on the presentation of the child.

The inotropes should ideally be given through a second intravenous line (preferably an IO or central line for adrenaline).

Management of arrhythmias

Tachycardias

Most tachyarrhythmias are variations of SVR due to aberrant intracardiac conduction pathways that allow self-sustaining circuits to override the usual conduction pathway. It is crucial to decide whether the rate is well tolerated physiologically or not. Then distinguish between a narrow and a broad complex tachycardia. The former is always supraventricular in origin, the latter may be supraventricular or ventricular in origin. A QRS complex longer than 0.12 seconds is considered 'broad'.

The first line of management should involve the initial management detailed in Chapter 4.

The flow chart in Figure 6.6 gives an appropriate management path.

Bradycardia

A bradycardia is a rate of:

- slower than 90 bpm in an infant
- slower than 80 bpm between the ages of 5 and 11
- slower than 60 bpm in an older child.

The first stage in treating a bradycardia is to check that it is not secondary to a systemic illness or a sign of imminent collapse. Bradycardia is an agonal rhythm in the critically ill or hypoxic child. Other causes of bradycardia include hypertension, raised intracranial pressure or physical training in the teenager.

As with adults, the blood pressure and conscious level of the child should be assessed in order to guide the next step. Once causative factors have been addressed atropine (20 μg/kg) should be given if the heart rate does not improve. Adrenaline 10 μg/kg may be used *in extremis*.

Heart block

The classification of heart block is the same for children as it is in adults. It is rare as a primary condition and most children who present will have a history of cardiac intervention or drug therapy. Assessment of the adequacy of the circulation is of prime importance in making decisions. Symptomatic heart block is treated temporarily with intravenous isoprenaline or external pacing if the equipment is available. Consultation with a paediatric cardiologist is essential to guide management in these children.

The 'spelling' child with tetralogy of Fallot

Spelling occurs when the infundibulum goes into spasm. The spell may be secondary to fever, dehydration or another intercurrent illness. It can occur in children from birth until they undergo surgical repair. Children with ToF typically present to their local hospital with an exacerbation of cyanosis. These episodes of acute desaturation may get worse as the child gets older.

The mainstay of treatment is to relieve anxiety and try to decrease the quantity of blood shunted (right to left) across the VSD. This is done by:

- trying to relax the muscle of the infundibulum
- increasing right ventricular filling
- improving the balance between SVR and PVR to reduce the shunt across the VSD.

Oxygen, the knee–chest position, morphine, fluid loading and vasoconstrictors are the mainstays of treatment. In extremes, ventilation, vasoconstrictor infusions and cooling (to minimize oxygen consumption) are used prior to emergency surgery (see Figure 6.7).

Problems with known/treated/palliated CHD

The parents of children in the cardiac outpatient population will have a good idea of their child's usual SaO_2 and activity level. The children are likely to present to ED with a

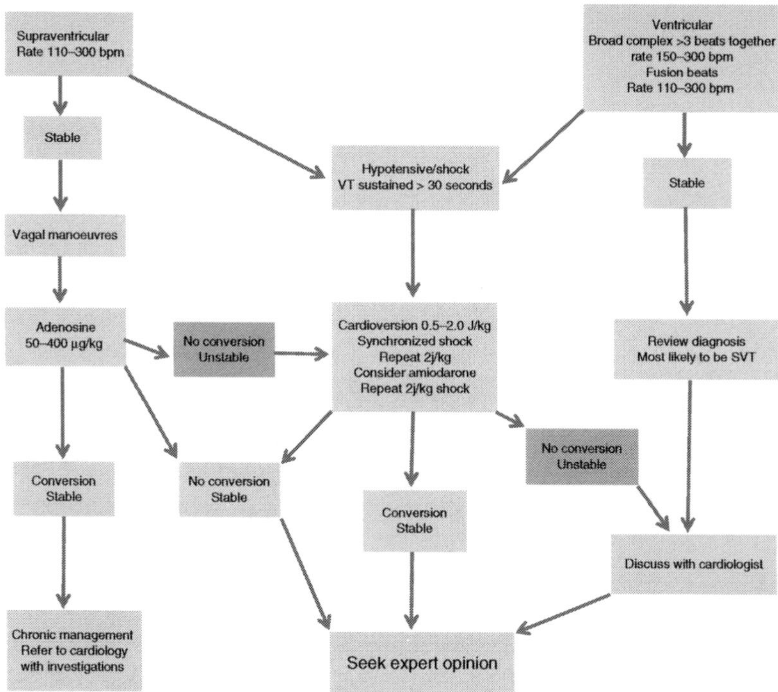

Figure 6.6. Management of tachycardia.

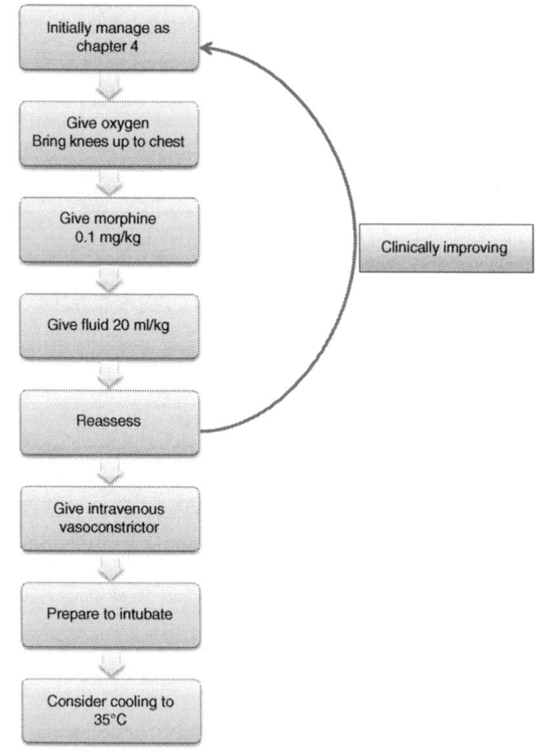

Figure 6.7. Management of a child with ToF who is spelling.

common paediatric illness which has been made more severe by their underlying CHD. The child with CHD may also present with worsening of their underlying cardiac condition.

Worsening cyanosis

This may be unforeseen or develop ahead of the cardiologist's expectations. A full physical examination should be performed in order to exclude intercurrent pulmonary or other diseases. In the absence of a clear secondary cause of the cyanosis, referral back to the cardiac centre is appropriate. The finding of a large pleural effusion in this context may present difficulties as drainage will be required to improve respiratory function but the sedation or anaesthesia required for drainage may cause severe instability. Beyond the neonatal period PgE has no role.

Heart failure

This may be a consequence of either an arrhythmia or myocardial decompensation after previous surgical treatment. The assessment of cardiac function and related arrhythmias needs to be thorough. The management should be as above, with advice from the child's cardiac centre.

Syncope

This may be a consequence of a tachycardia/bradycardia or worsening cardiac function. It may be the result of the progression of disease or the complications of surgery.

Palpitations

This may be the symptom of an arrhythmia that can be detected clinically. It might be an anxiety symptom but should be investigated in the usual way and will merit referral back to the cardiology clinic.

Infective endocarditis

Non-specific symptoms in a child with a known structural cardiac disease should alert the admitting physician to the possibility of infective endocarditis. Clinical assessment of the circulation will guide the intensity of therapy but crucial in the management of such a child is a microbiological identification of the infective organism. Unless there is a clear reason for urgent treatment, antibiotics should not be started empirically.

Summary

Managing children with CHD can be an intimidating task. Although this chapter has explained the details of their management, it should not be forgotten that the initial management is the same as for all other emergency conditions. The main difference is that prostaglandin therapy should always be considered in a sick neonate and a low threshold should be held for its use.

Golden rules when managing children with CHD

- Ask the parents what the saturations are normally – aim for the saturations given
- Children with CHD still suffer from common illnesses
- When other factors have been ruled out consider cardiac decompensation
- Always perform an ECG in a child with CHD to look for arrhythmias

Further reading

Biarent D, *et al.* European Resuscitation Council Guidelines 2010, Section 6. Paediatric life support. *Resuscitation* 2010;**81**:1364–1388.

Marino B, Fine K, McMillan J. *Blueprint Paediatrics*. Blackwell, 2006.

Wren C, O'Sullivan JJ. Survival with congenital heart disease and need for follow up in adult life. *Heart* 2001;**85**:438–443.

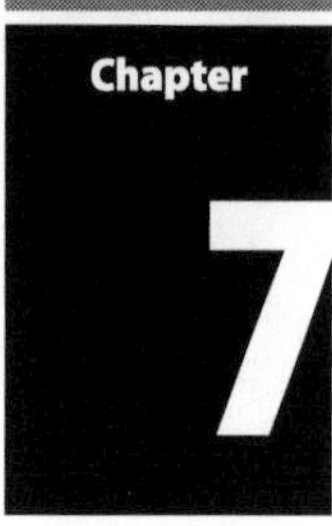

The child with shortness of breath

Brian Shields and Benjamin Stanhope

Introduction

Respiratory disease makes up approximately 35% of all unplanned PICU admissions in the UK. The commonest causes are:

- bronchiolitis (41%)
- pneumonia/lower respiratory tract infection (LRTI) (21%)
- croup (6.8%)
- asthma (6.5%).

Shortness of breath can be the presenting feature of a host of problems. This chapter primarily aims to cover the pulmonary causes. Asthma is covered in Chapter 8.

How respiratory pathology differs in children

Children have a greater initial capacity to respond to physiological stress than adults. Exceptions to this include small neonates and children with chronic illness. When children become exhausted they can decompensate suddenly and precipitously.

Pathology

Children are more prone to virally mediated chest problems such as bronchiolitis and viral-induced wheeze than adults. This is due to:

- mucous plugging
- inflammation of their much smaller airways having a greater impact
- relative immaturity of immune development.

Increasingly, children with an extensive history of chronic lung disease due to prematurity and mechanical ventilation are presenting to the ED. These children are particularly susceptible to all forms of chest infection.

Physiology

There is evidence to suggest that children younger than 1 year old with bronchospasm do not respond to standard medications such as β_2-agonists, presumably due to lack of airway receptor development.

Managing the Critically Ill Child, ed. Richard Skone *et al.* Published by Cambridge University Press.

What are the warning signs that a child is really sick?

To doctors unfamiliar with managing children, it can be very difficult to differentiate those with a simple chest infection from those who are critically ill. For many children the results of giving fluid, paracetamol and cooling by removing clothes can be dramatic. However, Table 7.1 lists some signs that should cause concern in any child.

Table 7.1.

	Intermediate risk	High risk
Respiratory rate (RR)	Age < 12 months and RR > 50 breaths/min Age > 12 months and RR > 40 breaths/min	RR > 60 breaths/min
Other respiratory features	Nasal flaring Crepitations (pneumonia or bronchiolitis) SaO_2 < 95% in air	Apnoea Grunting Moderate or severe chest indrawing Head bobbing SaO_2 < 90% on air
Colour	Pallor reported by parent/carer	Pale/mottled/ashen/blue
Activity[b]	No response to normal social cues[a] Wakes only with prolonged stimulation[a] Decreased activity[a]	No response to social cues[a] Unable to be roused, or if rousable does not stay awake[a] Appears ill to healthcare professional[a] Confusion/altered mental state Unable to speak in sentences
Hydration/feeding	Poor feeding in infants (less than 50% of normal fluid intake in preceding 24 hours) Dry mucous membranes Reduced urine output Capillary refill time > 3 seconds	Reduced skin turgor Unable to feed
Temperature	Fever > 5 days duration	Age < 3 months and temperature > 38°C Age 3–6 months and temperature > 39°C

[a] Activity and appearance are highly subjective and are considered poor markers of severity by some experts.
Data adapted from: British Thoracic Society, 2002; SIGN, 2006; NICE, 2007. http://www.cks.nhs.uk/cough_acute_with_chest_signs_in_children/management/detailed_answers/assessment.

Specific conditions causing shortness of breath

Bronchiolitis

Bronchiolitis is a condition caused by inflammation of the small airways (bronchioles) of the lungs. It is most common in children aged 2–6 months, and is uncommon in children over 1 year old. It is usually caused by respiratory syncytial virus (75%), but can also be caused by parainfluenza, influenza and adenoviruses.

Bronchiolitis usually has a gradual onset with coryzal symptoms and mild fever followed by cough and increasing respiratory distress. Disease severity peaks at around 4–5 days and then gradually improves. Approximately 9% of all hospital admissions with bronchiolitis require admission to PICU.

In bronchiolitis, the bronchiolar epithelial cells are invaded by virus, resulting in:

- ciliated cell death
- sloughing of dead cells into the airway
- increased mucus production
- proliferation of non-ciliated cells.

This results in reduced mucus removal, air trapping and reduced gas exchange. The end result is an obstructive airway disease similar to asthma.

Children who are admitted to hospital will initially receive supportive care with humidified oxygen, nasogastric or IV fluids, or observation. They can usually be managed on 'general' paediatric wards with continuous pulse oximetry monitoring and regular observations.

Identifying the sicker children with bronchiolitis

Although many children with bronchiolitis will look quite unwell, Table 7.2 highlights the main signs that should prompt admission to hospital. Table 7.3 lists patients who are at high risk of getting severe bronchiolitis and in whom a lower threshold for admission should be practised.

Table 7.2. Signs of bronchiolitis that should warrant admission to hospital.

Poor feeding (< 50% of usual fluid intake in preceding 24 hours)
Lethargy
Apnoea
Respiratory rate > 60/min
Nasal flaring and/or grunting
Severe chest wall recession
Cyanosis
Oxygen saturation ≤ 94% in air
Uncertainty regarding diagnosis
High-risk factors (see above)

Table 7.3. High-risk patients with bronchiolitis.

Prematurity < 35 weeks
Chronic lung disease (cystic fibrosis, bronchopulmonary dysplasia)
Age less than 12 weeks
Congenital heart disease
Hypotonia (e.g. trisomy 21 or neuromuscular disease)
Immunocompromised
Anatomical airway abnormalities

Signs of a deteriorating child

Children who appear to be worsening should receive regular capillary blood gases. As the child's work of breathing becomes greater, and they tire, the $PaCO_2$ will rise. If there is a trend towards a rising $PaCO_2$ (especially if the child is on CPAP – see below) then intubation is likely to be needed.

Apnoeas are relatively common in younger babies suffering from bronchiolitis. The majority are brief (less than 5 seconds) and self-terminating. However, the signs that a child having apnoeas might need intubation include:

- prolonged apnoeas
- needing stimulation to terminate apnoeas
- increasing frequency of apnoeas
- apnoeas associated with episodes of hypoxia and bradycardia.

Targeted treatments for bronchiolitis

Oxygen

Humidified oxygen is usually delivered via an appropriately sized headbox, with adequate gas flow to avoid CO_2 build-up inside the box. The oxygen needs to be humidified because of the build-up of secretions that would otherwise dry up and worsen the condition. Face masks or nasal prongs may be used although they are sometimes poorly tolerated.

Fluid management

Children who are unable to feed effectively should receive nasogastric feeds. Those who have severe respiratory distress may require intravenous fluids instead.

Intravenous fluids should be restricted to two-thirds of usual maintenance in severe bronchiolitis (see Chapter 32). This is because of the risk of syndrome of inappropriate antidiuretic hormone secretion (SIADH) and hyponatraemia (which can be severe enough to cause convulsions). However, some children may be hypovolaemic due to reduced intake and may need fluid boluses. Clinical assessment will dictate the appropriate management.

Ventilatory support

Continuous positive airway pressure (CPAP) or mechanical vertilation (IPPV) may be needed for infants exhibiting:

- apnoeas (see above)
- hypoxaemia refractory to oxygen therapy

- hypercapnia
- moderately increased work of breathing.

CPAP in bronchiolitis aims to improve gas exchange by preventing alveolar collapse. Because of the obstructive nature of the pathology, CPAP actually reduces the $PaCO_2$ in bronchiolitis by keeping airways open and decreasing the work of breathing. CPAP also helps to minimize apnoeas by stimulating breathing in children.

IPPV in bronchiolitis initially requires high inspiratory pressures and long inspiratory times. Once alveoli are recruited pressures can be gradually weaned. When ventilating bear in mind similar principles to those of ventilating a child with asthma (see Table 7.4).

Table 7.4. Ventilation strategy in bronchiolitis.

Use a protective lung strategy (tidal volume of 5–10 ml/kg)
Allow enough time for expiration to avoid 'gas trapping'
Keep peak inspiratory pressure below 30 cmH_2O (or plateau pressure depending on measurement)
Use high PEEP values (up to 10 cmH_2O) to overcome airway collapse – titrated to optimize compliance
Use longer inspiratory times to allow air to flow through the high resistance airways (0.75–1 second, depending on size and age)
Tolerate moderate hypercapnoea (to a pH of 7.2)
Suction the ET tube regularly as secretions may build up rapidly

Antibiotics

Secondary bacterial infection in bronchiolitis may affect as many as 40% of patients who require intubation. Patients at high risk of severe bronchiolitis are also at increased risk of secondary bacterial infection. Antibiotics should be considered in high-risk patients, or if there is strong clinical suspicion of bacterial infection (high temperature or lobar changes on CXR).

β_2-Agonists, adrenaline and corticosteroids

Use of these agents is not supported by the current literature.

Potential pitfalls when managing children with bronchiolitis

- Apnoea can occur without preceding signs of severe respiratory distress.
- Symptoms will peak at around 4–5 days so be aware that children in the first few days of illness are likely to get worse.
- Bronchodilators are ineffective.
- Secondary bacterial infections or collapse/consolidation can complicate bronchiolitis and prolong PICU stays.

Wheeze in pre-school children ($\leq$ 5 years)

Wheeze in pre-school children is a common presentation. It should be distinguished from wheezing episodes in older children as the majority of pre-school wheezers will not go on to develop asthma. Wheeze in pre-school children has been described in two main categories:

- episodic (viral) wheeze – wheeze following upper respiratory tract infection (URTI) lasting 2–4 weeks but the patient is otherwise well
- multiple trigger wheeze – wheeze following URTI plus interval symptoms and/or wheeze due to other triggers. There may be a personal or family history of atopy.

The vast majority of these children will not have severe problems unless they have a past history of chronic lung disease or atopy.

Targeted treatments for pre-school wheeze

Inhaled β_2-agonists

These form the mainstay of treatment of acute wheeze, although inhaled salbutamol has been shown often to have no effect in children less than 1 year of age.

Inhaled steroids

These are not effective in the acute setting. However, long-term inhaled corticosteroids may reduce severity of future wheeze episodes in children with multi-trigger wheeze.

Oral steroids

Steroids have been shown to be ineffective in non-atopic children with episodic (viral) wheeze. In atopic children they may be of some benefit.

Severe wheeze

Intravenous salbutamol, aminophylline and magnesium sulphate can all be considered in severe cases. They can be used for the same recommendations and dosing regimens as for asthma. The indication and strategies for ventilation in these children will be similar to those for asthma also (see Chapter 8).

Potential pitfalls when managing pre-school children with wheeze

Always reassess the child after their initial treatment to ensure that the bronchodilators are effective. Symptoms can return suddenly after initial improvement, so patients should be monitored carefully.

Pneumonia

Causes

The most common bacterial organism that causes community-acquired pneumonia (CAP) in children is *Streptococcus pneumoniae*, with *Mycoplasma pneumoniae* and *Chlamydia* infection being less common. *Bordetella pertussis* infection can occur in non- or partially immunized children.

Respiratory syncytial virus is the commonest viral pathogen in paediatric pneumonia. Other viruses that cause CAP include parainfluenza, adenovirus, rhinovirus, varicella zoster virus, influenza, cytomegalovirus, herpes simplex virus and enteroviruses. Viruses account for 14–35% of CAP cases in childhood. There may be mixed bacterial/viral infection in up to 40% of cases.

Viral causes are more common in pre-school-age children.

Clinical features

Symptoms and signs of pneumonia may include:

- tachypnoea
- tachycardia
- use of accessory muscles
- nasal flaring
- subcostal/intercostal recession
- cough with sputum production
- fever
- chest pain
- dyspnoea.

Bacterial pneumonia should be considered in children aged up to 3 years when there is a combination of:

- fever of $> 38.5°C$
- chest recession
- respiratory rate of > 50 breaths/min.

If wheeze is present in a pre-school child, primary bacterial pneumonia is unlikely. For older children a history of difficulty in breathing is more helpful than clinical signs.

Targeted treatments for pneumonia

When managing children with severe pneumonia, there is significant overlap with that of sepsis (see Chapter 5).

Antibiotics

Amoxicillin is the first-choice antibiotic therapy in children under the age of 5 years because it is effective against the majority of pathogens that cause CAP in this group. Local guidelines should be followed for any other choices. Macrolide antibiotics may be used as empirical treatment in children above 5 years of age because of the higher incidence of *Mycoplasma pneumoniae* infection.

Physiotherapy

There is no evidence to support the use of physiotherapy for pneumonia in otherwise healthy children. Physiotherapy may be of benefit to children with neuromuscular or musculoskeletal disease who have difficulty clearing secretions on their own.

CPAP/ventilation

The decision of when to ventilate children with pneumonia will depend on similar factors to all those mentioned above, i.e.:

- hypoxia refractory to oxygen therapy
- rising $PaCO_2$
- a child who appears to be tiring/confused/irritable
- large fluid requirement and sepsis.

As a guide to whether a child is tiring, if they allow you to put in a cannula without crying or making a fuss, it is likely that they are very unwell.

CPAP is used in pneumonia in the same way as it is in adults. The major caveat to the use of CPAP is to not let a child deteriorate on it. If they do not respond quickly (within 30 minutes) then delaying intubation can be dangerous.

If a decision is taken to ventilate a child with pneumonia, be aware that they will desaturate very quickly on induction. Preoxygenate the child as much as possible, ventilate the patient with a bag and mask while waiting for the muscle relaxant to work, and do not take too long before abandoning an attempt at intubation if you struggle.

Pleural effusion and empyema

Infective causes of pleural effusion

The most common cause of empyema in the UK is *Streptococcus pneumoniae*. Other organisms include *S. pyogenes*, *Haemophilus influenzae* type b, *Mycoplasma pneumoniae*, *Pseudomonas aeruginosa* and other streptococcal species. In developing countries *Staphylococcus aureus* is the main cause and Gram-negative bacteria are more common.

There is a constant production and reabsorbtion of fluid within the pleural space. In pneumonia, parenchymal inflammation can lead to an increase in pleural fluid (effusion). If not reabsorbed, there will be an increase in inflammatory cells resulting in pus (empyema) and fibrin deposition causing loculations. If left untreated, the loculations will develop into thick and non-elastic bands, which may impair lung function and cause chronic problems.

Non-infective causes of pleural effusion

Rarely, an effusion is the presenting sign of an underlying malignancy in a child. Many of the other secondary causes of pleural effusion occur in children with a known underlying condition such as congenital heart disease, renal disease, connective tissue disorders and trauma, which includes post-cardiothoracic surgery.

Differences between adults and children

It is uncommon for children to have pre-existing lung disease, therefore the final outcome of pleural effusion and/or empyema is almost always excellent. This is in contrast to adults, where empyema is a cause of significant morbidity and mortality (20%) due to co-morbidities.

Targeted treatments of pleural effusion/empyema

Antibiotics without chest drain

If the effusion is small and the child is well then conservative antibiotic therapy can be given, coupled with close observation. Signs of deterioration or failure to improve should prompt urgent consideration of drainage of the effusion (see Table 7.1).

Antibiotics with chest drain

Early intervention with drainage of effusions/empyemas has been shown to reduce length of stay. There is no evidence to indicate that large-bore chest drains confer any advantage over smaller. As with adults, remember the basic principles of chest drain management.

- All chest tubes should be connected to a unidirectional-flow drainage system (such as an underwater seal bottle) which must be kept below the level of the patient's chest at all times.
- A bubbling chest drain should never be clamped.
- A clamped drain should be unclamped immediately if a patient complains of breathlessness or chest pain, or deteriorates whilst being ventilated.
- The drain should be clamped for 1 hour after 10 ml/kg of chest fluid has drained as re-expansion pulmonary oedema is a potential problem.

Potential pitfalls when managing children with pleural collections

General anaesthesia and large-volume chest fluid aspiration pose a significant risk of sudden death in children with superior mediastinal obstruction related to malignancy. Aspiration of pleural fluid should therefore be of small volume (e.g. 5 ml) for diagnostic purposes only and general anaesthesia/sedation avoided under such circumstances.

Non-pulmonary causes of shortness of breath

Cardiac

Heart failure may present with tachypnoea. Patients would also have other signs of failure such as tachycardia, pallor, sweating, weak pulse and hepatomegaly. This may occur in children with a past history of cardiac disease or acutely in children with undiagnosed conditions such as large ventricular septal defect or viral myocarditis (see Chapter 6).

Metabolic

Hyperammonaemic states with associated, often profound, metabolic acidosis secondary to inherited metabolic conditions, such as urea-cycle disorders or organic acidaemias, can act as a respiratory stimulant and cause tachypnoea (see Chapter 12 for management).

Diabetic ketoacidosis (Chapter 11) and, less commonly in children, salicylate poisoning also present with a metabolic acidosis-driven tachypnoea.

If any of these conditions are suspected, initial investigation should include a blood gas, lactate and ammonia.

Monitoring and investigations

Pulse oximetry, ECG, blood pressure, temperature and blood glucose should be monitored in every child admitted to hospital. The tests below may aid in making a diagnosis and assessing the severity of disease.

Blood tests

Acute-phase reactants (full blood count (FBC), C-reactive protein(CRP), erythrocyte sedimentation rate (ESR))

These markers distinguish poorly between bacterial and viral infections in children and therefore should not be measured routinely. However, they may be helpful in monitoring response to treatment in severe bacterial infections and empyema (particularly CRP).

Blood gas measurement

Capillary blood gas measurement gives an acceptable indication of $PaCO_2$ and pH. It is less reliable in children with impaired peripheral perfusion (see Chapter 37).

Blood gases should be measured in children with signs of severe respiratory distress, apnoea or exhaustion. Ex-preterm infants with chronic lung disease may have a chronically raised $PaCO_2$ with metabolic compensation (similar to adults with severe COPD).

Sampling blood gases should not delay the institution of respiratory support in children with signs of severe respiratory distress, apnoea or exhaustion.

Serum electrolytes

These should be measured in children with severe respiratory distress or LRTI when SIADH cannot be excluded. Serum potassium should be monitored in children requiring IV salbutamol or aminophylline, or prolonged, frequent nebulized salbutamol.

Radiology

Chest X-ray

Chest radiography should not be performed routinely in children with mild uncomplicated acute LRTI or bronchiolitis. Instead it should be considered in:

- patients who are high risk
- patients not following an expected clinical course
- patients possibly requiring additional ventilatory support.

When interpreting paediatric CXRs, findings are poor indicators of aetiology; however, hilar consolidation is more likely to be associated with severe disease. A large effusion causing whiteout can be difficult to differentiate from severe collapse/consolidation on X-ray.

Ultrasound

Ultrasound can be helpful for:

- determining depth of an effusion
- differentiating effusion from consolidation in whiteout
- identifying loculations and density of fluid–suggesting empyema
- guidance when inserting chest drains.

CT scan

If a CT scan of the thorax is indicated in a child, it is worth discussing this with your local tertiary centre respiratory or PICU team, as small children may need an anaesthetic for the procedure. It may be possible, depending on how unwell the child is, to transfer them unintubated in order to have the scan performed in a specialist centre.

Microbiology

Blood cultures should be performed in all critically unwell children. Any pleural fluid obtained should be sent for Gram stain and culture. An anti-streptolysin O (ASOT) test should be requested for all patients with pleural effusion.

Nasopharyngeal aspirate (NPA)

Rapid direct immunofluorescent antibody testing can identify the causative virus in bronchiolitis. Whilst not necessarily affecting management, this information may be useful when nursing children in cohorts during winter epidemics of the disease.

Post-intubation management

Removing the work of breathing and applying PEEP can often improve the situation markedly in children with an isolated chest infection. In the absence of cardiovascular instability insertion of invasive monitoring such as a central or arterial line is not necessary.

A repeat CXR after intubation is essential in order to check ET tube placement.

If a child is failing to respond to ventilation and remains hypoxic then it is worth considering whether there is a mechanical problem or whether the diagnosis is correct.

Mechanical

The most common cause for a child to be difficult to ventilate is endobronchial intubation. This should be checked on a CXR as soon as possible. Another cause is mucus plugging. A suction tube should be passed down the ET tube with saline wash in order to remove any plugs.

Diagnosis

Failure to respond to therapy should raise suspicion about your diagnosis. Consider a pneumothorax (especially if a neck line has been sited, or high pressures have been used to ventilate). Also think about congenital cardiac disease (especially in neonates).

Other considerations

Once the child has been intubated and is stable attention should move to:

- optimizing ventilation (titrate to the blood gases)
- checking glucose and electrolytes
- checking temperature
- gaining further IV access (if needed).

Preparing for transfer

As with other chapters, preparation for transfer will need detailed, written, documentation of the history, clinical findings and lab results. Other items which should be arranged prior to transfer include:

- copies of any investigations/images to be taken or sent to the receiving hospital – pre- and post-intubation CXR should be available
- a copy of all of the blood gases taken throughout the episode
- ensure that the parents are aware of any plans why/and to where the child is being transferred.

Summary

Shortness of breath is a common mode of presentation for children. A methodical approach to its management is needed, as well as a decisive plan. If there is any doubt about the management of the patient, it is best to get the input of a PICU retrieval team sooner rather than later.

Golden rules

- The work of breathing for children is higher than that for adults
- Children can compensate for respiratory disease
- They also decompensate quickly
- Children with chronic disease will need closer monitoring and earlier intervention for common illnesses

Further reading

British Thoracic Society. 2005. *Guidelines for the management of pleural infection in children.*

Clark JE. Children with pneumonia: how do they present and how are they managed? *Arch Dis Child* 2007; **92**:394–398.

Yanney M, Vyas H. The treatment of bronchiolitis. *Arch Dis Child* 2008; **93**:793–798.

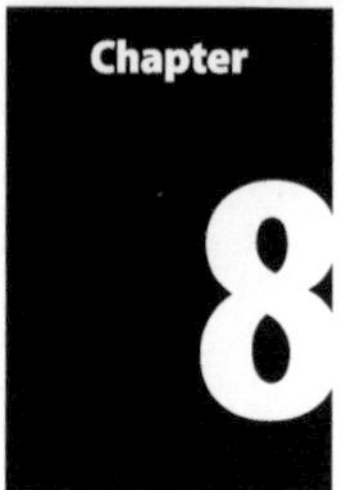

The child with asthma

Josephine Langton and Stuart Hartshorn

Introduction

The UK has one of the highest prevalence rates of childhood asthma worldwide; it affects 1.1 million children in the UK, equating to one in ten children.

Because of improved management, hospital admission rates for childhood asthma have decreased over the past 20 years. However, in 2009 12 children under 14 years of age died from asthma in the UK. A diagnosis of asthma is much more likely in young children, but fatal or life-threatening exacerbations are more common in adolescents.

Much of this chapter makes reference to sections of the British Thoracic Society (BTS)/ Scottish Intercollegiate Guidelines Network (SIGN) guidelines pertinent to the assessment and management of acute exacerbations of asthma in children.

Pathophysiology

Asthma is a chronic inflammatory condition associated with variable and reversible airway obstruction. It is characterized by recurrent episodes of cough, wheeze, chest tightness and difficulty in breathing. Asthma is known to be associated with a family history of atopy, exposure to certain environmental factors and intrinsic airway hyper-reactivity.

Exposure to specific triggers (e.g. viral upper respiratory tract infections, the cold, exercise or smoke) causes:

- airway oedema
- excess mucus production
- bronchoconstriction.

How asthma differs in children

Although asthma is a condition that affects both children and adults, there are age-related differences in presentation, investigation and management. The prevalence of asthma is much higher in children, and they are much more likely to present with acute exacerbations.

Assessing children with asthma

Asthma is a clinical diagnosis. A clinical assessment is, therefore, the best method to determine severity of an exacerbation. When assessing a child it is important to use age

Managing the Critically Ill Child, ed. Richard Skone *et al.* Published by Cambridge University Press.

specific parameters (Table 8.1). Tachypnoea and tachycardia are suggestive of respiratory distress. Bradypnoea and bradycardia suggest fatigue and imminent collapse.

Table 8.1. Age-specific normal values.

Age	Respiratory rate range (breaths per minute)	Heart rate range (beats per minute)	Systolic blood pressure range (mmHg)
< 1 year	30–40	110–150	70–90
1–5 years	20–35	90–120	80–100
5–12 years	15–25	80–120	90–110
> 12 years	15–20	60–100	100–130

Recession

Features of respiratory distress include intercostal, subcostal and sternal recession; if this is present in an older child (over 7 years) it suggests severe respiratory distress. Infants may also head bob and have nasal flaring. As children become tired from their increased respiratory effort, these clinical signs can become less apparent.

Wheeze

Assessing the amount and character of the wheeze is important; biphasic wheeze suggests increasing obstruction, while a silent chest indicates that the exacerbation is life-threatening.

Conscious level and speech

Inability to talk or a decrease in conscious level also signifies a severe or life-threatening exacerbation.

Regular review during their admission is essential as children who have previously appeared to be sick but stable can rapidly deteriorate. Clinical features for assessment of severity are listed in Table 8.3.

Presentation of acute asthma exacerbations

Children with an acute exacerbation of asthma typically present with a history of wheeze, worsening cough, chest tightness and increasing difficulty in breathing. Parents will often use the term 'wheezing' to describe any abnormal noise associated with breathing. It is therefore important to clarify exactly what they mean in order to rule out other diagnoses.

In order for children to be managed appropriately, the severity of their symptoms must be accurately assessed. When assessing the severity of the exacerbation it is useful to find out about:

- symptom duration
- exposure to known triggers
- medication used at home
- recent increase in use of their reliever.

Table 8.2 lists risks factors that would put a child at risk of having a severe exacerbation of asthma.

Table 8.2. Risk factors for severe exacerbations (adapted from BTS/SIGN guideline).

Previous life-threatening asthma, e.g. PICU or HDU admission
Previous admission to hospital for asthma within the last year
Repeated ED attendances for asthma within the last year
Treatment regimen consisting of three or more classes of asthma medication
Repeated use of β_2-agonist
'Brittle' asthma – multiple sudden severe exacerbations, poorly responsive to therapy
Non-compliance with treatment

Investigations

Two quick, non-invasive, investigations that can be used to provide information about the severity of the exacerbation are:

- pulse oximetry
- peak expiratory flow (PEF) compared to patient's own best value or best predicted value (in children over 6 years).

Chest X-ray

Chest X-rays are rarely useful as they typically show hyperinflation and atelectasis and tend not to affect patient management. They should be reserved for life-threatening cases not responding to treatment, or when there is persistent asymmetry of chest signs.

Blood gases

Blood gas analysis (typically capillary in children) should be reserved for those with severe or life-threatening symptoms or when ventilatory support is being considered. Blood gas abnormalities should not themselves be used as absolute indicators for intubation and ventilation; however, trends over time provide valuable additional information about the response of the patient to treatment.

Blood lactate level can signify severe hypoxia or poor perfusion. It can also increase with aggressive adrenoceptor stimulants such as salbutamol.

Table 8.3. Clinical features for assessment of severity (reproduced from BTS/SIGN guideline).

	Moderate asthma exacerbation	Acute severe asthma	Life-threatening asthma
Talking	Able to talk in sentences	Can't complete sentences in one breath or too breathless to talk or feed	Confused, exhausted
Oxygen saturations	≥ 92%	< 92%	< 92%
Peak flow	≥ 50% best or predicted	33–50% best or predicted	< 33% best or predicted
Heart rate	≤ 140/min in children (aged 2–5 years) ≤ 125/min in children (aged > 5 years)	> 140 in children (aged 2–5 years) > 125 in children (aged > 5 years)	Hypotension
Respiratory rate	≤ 40/min in children (aged 2–5 years) ≤ 30/min in children (aged > 5 years)	> 40 breaths/min (aged 2–5 years) > 30 breaths/min (aged > 5 years)	Poor respiratory effort
Examination			Silent chest Cyanosis

Management

Initial management

For acute exacerbation of asthma, the aim of treatment is to reverse bronchoconstriction and promote oxygenation. Current management of asthma is based on the BTS/SIGN guideline (Table 8.4). Initial therapy is well established with a large amount of evidence documenting both safety and efficacy.

Table 8.4. Management of acute asthma (reproduced from BTS/SIGN guideline).

Age 2–5 years			Age > 5 years		
Assess asthma severity			**Assess asthma severity**		
Moderate asthma • SpO_2 ≥92% • No clinical features of severe asthma **NB: If a patient has signs and symptoms across categories, always treat according to their most severe features**	**Severe asthma** • $SpO_2 < 92\%$ • Too breathless to talk or eat • Heart rate > 140/min • Respiratory rate > 40/min • Use of accessory neck muscles	**Life-threatening asthma** $SpO_2 < 92\%$ plus any of: • Silent chest • Poor respiratory effort • Agitation • Altered consciousness • Cyanosis	**Moderate asthma** • $SpO_2 \geq 92\%$ • PEF > 50% best or predicted • No clinical features of severe asthma **NB: If a patient has signs and symptoms across categories, always treat according to their most severe features**	**Severe asthma** • $SpO_2 < 92\%$ • PEF 33–50% best or predicted • Heart rate > 125/min • Respiratory rate > 30/min • Use of accessory neck muscles	**Life-threatening asthma** $SpO_2 < 92\%$ plus any of: • PEF < 33% best of predicted • Silent chest • Poor respiratory effort • Altered consciousness • Cyanosis
	Oxygen via face mask/nasal prongs to achieve SpO_2 94–98%			Oxygen via face mask/nasal prongs to achieve SpO_2 94–98%	
• β_2-Agonist 2–10 puffs via spacer ± facemask [given one at a time single puffs, tidal breathing and inhaled separately] • Increase β_2-agonist dose by 2 puffs every 2 minutes up to 10 puffs according to response	• β_2-Agonist 10 puffs via spacer ± facemask or nebulized salbutamol 2.5 mg or terbutaline 5 mg • Soluble prednisolone 20 mg or IV hydrocortisone 4 mg/kg • Repeat β_2-agonist up to every 20–30 minutes according to response	• Nebulized β_2-agonist: salbutamol 2.5 mg or terbutaline 5 mg plus ipratropium bromide 0.25 mg nebulized • Oral prednisolone 20 mg or IV hydrocortisone 4mg/kg if vomiting **Discuss with senior clinician, PICU team or paediatrician** • Repeat bronchodilators every 20–30 minutes	• β_2-Agonist 2–10 puffs via spacer • Increase β_2-agonist dose by 2 puffs every 2 minutes up to 10 puffs according to response • Oral prednisolone 30–40 mg **Reassess within 1 hour**	• β_2-Agonist 10 puffs via spacer or nebulized salbutamol 2.5–5 mg or terbutaline 5–10 mg • Oral prednisolone 30–40 mg or IV hydrocortisone 4 mg/kg if vomiting • **If poor response** nebulized ipratropium bromide 0.25 mg • Repeat β_2 agonist and ipratropium up to every 20–30 minutes according to response	• Nebulized β_2-agonist: salbutamol 5 mg or terbutaline 10 mg plus ipratropium bromide 0.25 mg nebulized • Oral prednisolone 30–40mg or IV hydrocortisone 4mg/kg if vomiting **Discuss with senior clinician, PICU team or paediatrician**

• Consider soluble oral prednisolone 20 mg **Reassess within 1 hour**	• **If poor response** add 0.25 mg nebulized ipratropium bromide		• Repeat bronchodilators every 20–30 minutes
Assess response to treatment		**Assess response to treatment**	
Record respiratory rate, heart rate and oxygen saturation every 1–4 hours		**Record respiratory rate, heart rate, oxygen saturation and PEF/FEV every 1–4 hours**	
Responding • Continue bronchodilators 1–4 hours prn • Discharge when stable on 4 hourly treatment	**Not responding** • **Arrange HDU/PICU** transfer Consider: • **Chest X-ray and blood gases**	**Responding** • Continue bronchodilators 1–4 hours prn • Discharge when stable on 4 hourly treatment	**Not responding** • **Continue 20–30 minute nebulizers and arrange HDU/ PICU transfer** • Consider: **Chest X-ray and blood gases**
• Continue oral prednisolone for up to 3 days **At discharge** • Ensure stable on 4 hourly inhaled treatment • Review the need for regular treatment and the use of inhaled steroids • Review inhaler technique • Provide a written asthma action plan for treating future attacks • Arrange follow up according to local policy	• **IV salbutamol** 15 µg/kg bolus over 10 minutes **followed** by continuous infusion 1–5 µg/kg/min (dilute to 200 µg/ml) • **IV aminophylline** 5 mg/kg loading dose over 20 minutes (omit in those receiving oral theophyllines) **followed by** continuous infusion 1 mg/kg/hour	• Continue oral prednisolone 30–40 mg for up to 3 days **At discharge** • Ensure stable on 4 hourly inhaled treatment • Review the need for regular treatment and the use of inhaled steroids • Review inhaler technique • Provide a written asthma action plan for treating future attacks • Arrange follow up according to local policy	• **Consider risks and benefits of:** • **Bolus IV salbutamol** 15 µg/kg if not already given • Continuous **IV salbutamol** infusion 1–5 µg/kg/min (200 µg/ml solution) • **IV aminophylline** 5 mg/kg loading dose over 20 minutes (omit in those receiving oral theophyllines) **followed by** continuous infusion 1 mg/kg/ hour • **Bolus IV infusion of magnesium sulphate** 40 mg/kg (max 2 g) over 20 minutes

Oxygen

Oxygen should be given when SaO_2 is less than 94%.

Inhaled bronchodilators

Inhaled β_2-adrenoceptor agonists, such as salbutamol or terbutaline, are the first-line therapy irrespective of severity. β_2-agonists can be administered via an inhaler, a spacer or a nebulizer. Ten puffs of an inhaled bronchodilator given via a spacer has the same therapeutic effect as the nebulized route, as long as the patient is able to use the inhaler properly. Nebulized treatment should be reserved for those with severe or life-threatening exacerbations.

Ipratropium bromide, when used in combination with β_2-agonists, has been shown to reduce the need for hospital admission in those with severe exacerbations.

Steroids

Systemic corticosteroids are important and should be given early. Evidence shows that this will reduce the need for admission and prevent symptom relapse. Oral and IV steroid therapy have similar efficacy, so IV treatment should only be used in children who are vomiting or unable to swallow.

Life-threatening asthma

In patients failing to respond to optimal first-line treatment or those with features of life-threatening asthma, it is crucial to involve the intensive care team early.

In contrast to the extensive evidence about initial management of acute asthma, there is relatively little guidance for second-line therapy in those who are not responding. The options available are detailed below, with the treatment of choice often determined by local hospital guidelines.

Intravenous salbutamol

This should be considered when there is poor response to inhaled β_2-agonists as there is evidence to suggest that it reduces the duration and severity of severe exacerbations of asthma. It should be given as below:

- loading dose of 15 μg/kg over 10 minutes
- followed by a continuous infusion of 1–5 μg/kg/min, dose-adjusted according to response and heart rate.

Aminophylline

This should only be used in severe or life-threatening exacerbations that are failing to respond to conventional therapy. There is limited evidence for its efficacy. It may improve lung function, but there is no evidence to confirm a reduction in acute symptoms or need for intubation. Evidence about impact on duration of admission is unclear.

There is a significant risk of vomiting and cardiac arrhythmias. Cardiac monitoring is essential.

- Loading dose of 5 mg/kg over 20 minutes (omit if on oral theophylline).
- Followed by a continuous infusion of 1 mg/kg/h.

Magnesium sulphate

Evidence confirms that this is a safe therapy in asthma but the therapeutic benefit remains unclear. It may reduce the rate of intubation and ventilation. Studies do suggest that in severe exacerbations there is a reduction in admission rate and improved lung function.

- Doses of up to 40 mg/kg (maximum 2 g) over 20 minutes.
- Hypotension can be a complication.

Intubation and initiating intensive care

Most children with acute exacerbations of asthma respond to early and aggressive medical treatment, but those who fail may require intubation and ventilation. Prior to considering intubation all other therapies should be maximized.

Indications for ventilation

The decision to ventilate a child in status asthmaticus is a clinical one. The mortality in ventilated children is approximately 4%. It remains unclear whether ventilation contributes to this mortality rate, or whether it simply represents the chance of dying in children with asthma severe enough to warrant ventilation.

Failure to initiate ventilation in a timely manner may put a child at undue risk. Indications for mechanical ventilation in children with status asthmaticus include:

- altered sensorium
- progressive exhaustion
- severe hypoxia despite maximal oxygen therapy
- failure to reverse a respiratory acidosis
- a silent chest
- cardiac or respiratory arrest.

Induction of anaesthesia

As with any of the conditions detailed in this book, intubation is a risky phase of management. When intubating a child in status asthmaticus it is important to anticipate:

- rapid desaturation
- reflux/vomiting (especially if on aminophylline)
- cardiovascular instability
- the potential to cause a pneumothorax as positive-pressure ventilation is initiated.

Ketamine is routinely used on PICU as an induction agent (1–3 mg/kg depending on the state of the child). It is ideal for asthma due to stimulation of the sympathetic system and bronchodilator effect. Suxamethonium or rocuronium are used as first-line muscle relaxants.

Choice of ET tube

A cuffed ET tube can be used, even in small children, in order to manage the high airway pressures used for ventilation. A cuffed ET tube will obviate the need for a tube change to minimize a leak.

Sedation

Morphine and midazolam are still used as sedative agents in status asthmaticus, although in severe cases a ketamine infusion can be used (instead of morphine) in order to promote bronchodilatation. Ketamine is given at a rate of 0.5–2 mg/kg/h.

All patients ventilated for asthma should receive a muscle relaxant infusion, e.g. rocuronium at 1mg/kg/h.

Factors complicating ventilation in asthma

Two principal factors that influence ventilation in asthma are 'gas trapping' and 'auto-PEEP'.

Gas trapping (breath stacking)

If the ventilator is set with too short an expiratory time (e-time) then the resistance of the airways will not allow the air blown in during the inspiratory phase to escape during expiration. If there is a part of the tidal volume left behind with each breath, the lung volume at end-expiration will increase with each cycle.

Eventually this will reach a point where the lung volume at end-expiration will reach the plateau portion of the lung compliance curve. The ventilator will continue to deliver positive pressure, and the intrathoracic pressure will increase. This can lead to severe cardiovascular compromise.

Auto-PEEP

The gas that remains in the alveoli from 'gas trapping' will exert its own positive pressure, above atmospheric pressure. This is auto-PEEP.

Setting a ventilator in asthma

Ventilation strategies for children with asthma follow the same principles as for adults. Asthma is an obstructive lung pathology that restricts the movement of gases. It is reasonable to start ventilation with a lung-protective strategy (see Chapter 4 for settings), but rapid titration will be needed which takes into account the need for:

- long expiratory times – to allow air to move out and prevent gas trapping
- long inspiratory times – to allow adequate gas exchange
- high airway pressures – much of which will not be transmitted to the alveoli
- positive end-expiratory pressure – to overcome the tendency of airways to collapse.

Inspiratory pressure

Inspiratory pressures in children are the same as adults. A pressure of 30 cmH_2O is considered the maximum, which should only be exceeded if there is no other option. The pressure should be titrated to deliver a smaller tidal volume of 5–7 ml/kg, if possible.

Inspiratory and expiratory times

Long inspiratory times (i-times) will be needed to allow the pressure of ventilation to overcome the resistance of the airways. Teenagers should have settings similar to those of adults (assuming they are a normal size). Infants will need i-times set at 0.75–1.0 second initially. This can be increased as necessary.

The limiting factor for the e-time is the respiratory rate. Most children can tolerate a relatively low respiratory rate of 10–12 breaths per minute. This is because a paralysed child will produce considerably less CO_2 than an awake child.

Ventilators capable of displaying the ventilation flow loops are ideal for demonstrating that a child is managing to breathe out completely. If the expiratory flow does not return to a baseline, then the e-time should be lengthened (respiratory rate lowered).

Positive end-expiratory pressure (PEEP)

There are two schools of thought regarding the use of PEEP in asthma. Most people hold with the theory that the PEEP should be set to match the patient's own intrinsic PEEP (auto-PEEP). This will optimize the airway opening and allow the greatest degree of gas transfer.

It can be found by gradually increasing the PEEP until the tidal volume no longer increases with each breath.

Others opt not to use any PEEP on the grounds that it allows for a larger difference between inspiratory and expiratory pressures (thus increasing the tidal volume).

Carbon dioxide

Permissive hypercapnoea is practised in status asthmaticus. A much higher than normal $PaCO_2$ may have to be tolerated (seek expert advice at this point). Treating the acidosis with sodium bicarbonate is counter-productive due to the increased carbon dioxide load.

Potential problems with ventilation

Hypoxia

If hypoxia persists on the ventilator, increase the FiO_2 and request an urgent CXR. Examine the child, looking for signs of:

- pneumothorax
- endobronchial intubation.

In the absence of either, increase the drug regime, i.e. salbutamol and ketamine, and consider the use of volatile agents.

Cardiovascular instability

If a child's blood pressure drops while being ventilated, give a fluid bolus and rule out a tension pneumothorax clinically.

Preparing the child for transfer

As with other chapters, the mainstay of preparing a child for transfer is first to stabilize the child, then ensure that the child is optimized, i.e. adequate intravenous access, and a secured airway.

Details of the treatment given and history should be documented, and all radiological investigations available for transfer. Blood gases should all be available and labelled relative to the child's condition at the time of taking, i.e. 'pre-intubation' or 'after starting aminophylline'.

Summary

Asthma still carries a significant mortality rate. It should never be underestimated. Although the majority of children improve with medication, it is still necessary to ventilate the sickest children. If in doubt, contact the local PICU retrieval team for advice at any point along the treatment algorithm.

Golden rules

- A child who is getting quieter may be becoming sicker
- Regular repeated observations are essential
- Don't be afraid to ventilate a child if they fail to respond to medical management
- Difficulty in ventilating a child may be due to a pneumothorax
- Discuss any child that you are concerned about with PICU

Further reading

British Guideline on the Management of Asthma. A national clinical guideline. May 2008, revised January 2012: British Thoracic Society/SIGN.

Browne G, Lam L. Single-dose intravenous salbutamol bolus for managing children with acute severe asthma in the emergency department: reanalysis of data. *Pediatr Crit Care Med* 2002;**3**(2):117–123.

Cheuk DKL, Chau TCH, Lee SL. A meta-analysis on intravenous magnesium sulphate for treating acute asthma. *Arch Dis Child* 2005;**90**:74–77.

Ciarallo L, Brousseau D, Reinert S. Higher-dose intravenous magnesium therapy for children with moderate to severe acute asthma. *Arch Pediatr Adolesc Med* 2000;**154**:979–983.

Mitra A, *et al.* Intravenous aminophylline for acute severe asthma in children over two years receiving inhaled bronchodilators. *Cochrane Collaboration* 2009.

Partridge R, Abramo T. Acute asthma in the pediatric emergency department. *Pediatr Emerg Med Pract* 2008;**5**(11).

Roberts G, *et al.* Intravenous salbutamol bolus compared with an aminophylline infusion in children with severe asthma: a randomised controlled trial. *Thorax* 2003;**58**:306–310.

www.asthma.org.uk.

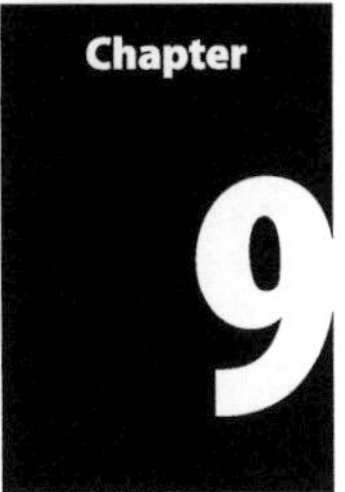

The child with decreased consciousness and coma

Mark D. Lyttle

Introduction

Consciousness is a measure of a child's ability to interact with their environment and other people. Decreased consciousness may be due to any disease in its most severe form. Although non-traumatic causes are less frequent, they carry a higher mortality rate of almost 50%.

The annual incidence according to cause is:

- trauma 338/100 000 in children 0–15 years old
- non-traumatic 160/100 000 in the first year of life
- non-traumatic 30/100 000 in all children

The aim of immediate management is to minimize any neurological damage whilst making a definitive diagnosis. Therefore, therapeutic measures must take place at the same time as diagnostic procedures.

After initial assessment and stabilization, management centres on determining the specific diagnosis. However, 14% of children presenting with coma remain undiagnosed after hospital discharge or post-mortem examination. With appropriate assessment and investigation, the risk of missing important diagnoses is reduced, and potentially lifesaving therapy can be initiated without delay.

How decreased consciousness differs in children

Assessment

An identical stimulus will cause a range of responses in different children, and reactions are often different from those seen in adults. A modified version of the GCS is used in younger children in order to take into account their developmental abilities (see Chapter 35). Assessment is most difficult in preverbal children and infants, as the symptoms and signs are often non-specific, and poor differentiators of the underlying cause. In babies there may be excessive sleepiness, decreased feeding or irritability.

Many children have an underlying condition causing a baseline conscious level that would not be seen as normal in other children. While clinicians will be able to detect gross abnormalities, care-givers will appreciate subtle variations, and they should be involved in the assessment of such children if possible.

Managing the Critically Ill Child, ed. Richard Skone *et al.* Published by Cambridge University Press.

Causes

The incidence of head injury increases throughout childhood, peaking in adolescence. Non-traumatic coma has a bimodal distribution, being most common in infants and toddlers, with a smaller peak in adolescence. It is secondary to a diffuse metabolic insult in 95% of cases, and structural lesions in 5%. Some conditions are much less common in children than in adults, notably hypertensive encephalopathy and cerebrovascular accidents.

The features of each condition are discussed later in this chapter. Table 9.1 outlines some of the more common causes by age of presentation

Table 9.1. Common causes of decreased consciousness by age of presentation.

Age range	Cause	Additional information
Infant (0–1 year)	Infection	More common in infants Nonspecific presenting features
	Non-accidental injury (NAI)	Consider in all cases of decreased consciousness with no clear cause
	Hypoglycaemia	May be due to congenital cause, poor feeding, or underlying cause, e.g. infection
	Raised intracranial pressure	May be due to congenital malformations Often slowly increasing, head circumference expanding due to open sutures
	Inherited metabolic disease (IMD)	Present with first illness
Young child (1–5 years)	Infection	Compared with infants, classic features of infection tend to be present
	Traumatic causes	Usually due to exploratory behaviour Consider NAI
	Toxin ingestion	Usually accidental due to exploratory behaviour
	Raised intracranial pressure	More acute than infants as sutures closed
	Hypoglycaemia	May be lack of substrate May be inherited metabolic disease
	Inherited metabolic disease	May never have had illness as infant
Older child (5–12 years)	Infection	Classic signs of infection generally present
	Metabolic/endocrine disease	First presentation of endocrine disorders
Adolescent (over 12 years)	Traumatic causes	Risk-taking behaviour Multisystem and isolated head trauma
	Diabetic ketoacidosis	Most commonly presents in adolescence Often due to poor compliance
	Toxin ingestion	Often deliberate May be deliberate self-harm or recreational

Investigations and management

Overarching principles

As mentioned above, history-taking, examination, investigation and therapeutic measures must occur simultaneously. Many of the conditions in Table 9.1 require early, and aggressive, intervention.

Treating life-threatening causes concurrently at the beginning of the clinical course while simultaneously conducting investigations to determine the diagnosis is often the best management strategy, as no individual cause is more important, and several may coexist in the same child.

Early liaison with specialist teams at a tertiary centre is often important to optimize care, especially if a particular diagnosis becomes likely. This may involve contacting general paediatricians, intensivists, neurologists, specialists in metabolic medicine, endocrinologists, cardiologists or toxicologists.

Investigations

Several causes of decreased consciousness may be recognized clinically but require further investigation, whereas some diagnoses can only be made through laboratory testing. The rarity of many of the causes adds to the diagnostic difficulty. In children in whom the cause is clear, including those with trauma or recurrent episodes of decreased consciousness, it is acceptable to perform directed investigations. In children who are post-ictal it is acceptable to adopt a watch-and-wait approach for the first hour provided they have a normal blood sugar.

Initial investigations for all children

Children with decreased consciousness of unknown cause should have the investigations listed in Table 9.2 performed at the earliest opportunity. These will identify all immediately treatable problems, and include those samples that can aid diagnosis at a later stage.

Table 9.2. Initial investigations in a child with decreased consciousness.

Capillary and laboratory blood glucose
Blood gas
Urea and electrolytes
Liver function tests
Plasma ammonia
Full blood count and film
Coagulation studies
Blood culture
1–2 ml of plasma to be separated, frozen and stored for later analysis
1–2 ml of plain serum to be saved for later analysis
Urinalysis for ketones, glucose, protein, nitrites and leucocytes
10 ml of urine to be saved for later analysis
ECG

Further investigations

The additional tests in Table 9.3 should be requested if the cause remains unknown after the initial investigations or if confirmation of a suspected diagnosis is needed.

Table 9.3. Further investigations to consider in a child with decreased consciousness.

CT brain
- Especially if the working diagnosis is raised intracranial pressure (ICP), intracranial abscess, or cause unknown

Lumbar puncture (check for contraindications first)
- Microscopy, Gram stain, culture and sensitivity, glucose, protein
- PCR for herpes simplex with/without pneumococcus/meningococcus, other viruses
- Other tests may be performed in individual cases

Urine and blood toxicology
Urine organic and amino acids
Plasma lactate

Advanced investigations

If the cause remains unknown after the initial investigations, CT brain and lumbar puncture results, the following should be performed:

- EEG for non-convulsive status epilepticus
- acyl carnitine profile and plasma amino acids
- ESR and autoimmune screen
- thyroid function test and thyroid antibodies.

General management

Attention should be given to the basics of resuscitation prior to establishing the underlying cause of the decreased consciousness (see Golden rules at the end of the chapter and Chapter 4). This will ensure that if the cerebral insult is due to reduced cerebral blood flow or hypoxia it will not be worsened. Some simple interventions may improve the conscious level. Decreased consciousness usually represents disease in its most severe form. Senior assistance should be sought immediately in order to intervene early to manage problems such as hypovolaemia, hypoglycaemia and raised ICP.

Intubation

The selection of drugs for induction should be based on the underlying condition and pre-existing pathology, and they should be given judiciously. Some children will present a difficult airway, whether expected or unexpected, and this should be anticipated. Even with these precautions, the patient may deteriorate rapidly, especially if they have elevated ICP or severe sepsis. It is, therefore, sensible to have resuscitation drugs prepared.

In patients selected for intubation it is vital to clearly document both the neurological assessment immediately prior to intubation, and the progression of conscious level in the time preceding intubation. It will be possible to continue to monitor the response to treatment in certain underlying conditions such as hypovolaemia, but others, such as intractable seizures, may require additional equipment. Patients will still require adequate sedation in the normal manner once intubated.

Abbreviated neurological assessment

If time permits, a full neurological assessment should be performed. However, in an emergency, important signs that can be assessed quickly include pupil size and symmetry and response to stimulus. Supraorbital pressure should be used as the painful stimulus as this is

Table 9.4. Management of a child with decreased conscious level.

Phase of management	Assessment	Action
Initial phase On presentation of the child Also see Chapter 4	Manage airway and assess for need to intubate • GCS/pupil size and symmetry • Hypoxia refractory to oxygen • Rising CO_2 • Poor respiratory effort • Inability to maintain airway • Concerns about raised ICP • Cardiovascular shock Assess circulation for: • Signs of shock • Arrhythmias • Hypovolaemia Check blood glucose	Give oxygen • Ventilate by hand if needed Gain IV access • IO if more than three IV attempts Give fluid bolus • 20 ml/kg of crystalloid Take blood including ABG, clotting and cross-match If situation allows collect a 'hypoglycaemic screen'
After initial assessment Once imminently life-threatening risks have been addressed	Assess response to phase 1 Assess neurology • Supraorbital painful stimulus • AVPU (alert, responds to voice, responds to pair, unconscious) / GCS • Record GCS every 15 minutes if < 12 • Every hour if > 12	Consider antibiotics Repeat blood gases to assess: Ventilation Electrolytes Acidosis If raised ICP suspected manage as in Chapter 19
Further stabilization Not immediately lifesaving procedures	Continue to reassess clinical condition and blood results Search for cause according to investigations mentioned above Definitive plan (transfer) Decide on further monitoring	Contact retrieval team Document and review results as they arrive Arterial line if: • Haemodynamic instability • Starting inotropes • Repeated blood gases CVC if: • More definitive access needed • Starting inotropes • Giving high concentration drugs Correct coagulopathy

replicable between observers, and avoids any confusion caused by paraesthesia or hemiplegia. During initial assessment AVPU or modified GCS assessments are appropriate. For subsequent assessments the modified GCS will reflect more subtle changes in consciousness

Hypoglycaemia

The blood glucose concentration should be determined immediately in all cases. Even if present, hypoglycaemia may not be the sole cause of decreased consciousness. It should therefore be corrected quickly and the patient should be reassessed once corrected.

If the blood glucose is less than 2.6 mmol/l the following should be performed:

- give 2 ml/kg of 10% dextrose
- maintain blood glucose between 4 and 7 mmol/l with an infusion of 10% dextrose
- request the following bloods as part of a 'hypoglycaemic screen':
  - lactate
  - insulin
  - cortisol
  - growth hormone
  - free fatty acids
  - β-hydroxybutyrate
  - acyl carnitine profile from the stored samples taken with initial investigations.

If the blood glucose is between 2.6 and 3.5 mmol/l then the laboratory glucose result from initial investigations should be reviewed urgently.

Management of specific conditions

As decreased consciousness is the end point of many disease processes, the individual causes are covered in detail elsewhere in this book. However, a specific cause is sometimes identified based on the clinical features. Targeted management should then be instituted.

The conditions below are mentioned in detail elsewhere in the book. Should the conditions be suspected please consult the relevant chapter.

Infection

Decreased consciousness may be secondary to central nervous system or systemic infection. Investigations should consist of those listed above, with a lumbar puncture if there are no contraindications. Because infection is common and treatable, commencement of broad-spectrum antibiotics with or without acyclovir should be considered in all children presenting with decreased consciousness with non-specific features, especially if there is:

- temperature > 38 or $< 35.5°C$
- tachycardia or tachypnoea
- white cell count $> 15\ 000\ mm^3$ or $< 5000\ mm^3$
- non-blanching rash.

When examining these patients older children tend to present with classical features; however, infants may only display non-specific features such as floppiness, poor feeding, lethargy, irritability. They may not be pyrexial either. See Chapter 5.

Toxin ingestion

It should be routine to ask family or friends about medicines, essential oils or recreational drugs kept in the house. In older children direct questioning may also reveal the problem. In young children naloxone should be given if there are opiates in the home, or signs of toxicity present. See Chapter 13.

Diabetic ketoacidosis (DKA)

Decreased consciousness may be the first presentation of diabetes mellitus. As well as the blood sugar and pH, urinary ketones must be checked if DKA is suspected. Drowsiness in children with DKA is a very serious sign of potential disaster as it is caused by cerebral oedema and raised ICP (as well as venous sinus thrombosis). See Chapter 11.

Seizures

Seizures may be subtle, especially if only autonomic signs are present. The worry in children with decreased conscious level is determining between the post-ictal state and ongoing seizures. The investigations should be carried out as above if the seizure is prolonged and there is no previous history of epilepsy. See Chapter 10.

Arrhythmias

Decrease or loss of consciousness may be the first presentation of cardiac disease or occur in children with a known background of cardiac disease. The arrhythmia may also be precipitated by electrolyte imbalance or toxin ingestion. An ECG should be performed in all children with decreased consciousness. See Chapter 6.

Hypertensive encephalopathy

Hypertension is defined as a systolic blood pressure above the 95th centile on two separate readings. In children it may be due to a number of pathologies. However, the most common cause is renal disease. Distinguishing hypertensive encephalopathy from hypertension secondary to raised ICP is crucial as it will guide management. Treating hypertension secondary to raised ICP can cause deterioration due to decreased cerebral blood flow. When intracranial causes have been ruled out, the hypertension should be corrected in a controlled way, especially if there is a longstanding history of hypertension.

Inborn errors of metabolism

These often present in infancy when precipitated by the child's first illness. A high index of suspicion is needed in order to detect them early. Once suspected, it is vital to liaise with the regional metabolic team. See Chapter 12.

Transfer

Even at the point of transfer, some children will not have a diagnosis. It is important to continue to improve their clinical status where possible, often treating multiple remediable causes simultaneously. Respiratory and cardiovascular status should be optimized, and normal temperature should be maintained. Normoglycaemia and electrolyte balance should be achieved by using isotonic solutions containing dextrose. The results of any investigations should be made available to the retrieval team in an organized manner. A decision should be made regarding who is responsible for following up outstanding investigations and informing the receiving team. In the case of neonates, if the mother is too unwell to travel, a sample of her blood should be sent in case it is required for analysis or cross-match.

Summary

Treating a child with a decreased conscious level is challenging. Performing the basics well and correcting remediable causes may be the sum total of management before the retrieval team arrives. If time permits, all of the above investigations should be performed, where indicated. They should also be written clearly in the notes, with any late results phoned through to the relevant team at the referral centre.

Golden rules

- Begin assessment and treatment concurrently, not sequentially
- Check for and treat hypoglycaemia and remember to start a dextrose infusion after the bolus
- When putting in a line or taking bloods, perform all investigations concurrently
- Lumbar puncture is useful, but ensure no contraindications are present
- Have a very low threshold for commencing antimicrobials
- Ensure hypertension is not secondary to raised ICP before aggressive treatment
- Remember NAI, especially in those < 1 year, and those with no obvious cause
- Have a low threshold for giving a trial of naloxone

Further reading

Advanced Life Support Group. *Advanced Paediatric Life Support: The practical approach*, 5th edition. Wiley-Blackwell 2011.

Avner JR. Altered states of consciousness. *Paediatr Rev* 2006;**27**(9): 331–338.

Kirkham FJ. Non traumatic coma in children. *Arch Dis Child* 2001; **85**:303–312.

NHS Health and Social Care Information Centre. *Hospital episode statistics.* Department of Health. 2005. London. www.hesonline.nhs.uk.

Paediatric Accident and Emergency Research group. The management of a child (0–18 years) with a decreased conscious level. An evidence based guideline for health professionals based in the hospital setting. Available at: http://www.rcpch.ac.uk/child-health/standards-care/child-health-guidelines-and-standards/guidelines-endorsed-rcpch-subspe-0#PAERG_decon.

Wong C, Forsyth R, Kelly T, Eyre J. Incidence, aetiology, and outcome of non-traumatic coma: a population based study. *Arch Dis Child* 2001;**84**(3):193–199.

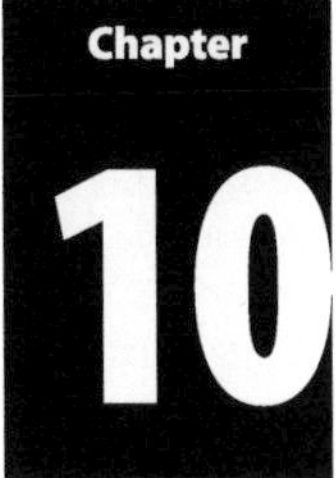

The child with seizures

Katie Z. Wright

Introduction

A fitting child is frightening for parents and carers. The management of a fitting child is also a challenge for health professionals, requiring a calm and structured approach with timely and specific interventions. This chapter covers the causes of fitting in different age groups. It also looks at specific points to elicit in the history and examination as well as the practical management of a fitting child.

Definitions and causes in children

A seizure can be defined as abnormal electrical activity of the cerebral cortex giving rise to signs and symptoms. Children presenting with seizures account for 5% of paediatric attendances to emergency departments.

Status epilepticus

Status epilepticus (SE) is divided into convulsive status epilepticus (CSE), which accounts for the majority of presentations, and non-convulsive status. SE is defined as a generalized convulsion lasting 30 minutes or longer, or when a patient fails to regain consciousness between successive fits over 30 minutes or longer. CSE is a life-threatening neurological emergency. It must be identified quickly and treated as it carries significant morbidity, and a mortality of approximately 4%. Neurological sequelae of SE include epilepsy, learning difficulties, behavioural problems and motor deficits. They occur more often in those under 1 year and can be devastating.

The first prospective population-based study on CSE was published in 2006. The north London study found the incidence of CSE in childhood to be 18–20 per 100 000 per year, nearly four times higher than reported in adults.

Non-convulsive SE, while alarming and in need of treatment, does not pose the same threat of immediate injury, specifically airway compromise. It is not treated with the same pathway. The priority for patients with prolonged absence or partial seizure activity is to seek expert advice from a paediatrician or paediatric neurologist as to which anticonvulsant agent to use.

Causes of seizures at different ages

Different aetiologies are more likely in different age groups; some common causes with age ranges are listed in Table 10.1. The treatment for CSE, however, remains constant.

Managing the Critically Ill Child, ed. Richard Skone *et al.* Published by Cambridge University Press.

Table 10.1. Causes of fitting at different ages.

Age	Possible cause of fitting
Neonate (up to 28 days)	Hypoglycaemia CNS infections,[a] predominantly meningitis Non-accidental injury (NAI) Metabolic conditions Electrolyte imbalance Pyridoxine deficiency
Infant	Hypoglycaemia CNS infection[a] Febrile illness Epilepsy NAI Metabolic condition Infantile spasms
Toddler	Hypoglycaemia Head injury Febrile illness Malignancy CNS infection[a] Accidental ingestion Epilepsy NAI
Child	Hypoglycaemia NAI Epilepsy Head injury Febrile illness Malignancy CNS infection[a] Accidental ingestion Deliberate overdose
Adolescent	Epilepsy CNS infection[a] Deliberate overdose Head injury Malignancy Alcohol intoxication or withdrawal

[a] Central nervous system (CNS) infection includes meningitis, encephalitis and cerebral abscess.

Neonates

The incidence of seizures is higher during the first 28 days of life than at any other time of life. During this period, seizures are likely to have an underlying pathology. They often do not present with the generalized tonic–clonic movements seen in older children and adults. The seizures may be subtle, with a combination of signs and symptoms, which may be motor, autonomic or behavioural. First-line management in this age range is phenobarbital with an IV loading dose of 20–40 mg/kg.

Fitting is seen with significant hypoglycaemia, usually when the blood glucose is less than 2 mmol/l. In neonates, this may be due to feeding difficulties, sepsis, or an underlying metabolic disorder. In these cases, rapid identification of the low blood sugar and its correction should prevent a seizure becoming prolonged. Treatment is with 2 ml/kg of 10% glucose intravenously (2.5 mmol/l for neonates), followed by a constant supply of glucose, i.e. maintenance fluid or NG feeding (see Chapter 32).

In neonates and babies, fitting may be the first indicator of a damaged brain from non-accidental injury (NAI). Subdural haematomas are not infrequently seen, as well as sub-arachnoid blood, cerebral contusions and diffuse axonal injury. There may be no outward signs of injury or abuse on initial assessment.

Febrile seizures

Febrile seizures (FS) are the most common cause of childhood seizure, affecting between 2% and 5% of all children. They can occur from 6 months to 6 years of age, with a peak incidence of a first febrile fit at 18 months of age. They are usually self-limiting, lasting less than 15 minutes. Up to 5% of children with febrile seizures will present with convulsive status epilepticus, and should be managed as detailed below (Figure 10.1).

Patients who have a tendency towards seizures will have a lower seizure threshold if they have an infection or fever, sometimes making the distinction between epilepsy and febrile convulsion difficult.

Infection

Meningitis is the most frequently seen central nervous system (CNS) infection in children. It must be considered in those with both a short-lived febrile fit and febrile CSE. If suspected, treatment should be according to local antibiotic policy, including cover for listeria in those younger than 3 months of age.

Poisoning and ingestion

Always consider ingestion and poisoning in children with a seizure of unknown cause, especially if they have become acutely unwell without a fever. Be persistent when questioning what medicines are in the household, both legal and otherwise, and how accessible they may be.

Epilepsy

Epilepsy is a term that covers a large collection of disorders of brain function, each manifesting with repeated and unprovoked seizure activity. While epilepsy is an important cause of seizures, not everyone with seizures has epilepsy. The overall incidence of epilepsy in the population is 0.5%, whereas it is estimated that up to 10% of individuals may experience at least one seizure in their lifetime.

In those with a diagnosis of epilepsy who are receiving anti-epilepsy drugs (AEDs) it is worthwhile checking compliance with medication, and that the dose is weight-appropriate. Fitting may be because they have had a recent change or withdrawal of medication, or the child may have 'outgrown' their current dose.

Complex children

Children with refractory seizures, or with complex care needs and seizure disorders, may be well known to their local emergency department and paediatric team. Some have a written management plan including details of seizure pattern, expected duration, recommended treatment and any side effects of medications. These may travel with the child or be held at the local ED. It is worth following the child's personal seizure treatment plan as they are often written by a process of iteration from previous episodes. If it does not work then a consultant neurologist should be contacted and intubation considered.

Whatever the cause of a generalized fit affecting the conscious level, if the seizure activity lasts longer than 5 minutes the emergency management is the same (Figure 10.1).

Management of a fitting child

After 30 minutes of seizure activity, the cerebral arterial autoregulation is lost and blood flow to the brain may become compromised. A vicious circle of anaerobic metabolism and lactic acidosis with cell death and oedema then develops, resulting in increased intracranial pressure. This in turn further reduces cerebral perfusion, exacerbating cell death. Systemic effects of prolonged seizures include leucocytosis, acidosis, disseminated intravascular coagulation, rhabdomyolysis and cardiac compromise with pulmonary oedema.

Many seizures are short-lived, resolving spontaneously within a few minutes. The treatment regime starts 5 minutes after the onset of the fit, to reduce the risk of medicating those who do not need it. For those who have stopped having seizures, airway management remains a priority.

For those seizures that continue beyond 5 minutes, many will continue for 20 or 30 minutes, and treatment should be started to stop the fit and prevent SE. Unless the child started fitting in the hospital, the first 5 minutes is likely to have passed at home or with the transporting ambulance crew.

History and examination

One of the challenges in managing a fitting child is taking a focussed history from those with the child while simultaneously assessing and managing airway, breathing and circulation. Ambulance crews will give a handover, note the details of any drugs given in the pre-hospital setting and the time of administration. SE in children is most commonly seen in those with a known diagnosis of seizure disorder. For children who fit regularly, teachers, carers and parents may have given rectal diazepam or buccal midazolam. Always ask about allergies or drug reactions.

While the child's seizure is being managed, a quick and directed examination for signs of meningism, rash, fever, head trauma or signs of other injuries should be performed. A full and thorough examination can be completed after the patient has been stabilized. This should include looking for a source of infection and full neurological assessment including fundoscopy. Any injuries should be documented, including photography if possible, and communicated to the admitting team.

Management of the seizure

While talking to the family or paramedic crew, airway assessment is the first priority. If not patent, use airway opening manoeuvres and adjuncts. The nasopharyngeal (NP) airway is particularly useful in this situation (unless the seizure is secondary to head injury), as:

- it can be used even if the teeth are clenched
- it is better tolerated than an oropharyngeal airway as the patient's conscious level improves.

If the airway remains compromised, or there is obvious respiratory depression that is not improving, consider early intubation.

While airway management is ongoing, another team member should simultaneously gain intravenous access. Blood samples should be drawn. The priority is a venous blood gas in order to measure blood glucose and electrolytes. A mixed metabolic and respiratory acidosis is the most common abnormality seen during or shortly after seizure activity. This should improve with cessation of seizure activity and a return to normal respiration. In addition measure the blood glucose with a bedside testing kit.

If IV access is proving difficult, consider IO access early.

Drug treatment

The updated, evidence-based consensus algorithm for the management of convulsive status epilepticus was published in the fifth edition of the *Advanced Paediatric Life Support Manual* in 2011 (Figure 10.1).

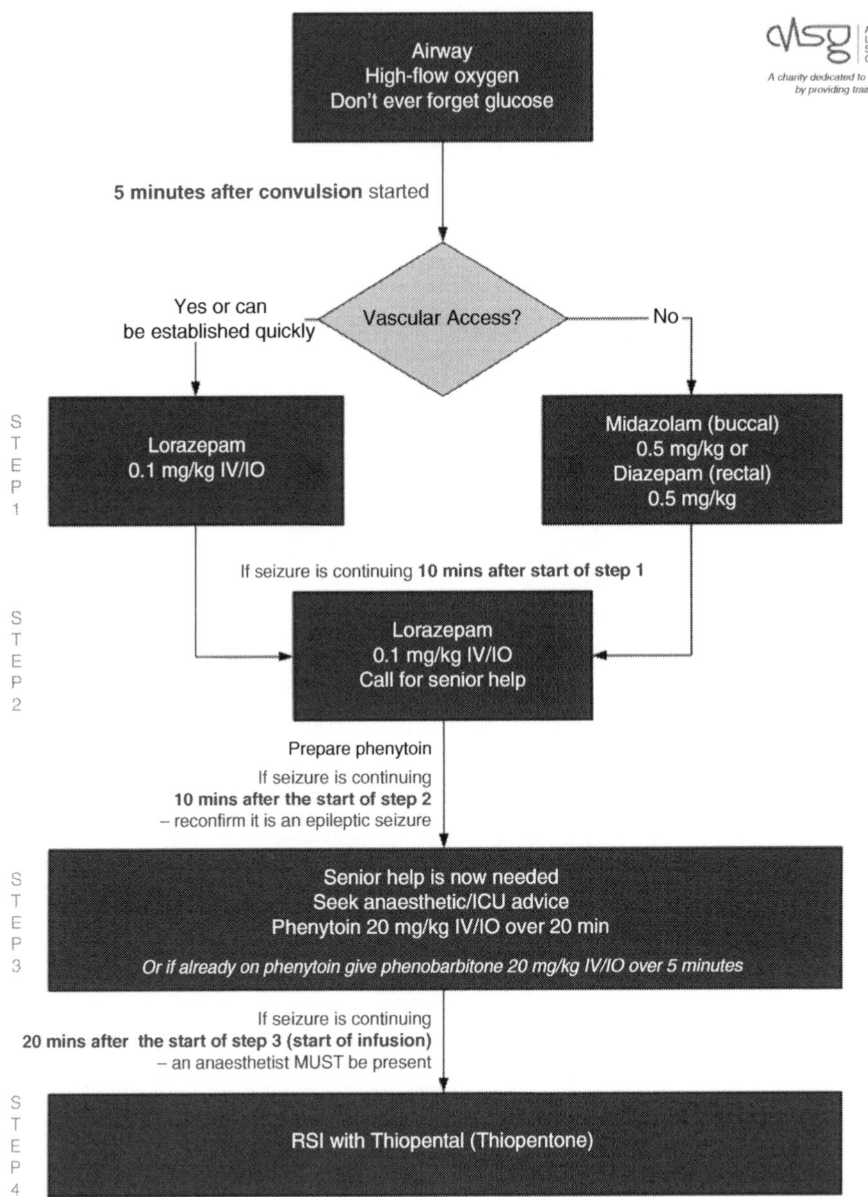

Figure 10.1. Status epilepticus treatment algorithm (reproduced with kind permission of the Advanced Life Support Group).

Following the algorithm

Steps 1 and 2

- If the seizure started 5 or more minutes ago, start at step 1 and proceed.
- If one initial dose of benzodiazepine (step 1) has been given before hospital, start at step 2 (assuming seizure activity continues past the 10 minutes).
- If lorazepam is not available use IV or IO diazepam as a substitute at 0.25 mg/kg.

No more than two doses of benzodiazepine should be given, which includes any pre-hospital medication. This should be enough to stop seizure activity in the majority of children.

Step 3

The majority of children (80% in some studies) should show a response to phenytoin within 20 minutes, and the anticonvulsant effect is relatively long-lasting; phenytoin has an average half-life of 24 hours.

The longer a fit continues, the more difficult it can be to terminate. In practical terms, this means the further down the algorithm you proceed without successfully stopping the fit, the more likely you are to need to intubate the child. Thinking ahead and having everything, and everyone, at hand is essential. This will include calling for senior anaesthetic help sooner rather than later, certainly at or before step 3. Colleagues will be happier to attend early and find a child who has stopped fitting than arrive after being called to a compromised, fitting child with evolving complications.

If the child is already on maintenance phenytoin, give phenobarbitone 20 mg/kg over 5 minutes for step 3 instead. Other alternatives if already taking phenytoin are levetiracetam (Keppra®) or sodium valproate, both of which can be used intravenously.

Rectal paraldehyde may also be used during step 3 with senior advice, at a dose of 0.4 ml/kg mixed with an equal volume of olive oil. It should not be left in a plastic syringe for more than a few minutes.

If 20 minutes after the start of the phenytoin infusion the seizure is persisting, proceed to a rapid-sequence induction (RSI) with thiopentone.

Intubation of the child with seizures

Intubation may be required for a number of reasons, including:

- airway obstruction
- control of seizures with thiopentone
- prolonged respiratory depression as a result of benzodiazepines.

If steps 1–3 of the algorithm and all other measures have failed to control seizure activity then a rapid-sequence induction (RSI) with thiopentone at 2–5 mg/kg is the fourth and final step of the treatment algorithm (Figure 10.1).

Ongoing sedation of the child

The child should be sedated with morphine and midazolam. In this instance it is reasonable to use midazolam in younger babies, but care should be taken as it may lead to significant hypotension. A short-acting muscle relaxant should be used initially in order to minimize the chance of missing movement associated with seizures. An infusion can always be started by the retrieval team.

The main problem with looking after a child who is ventilated is the false reassurance gained from muscle relaxants. Seizures may continue, or recur, even after the administration of thiopentone. Sudden changes in heart rate, blood pressure or pupil size may be the only signs of seizures.

If the child continues to fit after intubation a discussion should be had with your local PICU. They may suggest repeat doses of some of the drugs or a change of anticonvulsant. However, in the meantime give a bolus 0.5 mg/kg of midazolam and double the rate of the infusion.

Reassess the child

Once a child who has been in CSE is intubated the main aim of management is to reassess the patient and correct any factors that may have triggered or exacerbated seizures. This will include:

- treating any underlying infections
- correcting electrolyte or glucose abnormalities
- deciding on further investigations, e.g. CT scan
- ensuring adequate sedation
- sending off any investigations not done so far, e.g. blood cultures
- passing a NG tube.

The same measures for prevention of secondary brain damage in trauma can be employed for those intubated due to CSE (see Chapter 19). The main aims are:

- ensure normothermia
- aim for normocarbia
- aim for normoglycaemia
- maintain a 30-degree head-up position.

Once the seizures have been stopped the child should be relatively stable. If there are cardiovascular problems consider another diagnosis as a cause of seizures, e.g. sepsis or NAI. If there is any problem with ventilation perform a CXR. Check the ET tube position and look for signs of aspiration.

Extubating a child

If the child is known to have a seizure disorder or a cause of fitting which is easily corrected it may be considered best for the patient and their family to extubate them in the referring hospital rather than transfer them to another hospital. This should be done after discussion with the tertiary hospital.

In order to wake a child up and extubate them the team need to be certain that they are happy to do so. This will include factors such as:

- the age of the child
- the cause of the seizure
- the ease of intubation
- an appropriate ward for looking after a child who has had an anaesthetic
- medical cover out of hours.

Preparation for transfer

As with many of the other conditions the child should be prepared in a way that minimizes delays to transfer. This will mean making sure that there is a thorough written history of what has happened, including timings of the seizure. There also needs to be documentation of test results and radiological images should be available to transfer.

Summary

Managing seizures in children has become highly protocolized. Once the protocol has been followed it is important to get advice from your local PICU retrieval team. Decisive and timely intervention is important in order to prevent long-term injury. Don't ever forget the glucose.

Golden rules

- The management of seizures is highly protocolized
- Children with repeated seizures may have personalized protocols
- Perform a blood gas early and correct simple pathologies such as hypoglycaemia

Further reading

Advanced Life Support Group. *Advanced Paediatric Life Support: The Practical Approach*, 5th edition. Wiley-Blackwell. 2011.

Convulsive status epilepticus. *Arch Dis Child* 2007;**92**:28.

Stephenson JBP. Incidence, cause, and short-term outcome of convulsive status epilepticus in childhood: prospective population-based study. *Lancet* 2006;**368**:222–229.

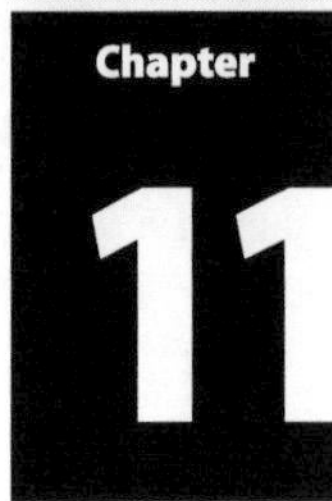

The child with diabetic ketoacidosis

Ian Jenkins

Introduction

Diabetic ketoacidosis (DKA) is defined biochemically as:

- ketonaemia and ketonuria
- hyperglycaemia (> 11 mmol/l)
- venous pH < 7.3.

The peak age for diagnosis of type 1 diabetes mellitus (T1DM) in the UK is 10–14 years old, although this peak is moving towards occurring younger (there has been a steep rise in patients under 5 years old presenting with DKA).

In the USA, 30–40% of new T1DM patients present with DKA. The mortality rate for these patients is 2–5%. Perhaps surprisingly, 5–25% of children with type 2 DM present with DKA at first diagnosis.

This chapter focusses on assessment and management of the infant or child suffering from DKA. It also aims to highlight the difference in management from that of adult DKA.

How does DKA differ in children?

The occurrence of cerebral oedema is the 'stand out' complication that makes this condition different in children compared to the presentation in adults. Cerebral oedema is more common in children under 5 years old, with its incidence decreasing markedly after puberty.

Cerebral oedema occurs in up to 1% of all childhood DKA and accounts for about half of the DKA-related mortality. It has a bi-modal appearance after DKA presentation; the first peak is at 3–6 hours, the second at 9–15 hours.

The approach to the management of childhood DKA has evolved quite distinctly from that of adults, particularly in respect of insulin and fluid administration. It may seem uncomfortable for most physicians, but the replacement of fluid in children with DKA (in the absence of significant shock) should occur over 48–72 hours. This reflects the fact that onset of DKA is a gradual process.

The aim of treatment is to correct the metabolic derangement over a similar period to which it came on. The British Society of Paediatric Endocrinology and Diabetes

Managing the Critically Ill Child, ed. Richard Skone *et al.* Published by Cambridge University Press.

(BSPED) have a website with an interactive page that guides doctors through each step of management.

Why does cerebral oedema occur?

The evidence for any one factor causing cerebral oedema in children is circumstantial. Some of the mechanisms listed below have been considered as mechanisms for cerebral oedema in DKA; however, the presence of cerebral oedema in these children before the initiation of treatment effectively rules many out. It is probably worth considering the clinical findings below as 'risk factors' for cerebral oedema rather than causative mechanisms.

Aggressive use of insulin

Insulin is necessary for sodium pumps to work at the blood–brain barrier. In animal models giving insulin exacerbates cerebral oedema.

Low $PaCO_2$

Hypocapnoea at presentation suggests greater derangement of physiology and thus greater propensity to further complications.

High serum urea nitrogen

Although this is associated with poorer outcomes, it may be just a marker of the underlying derangement.

Treatment with sodium bicarbonate

Sodium bicarbonate administration has been associated with increased mortality in DKA, but it is unclear whether the perceived need to use this simply makes it a marker of severe metabolic derangement. Acutely raising the pH has the same deleterious effect as hyperventilation on cerebral blood flow and haemoglobin dissociation; for this reason bicarbonate is rarely used and only in cases where myocardial function appears to be compromised.

Slow rate of rise of sodium

As the management of DKA progresses the serum sodium concentration should increase. Failure to observe this may be due to giving hypotonic fluids or the release of stress hormones (antidiuretic hormone is released in DKA). This is one reason why 'rehydration' should be gradual and comprise 0.9% saline.

What are the warning signs that a child is really sick?

Observations should be carried out as detailed in Table 11.1.

Table 11.1. Timing of observations in DKA.

Item	Hourly	2–4 hourly
Fluid balance	✓	
Heart rate (HR), blood pressure (BP), respiratory rate	✓*	
Neurological observations (see text)	✓*	
Capillary glucose	✓*	
Electrolytes (Na, K, Cl, urea, Ca, Mg, PO_4)		✓§
Blood gases and lactate		✓§
Blood and urine ketones		✓§

In the early phase, e.g. the first 24 h, the intervals above would be maintained. With resolution of the child's ketoacidosis, items marked as * could be put back to 2 hourly, items marked § could go 4 hourly. Note that raised intracranial pressure (ICP) can be a delayed phenomenon (second peak at 9–15 h).

Contacting PICU

The British Society of Paediatric Endocrinology and Diabetes recommend discussing with PICU any child who is younger than 2 years of age, or who demonstrates:

- a pH of less than 7.1, along with marked hyperventilation
- severe dehydration with shock
- depressed sensorium with risk of hypoventilation or aspiration.

Although the child may not be transferred to PICU it is worth discussing these cases in order to speed up any future involvement should the child develop neurological signs.

Lack of response to 30 ml/kg fluid boluses

This implies circulatory failure that may not be explained by DKA alone. There may be coexisting pathology, such as sepsis, and the child may need inotropes, together with invasive monitoring and central venous access.

Signs of raised ICP

All patients with DKA should be monitored using age-appropriate Glasgow coma scoring (hourly during the initial phase). This should not be used as a sole guide of management though. Other markers of raised ICP include:

- symptoms such as irritability, drowsiness, headache, incontinence
- specific neurological signs (cranial nerve palsies, abnormal posturing)
- rising blood pressure and slowing heart rate.

Targeted treatments in the management of DKA

The management of DKA in children can be found described in prescriptive form on the British Society of Paediatric Endocrinology and Diabetes (BSPED) website. This will help guide management in a step-by-step fashion. The main points of management are detailed below.

Fluid therapy

Slow rehydration over 48 to 72 hours

Historically, the need to maintain or increase serum osmolality was not as well appreciated and rapid fluid replacement was the norm.

'Rehydration' is perhaps a misleading term, implying a water shortage, whereas in fact significant whole body shortages of electrolytes such as sodium, potassium, chloride and phosphate exist along with water.

Gradual rehydration has not been shown experimentally to be associated with decreased incidence of cerebral oedema. Nonetheless, as part of the general approach to managing childhood DKA it is advised that 'rehydration' should take place over 48 hours (or 72 hours in the more severe cases).

Treat shock

Use 10 ml/kg boluses of normal saline up to a maximum of 30 ml/kg. If you feel more should be given perhaps there is underlying sepsis and consideration should be given to better access and inotropes.

Any 'resuscitation' fluid should be deducted from the calculated deficit (see below). This is not true of the International Guidelines (see Further reading below.)

Steps in calculating fluid replacement

1. Calculate the percentage dehydration, using 8% as the maximum (see BSPED website). Use the equation below to calculate fluid deficit:

   $10 \times \%$ dehydration $\times$ body weight (kg) $=$ total fluid deficit in ml.
   e.g. for a 10 kg child at 5% dehydration, this $=$ 500 ml.

2. Calculate maintenance fluid requirement (see BSPED website).
3. Add the total maintenance for 48 hours (or 72 hours depending on condition) to the deficit.
4. Subtract the resuscitation fluid already given. This volume should then be replaced over 48 (or 72) hours.

The initial fluid of choice is normal saline (with potassium 40 mmol/l).

When to change fluid

When glucose levels do drop, avoid the temptation of decreasing the insulin rate below 0.05 units/kg/h. Insulin is the key therapeutic agent and is needed to clear ketones.

Glucose (5%) should be added to the IV fluids when the glucose drops to 14 mmol/l. Pre-prepared fluids of 5% glucose in 0.9% saline should be available in hospitals with paediatric units.

Insulin

Continuous insulin infusion

Insulin is started at a maximum of 0.1 units/kg/h (research indicates that it might not be necessary to exceed 0.05 units/kg/h).

When the blood sugar comes down to 14 mmol/l then the lower rate of 0.05 units/kg/h should be employed.

Insulin should not be stopped when the blood glucose normalizes. Instead, dextrose should be added to the maintenance fluid.

Electrolytes and osmolality

Managing sodium and osmolality

Keeping the serum sodium concentration elevated is considered to be neuroprotective, as is maintaining serum osmolality.

There are important considerations in the interpretation of the laboratory level of the measured serum sodium in DKA. The measured sodium level is depressed by the high level of glucose that draws water into the extracellular space. The patient's true sodium concentration will be higher than that seen on a blood gas or lab sample when the glucose level is corrected and returns to normal. The corrected sodium level can be calculated as below:

$$\text{corrected Na} = \text{measured Na} + 2[\text{plasma glucose} - 5.6]/5.6 \text{ mmol/l}$$

'effective osmolality' ('eOsm') can be calculated as:

$$\text{eOsm} = 2 \times [\text{Na} + \text{K}] + \text{plasma glucose} + \text{urea mOsm/kg}$$

Potassium must be supplemented from the outset at 40 mmol/l in all non-bolus IV fluids (maintenance and replacement) as treatment may precipitate hypokalaemia.

Although phosphate levels do drop (as a consequence of renal and metabolic depletion) replacement has not been shown to benefit children, and doing so may cause inadvertent hypocalcaemia.

Intubation

The advantage of not intubating a child with DKA is that the neurology can be assessed at any point. However, there are occasions when intubation must be performed. They include:

- need for neuroprotection – obvious signs of raised ICP (see above and Chapter 19)
- a child who is tiring of the massive ventilatory effort
- protection of the airway in a drowsy child.

Treatment of raised ICP in DKA

A careful balance in DKA has to be struck between keeping the patient awake for careful neurological monitoring and sedating and ventilating them for neuroprotection and airway safety. Once a decision has been made to ventilate a child with raised ICP, management follows similar principles to that of head injuries (see Chapter 19).

Intervention for acutely raised ICP

Once all of the simple manoeuvres for minimizing ICP detailed in Chapter 19 are employed osmotic therapy can be used in DKA:

- mannitol 0.5–1.0 g/kg over 20 min
- 3% hypertonic saline 5 ml/kg over 10 min.

If ICP becomes a major problem then fluids should be restricted even further by halving the maintenance rate and extending the correction of the deficit to 72 hours. This means that inotropes or vasopressors may become necessary to maintain the cerebral perfusion pressure.

Radiological imaging

If a child begins to show signs of neurological deterioration, then a CT scan of the head should be arranged as an emergency. The aim of the scan is to detect any coexisting pathology, which may be incidental or related to the hypercoagulable state, e.g. venous sinus thrombosis.

Other treatments to consider during management

Heparin therapy (prophylactic)

The BSPED guidelines (see Further reading) recommend anticoagulation due to the dehydrated and hyperviscous state of the patient's blood, especially if femoral lines are used. Local guidelines should be used to guide systemic heparinization, e.g. > 20 units/kg/h, if the risk of thrombosis is deemed to be significant.

Antibiotics – if sepsis present or suspected

Take cultures of blood, urine and any other sample as indicated (including tracheal aspirate if intubated). If meningitis is suspected, treat accordingly, deferring dural puncture until the child has recovered from the DKA, when CSF PCR can be performed.

What do I need to do after intubation?

Neuroprotection

Once the child is intubated, assessing progress of the ICP becomes problematic. However, regular neurological observations (see Table 11.1) should be undertaken, as rapid deterioration and coning can occur (see Chapter 19 for further management).

Hyperventilation

There is evidence that in DKA cerebral autoregulation is diminished and keeping the $PaCO_2$ at pre-intubation levels will cause least disturbance. This is a contentious subject because hyperventilation will cause further cerebral vasoconstriction and ischaemia, whereas hypoventilation can cause cerebral vasodilatation and a rise in intracranial pressure.

A lung-protective strategy may make keeping the $PaCO_2$ at pre-intubation levels impossible. The result is that a compromise has to be struck between causing lung damage and managing the ICP (depending on how severe each problem is at the time). The target $PaCO_2$ should be discussed with PICU before intubation.

Imaging

Unless already done a CT scan should be considered immediately after intubation, mainly to exclude venous sinus thrombosis, infarction or haemorrhage.

Measuring blood ketone levels

This has become recommended in the last few years as a good marker of whether the pathological ketogenic process is being switched off. In the absence of this assay, urinary ketones should be monitored.

Preparing a child for transfer

The decision of whether a child should be retrieved by the retrieval service or transferred by the local team should be taken in conjunction with the PICU retrieval team (see Chapter 24).

The preparations for acute transfer should include everything detailed in Chapter 24, with the additional considerations of:

- frequent blood monitoring – ideally an arterial line or CVC should be sited to aid with regular blood sugar and electrolyte checks
- because of the bi-modal presentation of cerebral oedema there is a significant risk of an acute change in ICP, therefore hypertonic saline or mannitol should be available for the transfer
- 10% glucose should be available as a rescue treatment should the blood glucose level drop unexpectedly.

Documentation should be prepared before transfer, and should include:

- a detailed history including:
  - any precipitating factors: stress, infection, poor compliance
  - investigations to date
  - previous treatment regimen if a known diabetic
- a timeline of treatment including:
  - when the child presented
  - when insulin was started
  - exactly how much fluid has been given
  - whether it was incorporated into the calculated deficit
- blood results, including timing of samples, in order to track the rate of change.

As with all other conditions diagnostic imaging should be available for transfer, either as hard copies or via secure link.

Summary

Administration of fluids to children suffering from DKA can cause a lot of problems. The risk of cerebral oedema is sufficiently high to warrant developing different management protocols for children. Whereas early, aggressive therapy is the mainstay for most conditions this is one of the few disease processes that benefits from more controlled patient resuscitation.

Golden rules

- Discuss early with PICU
- Avoid bicarbonate administration for acidosis

- When blood sugars drop, add in glucose, do not stop the insulin infusion
- ICP can increase suddenly, even hours after treatment starts
- Avoid hypotonic fluids
- Be aware that intubation will mask signs of raised ICP
- Be careful to avoid missing sepsis as a cause of shock

Further reading

BSPED. British Society of Paediatric Endocrinology & Diabetes DKA Guideline 2009. http://www.bsped.org.uk/professional/guidelines/docs/DKAGuideline.pdf (accessed 17 June 2011).

Levin DL. Cerebral edema in diabetic ketoacidosis. *Pediatr Crit Care Med* 2008;**9**:320–329.

Wolfsdorf J, Craig ME, Daneman D, *et al.* Diabetic ketoacidosis. *Pediatr Diabetes* 2007;**8**:28–43.

Section 2 Clinical Conditions

Chapter 12

Inherited metabolic conditions

Saikat Santra

Introduction

Inherited metabolic disorders (IMD) are a diverse group of conditions caused by inherited deficiencies in one or more enzymes of key metabolic pathways in the body. Some conditions present very early in the newborn period whilst others lead to more slowly progressive disease. While some conditions have no effective treatment, others are manageable with appropriate medical and dietary interventions.

Many IMD conditions put the child at risk of serious and rapid metabolic decompensation, particularly when the body is already stressed, for example during infections. It is these conditions that will be concentrated upon in this chapter.

The acute management of most metabolic conditions is very similar and a systematic approach can be followed for most children in this situation.

How the condition affects children

At their simplest, inborn errors of metabolism can be thought of as a problem in converting one chemical (the substrate) into another chemical (the product). Disease can occur because of the accumulation of toxic substrates or metabolites, deficiency in the product of a reaction, or both (Figure 12.1).

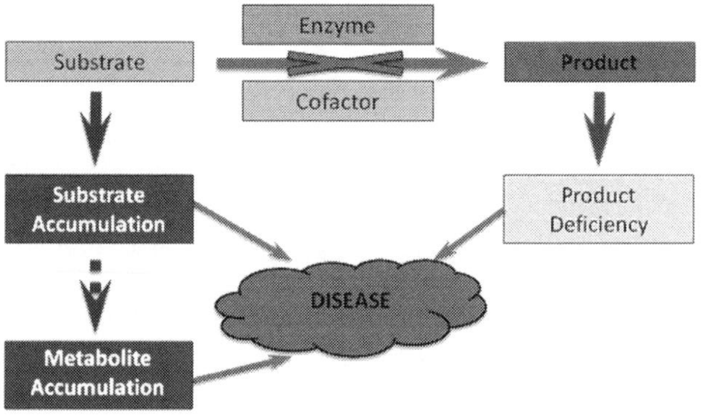

Figure 12.1. Potential ways in which metabolic pathway errors can lead to disease.

Managing the Critically Ill Child, ed. Richard Skone *et al.* Published by Cambridge University Press.

Examples of accumulating toxic metabolites include:

- ammonia
- amino acids such as leucine
- organic acids
- large molecules such as mucopolysaccharides.

Examples of product deficiencies include:

- hypoglycaemia
- energy deficiency.

The effects of IMDs are usually multisystem and often affect metabolically active organs. Features include encephalopathy, liver dysfunction/failure and cardiomyopathy. Mildly affected children, as well as those who are more severely affected but have survived the neonatal period, typically present to the ED during periods of stress to the body. These can include infections, pregnancy, prolonged fasting or high protein loads (for example GI bleeds). Sometimes the trigger is not always apparent. Gastroenteritis is a frequent trigger in childhood, as it causes increased energy demand and reduced nutrient absorption.

Specific inherited metabolic conditions

It is beyond the scope of this chapter to cover the presentations of all inborn errors of metabolism and at all ages. However, the commoner conditions in European populations that present acutely are detailed below.

Amino-acid-based conditions

Urea cycle disorders

The urea cycle is a pathway that removes excess nitrogen from amino acids by converting ammonia into urea, which is water-soluble and easily excreted.

The hallmark of all these conditions is an elevated ammonia level although the degree to which this occurs is variable between conditions and even between patients with the same condition. Severely affected infants typically present in the first week of life with severe hyperammonaemia and encephalopathy with plasma ammonia levels sometimes exceeding 1000 µmol/l.

Branched-chain organic acidaemias

Other steps in the breakdown of the branched-chain amino acids lead to one of the organic acidaemias namely:

- propionic acidaemia (PA)
- methylmalonic acidaemia (MMA)
- isovaleric acidaemia (IVA).

Severely affected infants typically present with encephalopathy and a severe metabolic acidosis from the accumulation of these organic acid intermediates. Hyperammonaemia is also seen as the organic acids cause a secondary inhibition of the urea cycle. Acute pancreatitis is a well-recognized complication of all three conditions and should be suspected if the child is particularly shocked or has severe abdominal pain. Metabolic strokes, especially affecting the basal ganglia, are a feared complication of decompensation.

Maple syrup urine disease (MSUD)

This condition is caused by an inherited deficiency of the enzyme complex which catalyses the second step of the breakdown of the three branched-chain amino acids: leucine, isoleucine and valine. Severely affected infants present with a progressive encephalopathy caused by the accumulation of leucine within the first 2 weeks of life. MSUD may lead to cerebral oedema (with a bulging fontanelle), seizures, cycling movements of the lower limbs and apnoeas.

There is no hyperammonaemia and the accumulation of ketoacids rarely causes metabolic acidosis but does cause ketonuria, which should raise suspicion of an inborn error of metabolism in a neonate. It is these ketoacids which also lend a characteristic odour of burnt sugar to the urine.

Enteral feeding (e.g. by nasogastric tube) with the appropriate amino acid mixture is preferable even in an emergency in children with MSUD. The amino acid mixture, in addition to carbohydrate, will enable the body to incorporate the excess branched-chain amino acids into protein (reducing the leucine levels in the brain).

Glutaric aciduria type 1

This condition, which is also an organic aciduria, occurs due to deficiency of one of the enzymes in the breakdown pathway of the amino acids lysine and tryptophan. These children are at risk of basal ganglia strokes during times of decompensation, particularly during the first 6 years of life. As with MSUD it is advisable to continue a lysine- and tryptophan-free amino acid mixture enterally to try and reduce the levels of these amino acids in the brain. An attempt should be made to use this even if intravenous fluids are required additionally. Carnitine supplementation is also necessary.

Fatty acid oxidation (FAO) disorders

This group of disorders includes patients with enzyme deficiencies of the carnitine cycle and of the fatty acid beta-oxidation pathway, such as:

- VLCAD deficiency — very long-chain acylCoA dehydrogenase
- LCHAD deficiency — long-chain hydroxyacylCoA dehydrogenase
- MCAD deficiency — medium-chain acylCoA dehydrogenase
- CPT1/CPT2 deficiencies — carnitine palmitoyl transferase
- CACT deficiency — carnitine acylcarnitine translocase.

These enzyme defects mean that children cannot mobilize fat as a source of energy. As a result they tend to present to hospital during times of catabolism, when the body is dependent on fat as a major source of energy. The more severe defects can cause a limited fasting tolerance, sometimes necessitating overnight tube feeding or cornstarch before bedtime. However, individuals who are less severely affected may only decompensate during times of stress.

The emergency treatment for all of these conditions is simply to administer sufficient carbohydrate to prevent the body from needing to draw on fat stores. This is usually provided as a glucose polymer drink/feed but if this is not tolerated then IV dextrose should be given. In these conditions the aim of treatment must always be to intervene before the blood glucose falls as hypoglycaemia is a late sign of decompensation. Hyperammonaemia is also seen in some children with acute decompensation of their FAO disorder.

Glycogen storage diseases

Children with these conditions are unable to release free glucose from glycogen (which accumulates in an enlarged liver). As a result, they are prone to hypoglycaemia after fasting. Depending on the condition this may occur as soon as 2 hours after feeding or only during times of illness. The management of these conditions is to provide sufficient glucose either enterally or, if not tolerated, intravenously to prevent hypoglycaemia.

Many of the intermediates in the glycogen pathway are metabolized to lactate. As a result children with these conditions can present with serum lactate levels up to 20 mmol/l. This will lead to a metabolic acidosis with its ensuing manifestations, e.g. tachypnoea. Bicarbonate treatment is usually not necessary as the lactic acidosis usually resolves quickly once glucose is being reliably delivered

Mitochondrial disorders

Children with defects in the components of the mitochondrial respiratory chain, or of enzymes leading to this such as Krebs-cycle defects and glutaric aciduria type 2 (multiple acylCoA dehydrogenase deficiency), present with energy failure (particularly affecting the metabolically active organs), especially during times of stress such as infection. In severe cases this can be fatal. In less severe cases the acute deterioration may be reversible with supportive care; however, most children will not recover to their previous level of functioning. Anaerobic stress manifests as lactic acidosis, which can be severe and in some cases responds to sodium dichloroacetate. There is much controversy about the use of so-called mitochondrial 'cocktails' of vitamins and co-factors in these conditions.

Table 12.1. Common complications of IMD with the specific diseases that cause them.

System	Organ system specific problems	Metabolic conditions in which they occur
Cardiovascular	Cardiomyopathy	Fatty acid oxidation disorders (especially long-chain) Mitochondrial disorders Some lysosomal and glycogen storage disorders (especially Pompe's) Organic acidaemias
Neurological	Encephalopathy Seizures Metabolic strokes	Organic acidaemias Urea cycle disorder Fatty acid oxidation disorder Mitochondrial disorders Organic acidaemias Urea cycle disorders MSUD Mitochondrial disorders Glutaric aciduria Organic acidaemias Mitochondrial disorders (Leigh syndrome)
Renal	Renal failure Renal tubular disease	Organic acidaemia Some lysosomal storage disorders (e.g. Fabry) Glycogen storage disease Mitochondrial disorders Tyrosinaemia type 1
Blood	Myelosuppression	Organic acidaemia Glycogen storage disorder (type 1b)
Liver	Liver dysfunction	Galactosaemia Tyrosinaemia (type 1) Urea cycle disorders Organic acidaemias Fatty acid oxidation disorder (especially longer-chain) Mitochondrial disorders (especially early-onset) Hereditary fructose intolerance Some lysosomal storage disorders (e.g. Wolman's, Niemann–Pick disease)
Other problems	Hyperammonaemia Rhabdomyolysis	Urea cycle disorder Organic acidaemias Fatty acid oxidation disorders Fatty acid oxidation disorders (especially long-chain, e.g. VLCAD)

When to suspect a metabolic condition

Almost all inherited metabolic disorders are inherited in an autosomal recessive manner. This means that both parents are usually asymptomatic carriers and therefore the suspicion of a metabolic disease should be raised when there is:

- parental consanguinity
- a family history of similar disease (including sudden, unexpected death in infancy).

In the newborn period, findings that should raise the suspicion of a metabolic disorder include:

- initial symptom-free period – during pregnancy accumulation of small molecules will be masked by placental removal
- severe metabolic acidosis
- hyperammonaemia – in all children an ammonia above 200 μmol/l requires investigation; levels above 100 μmol/l may still be significant outside the neonatal period
- rapidly progressive encephalopathy, liver disease and/or cardiomyopathy without clear alternative explanations
- characteristic odours such as those in MSUD (burnt sugar) or isovaleric acidaemia (sweaty feet).

The presentation of metabolic disease, particularly in neonates, can be nonspecific. It is important to consider inborn errors of metabolism in the differential diagnosis of all sick neonates, especially those being treated for suspected sepsis.

Targeted treatments for IMD

The emergency management of any sick metabolic patient can be considered under the following headings:

- ensure anabolism
- remove toxic precursors
- remove toxic metabolites
- give supportive treatment to maintain homeostasis
- reintroduce appropriate feeds.

Ensure anabolism

Decompensation usually occurs during periods of catabolism such as prolonged fasting or infections. The neonatal period is also a highly catabolic period. The first, and in some cases only, thing to do is to try and promote anabolism as much as possible. Giving carbohydrates will:

- provide calories for anabolism
- prevent the body breaking down muscle protein for fuel
- prevent the body breaking down fat for energy
- provide free glucose.

Wherever possible this should be given enterally. Most children with IMDs will have recipes for this provided by their metabolic dietician in an 'emergency regimen'. They should be encouraged to drink this regularly or be given it continuously through a nasogastric tube or gastrostomy. Glucose polymer solutions can be considered clear fluids from an anaesthetic perspective.

If oral solutions are not tolerated intravenous 10% dextrose should be given (lower concentrations may not provide a sufficient glucose intake to prevent catabolism). A glucose intake of 5–8 mg/kg/min should be sufficient in infants to suppress catabolism. Appropriate electrolyte supplementation should be given if intravenous fluids are to be used for some time.

If hyperglycaemia develops, add in a background insulin infusion rather than lower the glucose delivery. This will promote anabolism further. Rates of 0.05 unit/kg/h are usually sufficient.

An exception to this rule would be for patients with known disorders of mitochondrial function with lactic acidosis where excess glucose delivery could worsen lactic acidosis. In such conditions, 5% dextrose concentrations would be acceptable.

Remove toxic precursors

If hyperammonaemia is present, it is advisable in the short term to stop the child's natural protein-containing feeds during a decompensation in order to minimize ammonia production. The use of the emergency regimen (provided for each child) and intravenous fluids, if needed, should address this. In MSUD and glutaric aciduria type 1 it is important that the appropriate amino acid mixture is continued even if protein feeds are discontinued (see above).

Remove toxic metabolites

Drugs highly specific to children with IMD can be used to detoxify the body of specific metabolites such as ammonia. It is best to involve your local IMD team before starting treatment (unless a child has a pre-prepared management plan).

Hyperammonaemia causes stimulation of the respiratory centre, leading to tachypnoea and a respiratory alkalosis. At high levels, cerebral oedema is inevitable and urgent management to reduce the ammonia level is needed in order to try to avoid irreversible neurological damage. Levels greater than 150 μmol/l in an older child and 200 μmol/l in a neonate should be treated.

The appropriate medication, if started in time, can sometimes reduce ammonia levels quickly enough to prevent the need for more intensive treatment (see Chapter 36). In severe cases (e.g. when ammonia levels are over 500 μmol/l and/or are increasing despite medical therapy) haemofiltration or haemodialysis will be used on PICU to reduce ammonia levels quickly, in order to improve outcome.

Supportive treatment for homeostasis

During metabolic decompensation in many conditions, the pH can reduce dramatically – sometimes to less than 7.0. Remember that treating shock and promoting anabolism are more important than correcting acidosis – the parallels with DKA are useful to consider. In glycogen storage disease, for example, providing dextrose is sufficient to stop lactate production and the pH rapidly corrects with no other specific treatment.

Electrolyte imbalance should also be corrected, bearing in mind that many of the specialist drugs come as sodium salts and therefore have significant sodium content. This becomes more significant the younger the patient.

Reintroduce appropriate feeds

Children who receive no protein for a length of time can then become catabolic due to protein deficiency and this can worsen their metabolic condition. It is advisable, therefore, that some protein-containing feed is restarted within 72 hours at the latest. This will be taken care of in a specialist centre, after retrieval.

What do once the child is stabilized

Ammonia should be monitored at least every 4 hours until the levels are falling and stable. It is important to warn your clinical chemistry laboratory about this – as ammonia levels rise if samples are left standing for longer than 30 minutes. It is also useful at this point to ensure that the complications listed above such as coagulopathy or rhabdomyolysis are sought and acted on.

For children who do not have a known metabolic diagnosis, but in whom a metabolic disorder is suspected, it is important that samples for specialist tests are taken at the first opportunity. These will be advised by the regional IMD team on referral. The value of a first urine sample cannot be stressed highly enough.

Additional metabolic conditions to consider

There are also some other conditions where acute metabolic decompensation is not generally seen but attendance at the ED for other reasons can still occur.

Lysosomal storage disorders

These are a group of conditions where lysosomal enzymes are defective, leading to the accumulation of large molecules such as mucopolysaccharides. These children often have a number of structural problems affecting multiple organ systems. From an anaesthetic viewpoint there are several things to be aware of.

Table 12.2. Management of IMD.

Phase of management	Assessment	Action
Initial phase On presentation of the child	Manage initial phase as for all conditions (see Chapter 4)	Give oxygen • Ventilate by hand if needed Protect the airway Gain IV access • IO if more than two IV attempts Give fluid bolus • 20 ml/kg of crystalloid • Repeat as necessary
After initial assessment Once imminently life-threatening risks have been addressed	Ensure anabolism	Start IV 10% dextrose if oral rescue regime not tolerated (unless known mitochondrial disease) • Aim to give 5–8 mg/kg/min of dextrose Start insulin infusion if hyperglycaemic • 0.05 units/kg/h
Further stabilization Not immediately life-saving procedures	Remove toxic precursors Remove toxic metabolites Give supportive treatment to maintain homeostasis	Avoid giving amino acids (especially if hyperammonaemia) • Except MSUD and glutaric aciduria Contact IMD team for advice on specific drugs Manage the acidosis as in DKA, i.e. will resolve with management Look for complications such as coagulopathy and rhabdomyolysis

- Intubation may be very difficult due to a short neck, macroglossia, limited mouth opening and accumulation of storage material in the upper airway. A smaller ET tube is usually needed than would usually be estimated for the age of the child.
- Hypoplasia of the odontoid peg puts some children at risk of atlantoaxial subluxation especially in Morquio disease (MPS4). Storage material around the cervical spinal canal can also cause compression. Excessive flexion or extension of the neck during intubation can lead to permanent cervical cord damage.
- Many of these children have enlarged livers and spleens, increasing the risk of aspiration of gastric contents and making abdominal thrusts for resuscitation potentially dangerous.
- Skeletal abnormalities, especially pectus carinatum and kyphoscoliosis, may make resuscitation techniques difficult.
- These children often have cardiomyopathy and/or valvular heart disease.

Intubation should ideally only be attempted by experienced paediatric anaesthetists with expertise and equipment for a very difficult airway. It is also important that the airway of these patients is secured before any sedating medication is given.

Neurometabolic disorders

A large number of inborn errors of metabolism affect the brain. These children may attend the ED with seizures, dystonic spasms or encephalopathy. Although seizures in these conditions may require treatment with specific drugs, SE can usually be treated according to the standard APLS guidelines.

Summary

Although IMDs are complicated in their aetiology, the management of children with IMDs is quite straightforward. The most important priority is to get the child back into an anabolic state by providing substrate, i.e. rescue feeds or a crystalloid infusion that includes dextrose. For all children, early contact with the local IMD team is essential.

Golden rules

- IMD should be considered in any neonate who presents with sepsis
- Give dextrose-containing fluids early
- If IMD is suspected request a plasma ammonia level
- IMDs are multisystem diseases
- Seek expert advice early

Further reading

The British Inherited Metabolic Diseases Group has recently drawn up guidelines for the emergency management of most metabolic conditions, and advice for undiagnosed conditions. These guidelines are freely available to download from their website: www.bimdg.org.uk.

Hoffman GF, Zschocke J, Nyhan WL (eds.). *Inherited Metabolic Diseases: A Clinical Approach*. Springer, 2009.

Saudubray J-M, van der Berghe G, Walter JH (eds.). *Inborn Metabolic Diseases: Diagnosis and Treatment*, 5th edn. Springer, 2012.

Chapter 13

Paediatric toxicology

Marius Holmes

Introduction

Overdose in children is not uncommon. This is reflected in the fact that over a quarter of the telephone enquiries to TOXBASE in the year 2010/11 concerned children younger than 5 years of age. In many cases ingestion is proven to be benign and a period of observation is all that is required together with reassurance and home safety advice to parents. However, a history of ingestion should always be taken seriously.

This chapter will discuss the general management of children who have ingested poisons. It will also discuss specific drugs and toxins.

Important factors in paediatric overdose

History

Most paediatric poisonings are accidental, due to children's curiosity and exploration of their environment. It is important to take the ingestion of more unusual substances seriously, find out their ingredients (if a commercial product) and reference the product on databases such as TOXBASE.

There are some factors that need to be explored in detail when taking a history from a child who may have ingested a poison.

Toxin

Often in paediatric poisonings the agents are known. A clear history of where the child was and what other medications are available must also be taken. Remember in intentional overdoses to establish what other prescription drugs and over-the-counter medications there are in the home.

Dose ingested

Attempt where possible to estimate the maximum potential dose that could have been ingested. For instance, the parents may know that only one tablet is missing from a new blister pack. This is less easy with liquids or plant matter as the child is often found crying with the substance over their clothes and around their mouth. Always estimate the greatest amount possible, i.e. the dose per kg if a complete pack or bottle had been ingested.

Managing the Critically Ill Child, ed. Richard Skone *et al.* Published by Cambridge University Press.

Time of ingestion

The parents should know an approximate time when the ingestion could have taken place. It may have been witnessed or there could have been a time window when the child was not supervised. The timing of ingestion is important when calculating periods of observation, timing of drug levels and even the time to maximum toxicity.

If children are playing and one has taken something, remember to think that they might have shared it.

Presentation

The presentation of a poisoned child forms a continuum from a well child who needs no input through to an obtunded patient who is critically ill. Initial management is no different from any other seriously ill child (see Chapter 4) and is for the most part not dependent on the ingested agent in question.

Symptoms and signs

As mentioned above the history may not be that clear and you may be presented with an unconscious child. There are too many individual agents to mention within the scope of this chapter, but there are several common toxidromes (toxic syndromes) that may help you to think of different pharmaceutical groups. See Table 13.1.

Table 13.1. Common toxidromes.

	Sedatives, e.g. diazepam	Anti-cholinergics, e.g. tricyclic antidepressants	Cholinergics, e.g. organophosphates	Opiates	Sympathomimetics, e.g. cocaine	Serotonergics, e.g. SSRI
Consciousness	Reduced	Delirium	Reduced	Reduced	Excitation	Agitation
Pulse	–	Fast	Fast or slow	Slow	Fast	Fast
Blood pressure	Reduced	Increased	Increased	Reduced	Increased or decreased	Increased
Respiratory rate	Reduced	–	Increased	Reduced	Increased	Increased
Temperature	Reduced	Increased	–	Reduced	Increased	–
Skin	–	Dry	Sweating	–	Sweating	Sweating
Pupils	–	Large	Small	Small	Large	Large
Other features	Ataxia	Urinary retention, broad QRS, dry mouth, clonus, delayed gastric emptying	Voiding, defaecation, vomiting, lacrimation, drooling	Response to naloxone (short lived)	Seizures, tremor and hyperreflexia	Clonus, hyperreflexia

Specific conditions

Some common substances that cause poisoning are listed below.

Carbon monoxide

Carbon monoxide has an affinity for haemoglobin 250 times greater than oxygen. Once bound it forms carboxyhaemoglobin, which has a half-life of 4 hours (reduced to 90 minutes in 100% oxygen). Carboxyhaemoglobin cannot transport oxygen to the body.

This condition presents with nonspecific signs and symptoms. When entire families are subject to this poisoning, children are often the first to show signs. These range from malaise through to coma. Carbon monoxide poisoning should always be suspected in nonspecific coma, but especially so during the winter months and when there are reports of flu-like symptoms in the family. The simplest way to detect carbon monoxide poisoning is to perform a blood gas test for carboxyhaemoglobin.

Monitoring of oxygen delivery in carbon monoxide poisoning is difficult for the following reasons:

- the absorption pattern of red light by carboxyhaemoglobin will give falsely high saturation readings on a co-oximetry probe
- the PaO_2 on a blood gas will only tell you the amount of oxygen dissolved in plasma. It will not tell you how much is being transported by haemoglobin, i.e. a high PaO_2 does not mean good oxygen delivery.

Therefore, other indicators of oxygenation such as lactate and cardiovascular stability will guide the need for intubation. Carbon monoxide levels greater than 25% should also prompt consideration of intubation.

If carbon monoxide poisoning is present remember to assess the rest of the family and ensure the house boiler or fireplace is serviced. Advice regarding carbon monoxide monitors should be given.

Paracetamol

Toxic overdoses of paracetamol are usually associated with ingestion of greater than 150 mg/kg. There are very few signs or symptoms in early overdose. Toxicity starts from about 8 hours. If presentation is after 8 hours and a potentially toxic dose has been ingested treatment with *N*-acetylcysteine should be started pending drug level results. Activated charcoal is only effective if presentation is within 1 hour of overdose.

N-Acetylcysteine treatment takes place over 21 hours and consists of three separate infusions with different concentrations over different times. It often causes mild symptoms related to histamine release such as an urticarial rash. Rarely, it can cause anaphylactoid reactions with airway swelling, bronchospasm and hypotension.

Staggered overdoses are complex and although levels are useful to show that some paracetamol has been taken any significant overdose should be treated. If the presentation is delayed there may be a need for early intensive care and specialist hepatology input.

Although many liver specialists would advocate monitoring coagulation as a marker for severity of liver injury, blood products should be made available for children. They may need to be given if the child starts haemorrhaging, or if procedures such as central line insertion need to be performed. There should be a low threshold for intubation in encephalopathic children who require transfer to a tertiary centre.

Iron

Iron supplements are readily available over the counter. The tablets are often an inviting red colour and can be sugar-coated. Ingestions of 20 mg/kg of elemental iron can be potentially toxic. Symptoms occurring within the first 6 hours are mostly gastrointestinal, ranging from nausea to melaena. In large overdoses (>150 mg/kg elemental iron) there may be:

- coma
- life-threatening gastrointestinal haemorrhage
- cardiovascular collapse
- pulmonary oedema
- death.

The iron preparation taken should always be worked out as an elemental dose and then worked out per kilogram body weight of the patient. An abdominal X-ray should be considered to estimate the number of tablets consumed.

Iron levels should be taken 4 hours after ingestion and levels checked on TOXBASE to aid further management, including the possible use of desferoxamine, an iron-chelating agent, as the body has no way of excreting iron. Desferoxamine itself is not without risk as it can cause pulmonary fibrosis and acute respiratory distress syndrome. Activated charcoal has no role in iron overdose.

Consideration should be given to haemodialysis and whole bowel irrigation in severe cases and endoscopy may be considered to remove a tablet concretion from the stomach.

Opiates

Management of acute ingestion of opiates includes airway support, ventilation and treatment with naloxone. Methadone is often dispensed as a sweet green liquid, which is quite attractive to young children, so it is worth asking parents about what drugs are available in the house. It has a long half-life and will require a naloxone infusion to manage it effectively. If the ingestion has led to a respiratory arrest then basic management should be as detailed in Chapter 4.

Oral hypoglycaemics

Oral hypoglycaemics are a common prescription medication found in households. Children are more prone to having hypoglycaemic episodes than adults. Many agents are long-acting so admission with regular blood sugar measurement and observation is needed.

Tricyclic antidepressants (TCA)

Doses as little as 15 mg/kg should be treated as life-threatening in children. To put that into perspective, five small 50 mg tablets could kill a 4-year-old.

Early intravenous access and blood gas measurement is important. The child should have ECG monitoring and the QRS and QT intervals should be formally measured. Any prolongation of these should be treated with intravenous sodium bicarbonate.

Intravenous alkalinization reduces the active unbound TCA and so can dramatically narrow the QRS complex, terminate arrhythmias and correct hypotension. Any seizures should be treated in the usual way. However, phenytoin should be avoided where possible in

TCA overdose, due to its possible effects on cardiac conduction. Agitation may be managed with small aliquots of benzodiazepine. Activated charcoal may be effective if given within 1 hour of ingestion.

Caustic ingestions

With ingestion of caustic chemicals like acids and alkalis the most obvious initial symptoms are burns to the oropharynx. Symptoms from this include pain, vomiting and drooling. Because the substances are so unpleasant, usually not much is swallowed. When they are swallowed, haematemesis and oesophagitis may follow, progressing to oesophageal perforation.

Swelling around the epiglottis may cause airway obstruction. As with thermal injuries, early elective intubation may be required in anticipation of worsening oedema. In all of these children, a difficult intubation should be anticipated (see Chapter 16 for difficult airways).

If the chemical is in powder form ensure that it is brushed off the patient as much as possible, as water may activate the powder, causing extensive injuries. No gastric aspiration or chemical neutralization should be attempted as both of these can worsen the situation.

Initial management

Initial management involves stabilization as detailed in Chapter 4 (see Table 13.2 also). The targeted treatment for overdoses should then be guided by databases such as TOXBASE and the patient's clinical condition.

Decision to ventilate

The decision to ventilate is unlikely to be driven by respiratory failure in these children. Instead it will be taken depending on:

- need for airway protection, i.e. vomiting or coma
- need for invasive intervention, e.g. central line insertion in small children
- encephalopathy
- carbon monoxide levels (especially if greater than 25%).

If the child seems to be in respiratory distress it is worth performing a blood gas as the respiratory rate may reflect:

- underlying metabolic acidosis
- direct stimulation by ammonia or salicylates
- aspiration
- pulmonary oedema.

Cardiovascular support

Cardiovascular support follows the same principles as in Chapter 4. Fluid boluses, followed by inotropes, if needed, form the mainstay of treatment. The only differences to consider are:

- some drugs lead to arrhythmias, which should be corrected (e.g. TCA)
- some drugs have direct myocardial depressant effects which will require inotropes
- some children will have taken antihypertensive drugs which need vasopressors.

Investigations and other supportive measures

When gaining intravenous access blood should be taken to check:

- renal profile
- full blood count
- clotting screen
- specific drug/toxin levels as history/poison dictates
- glucose
- blood gas (methaemoglobin, carboxyhaemoglobin, anion gap and electrolytes)
- the possibility of a cross-match.

Calculate the time when blood needs to be taken for plasma toxin levels, as often this is separate from the initial time of intravenous access. Others things to consider are investigations specific to the overdose. This may include an electrocardiogram in TCA ingestion, or an abdominal radiograph in metal overdose, e.g. iron.

Passage of a NG tube will aid in gastric decompression, but will also allow the administration of charcoal if needed or it can be used for whole bowel irrigation (specialist advice only). It is, however, debatable whether an NG tube should be passed at all in caustic ingestion. With the situation under control ensure the child is kept warm.

Child protection

Once initial priorities have been addressed it is always important to think of the safety of the child in the future and also the safety of other children/vulnerable adults in the same home. Depending on the circumstances a home visit from a health visitor may need to be organized to ensure that there are no underlying child protection needs or that this event is not a reflection of lack of appropriate supervision. The involvement of social services and the police may be required urgently. Any child who has taken an intentional overdose should have a psychiatric assessment at an appropriate time prior to discharge.

Preparation for transfer

As with other chapters, preparation for transfer will need detailed, written, documentation of the history, clinical findings and lab results. Timing of ingestions and therapeutic interventions should also be documented.

Table 13.2. Initial management of a poisoned child.

Phase of management	Assessment	Action
On presentation of the child	Assess ABC • Airway patency • Oxygenation and ventilatory effort/volume • Cardiovascular status • GCS • Blood sugar	Airway control Assisted ventilation with oxygen IV versus IO access Give fluid bolus as required
After initial assessment	History of event, potential agent and dose Reassess response to initial treatment Reassess need to intubate • Ensure no decline in respiratory function • Concern over high aspiration risk • Need for bowel irrigation Consider need for more fluid resuscitation and need for inotropic support ECG and careful blood gas interpretation	Reference toxin any antidote or suggested therapy Site NG tube and aspirate prior to intubation (unless caustic ingestion) When 40 ml/kg of fluid has been given prepare inotropes. Consider inotropes after 60 ml/kg of fluid Start any antidote or drug treatment needed Are there child protection concerns? Consider other children in the home
Further stabilization Not immediately lifesaving procedures	Close continued monitoring as required Definitive plan • Progression to intubation • Level of continued care needed on ward • Need for specialist unit transfer	**Resuscitation room monitoring** Contact retrieval team Consider invasive monitoring and central access

Summary

Most overdoses in children are accidental. It is important to be forthright and direct when asking about drug availability within the house in order to get a good picture of what the child may have ingested. Expert advice is advisable in most cases, to ensure the appropriate management is undertaken.

Golden rules

- Find out what other prescribed medicines are in the home
- Always check toxins on TOXBASE (some common household substances are surprisingly toxic)
- Check the blood sugar
- The toxicity is worked out per kilogram weight – the child needs to be weighed
- Check all the blood gas results, including anion gap, methaemoglobinaemia and carbon monoxide level
- Think of child protection/supervision issues

Further reading

http://www.hpa.org.uk/webc/HPAwebFile/HPAweb_C/1317130944236.

http://www.toxbase.org/.

Chapter 14

The child with anaphylaxis

Nick Sargant

Introduction

Anaphylaxis is defined as a severe, potentially fatal reaction of rapid onset that occurs after contact with an allergic trigger. It is the most serious manifestation of a continuum of immunoglobulin E (IgE) mediated allergic disease (type 1 or immediate hypersensitivity).

Anaphylaxis results from degranulation of mast cells and the release of inflammatory mediators in response to an allergic trigger. Any allergic reaction with the capacity to be life-threatening should be treated as anaphylaxis, including serious localized reactions such as angioedema obstructing the upper airway.

The frequency of admissions for anaphylaxis has risen in recent years. In the UK there are 1–3 deaths per million people (adults and children) annually. In children, anaphylaxis appears to be more common in males until the age of 15, after which females are more commonly affected. Children under 1 year are the most likely group to be admitted.

How anaphylaxis differs in children

Presentation

In up to 20% of cases a trigger allergen may be unknown or unclear. The first signs of an anaphylactic reaction are often cutaneous. However, up to 18% of childhood cases show no dermatological features.

Food protiens are the most common cause of anaphylaxis in children. The mode of delivery of the allergen means that these are more likely to present with respiratory compromise (intravenous drugs or insect bites are more likely to cause cardiovascular problems). Because of the incidence of food allergy and difficulty in isolating a trigger, anaphylaxis should be considered in any child presenting with sudden onset of asthma following exposure to a possible allergen.

Signs to look out for in anaphylaxis are detailed in Table 14.1.

Speed of onset

Reactions to IV drugs and insect stings tend to have a very rapid onset whereas food anaphylaxis can take hours, especially if the allergenic part of the food is coated in another foodstuff and only exposed to the immune system during digestion.

Managing the Critically Ill Child, ed. Richard Skone *et al.* Published by Cambridge University Press.

Hypotension tends to occur later in children than in adults. Therefore any child with tachycardia, respiratory distress, stridor, pallor, drowsiness or uncharacteristic quietness should be taken very seriously.

Life-threatening reaction

Risk factors for severe or life-threatening reactions are thought to include:

- history of asthma
- previous or increasingly severe allergic reactions
- concurrent treatment with β-blockers
- allergens including peanut, tree nuts, fish and shell fish.

Table 14.1. Clinical manifestations of anaphylaxis.

System	Mechanism	Effect
Upper respiratory tract	Angioedema of the larynx and upper airways	Hoarseness Stridor Cough Dyspnoea Obstruction Respiratory arrest
Lower respiratory tract	Bronchospasm Mucosal oedema	Wheeze Chest tightness Reduced peak expiratory flow (PEF) Tachypnoea Dyspnoea Hypoxia Respiratory arrest
Cardiovascular	Shock results from widespread vasodilatation and loss of intravascular volume due to capillary leak Possible direct myocardial suppression by allergic mediators	Tachycardia Hypotension Arrhythmias Cardiac arrest
Gastrointestinal tract	Mucosal oedema	Nausea Vomiting Abdominal cramps Diarrhoea Incontinence
Skin	Histamine and other inflammatory mediators cause extravasation of fluid into the dermis	Urticaria Flushing Erythema Pruritus
Brain	Usually as a consequence of cardiovascular and respiratory compromise although neurological symptoms have been reported as presenting features infrequently	Dizziness Hypotonia Syncope Seizures

Management

General principles

The main management priorities after this are early recognition, removal of the allergenic trigger (where possible) and immediate administration of intramuscular (IM) adrenaline. Studies have demonstrated increased morbidity and mortality with delay in IM adrenaline administration. In otherwise healthy children it is better to administer IM adrenaline (10 μg/kg) than risk clinical deterioration by holding off treatment. The adrenaline will help with respiratory and cardiovascular problems. It is also thought to stabilize mast cell membranes in order to minimize histamine release.

Intramuscular administration of adrenaline is the preferred route of delivery. Intravenous or intraosseous administration should be reserved for children with life-threatening features to whom IM adrenaline has been given multiple times or for those in cardiac arrest.

Table 14.2. Initial management of anaphylaxis.

Immediate actions	
Rapid assessment Oxygen IM adrenaline without delay Remove allergen if possible Place patient in a recumbent position and elevate lower limbs if evidence of cardiovascular compromise Sit upright if respiratory compromise and cardiovascularly stable	
Airway	
Partial obstruction: Repeat IM adrenaline if no response to initial dose Nebulized adrenaline Repeat IM and nebulized adrenaline every 10 minutes as required Hydrocortisone	Complete obstruction: Intubation Surgical airway
Breathing	
Wheeze: Repeat IM adrenaline if no response to initial dose Nebulized salbutamol Hydrocortisone Consider IV salbutamol or IV aminophylline	Apnoea: Bag–mask ventilation ET tube Repeat IM adrenaline if no response to initial dose of adrenaline Hydrocortisone
Circulation	
Shock: Repeat IM adrenaline if no response to initial dose Crystalloid bolus IV adrenaline infusion	No pulse: Advanced life support
Reassess ABC	

Table 14.3. Drugs used in anaphylaxis.

Drugs in anaphylaxis	<6 months	6 months–6 years	6–12 years	>12 years
IM adrenaline (in-hospital doses)	10 μg/kg 0.1 ml/kg of 1:10000 (infants or young children) ***OR*** 0.01 ml/kg of 1:1000 (older children – maximum 0.5 ml 1:1000)			
Crystalloid (e.g. 0.9% saline)	20 ml/kg IV bolus (can be repeated as required)			
Nebulized adrenaline	400 μg/kg 0.4 ml/kg of 1:1000 up to a maximum of 5 ml (dilute to 5 ml with 0.9% saline if necessary)			
Hydrocortisone (IV or IM)	25 mg	50 mg	100 mg	200 mg
IV chlorphenamine	(weight ÷ 4) mg	2.5 mg	5 mg	10 mg
Nebulized salbutamol	2.5 mg		5 mg	
IV adrenaline infusion	**Only to be used in a life-threatening anaphylaxis resistant to IM adrenaline or where multiple IM doses have been required** Commence at 0.1 μg/kg/min and titrate to effect			
Vasopressors	Potent vasopressors such as noradrenaline, vasopressin and metaraminol can be used in cases of anaphylaxis where there is hypotension refractory to an IV adrenaline infusion and fluid resuscitation. This should only be done after discussion with the regional paediatric intensive care unit (PICU) or paediatric retrieval team			

While waiting for the adrenaline to work, basic management as in Chapter 4 should be initiated.

Steroids are given at the start of anaphylaxis management. However, their main value is in minimizing the chance of a biphasic reaction. The mainstay of treatment remains supportive therapy along with intramuscular adrenaline.

Intubation and initiating intensive care

Intubation

Indications for intubation include:

- airway obstruction
- severe bronchospasm resulting in hypoxia or apnoea
- IV adrenaline infusion requirement (anaphylaxis resistant to IM doses)
- reducing consciousness level
- cardiac arrest.

Anaphylaxis is one of the indications for using cuffed ET tubes in children, especially if bronchospasm is a feature, as high ventilation pressures may be required.

Care needs to be taken at induction to use drugs that do not worsen the cardiovascular state, or cause further histamine release (e.g. atracurium or morphine). Anaesthetic agents with less propensity for histamine release include vecuronium and fentanyl. If an IV induction is planned, ketamine would be the agent of choice.

In cases where there is upper airway obstruction an experienced ENT surgeon should also be in attendance and an inhalational induction considered. Inhalational induction allows for the airway to be assessed at laryngoscopy while spontaneous breathing is maintained (see Chapter 16). If upper airway swelling is so severe that conventional intubation is impossible, then it will be necessary to perform tracheostomy or cricothyroidotomy.

Ventilation

Relative hypovolaemia is a problem in anaphylaxis. It may be worsened after intubation in children with bronchospasm, as positive-pressure ventilation will result in a fall in venous return. Air trapping from overly aggressive, rapid ventilation will also have the same effect. A relatively low respiratory rate should therefore be set on the ventilator and permissive hypercapnoea practised (as in asthma – see Chapter 8).

Cardiovascular

As with all cases fluid should be titrated to clinical need. Any child requiring an adrenaline infusion and intubation for anaphylaxis will also require central venous access and an arterial line for invasive blood-pressure monitoring. If this is difficult then an IO needle can be used for adrenaline infusions.

Acute investigations

Anaphylaxis is a clinical diagnosis and therefore no specific confirmatory investigations are required. Arterial blood gases and CXR should be performed prior to transfer in order to guide ventilation, check ET tube position and rule out a pneumothorax.

Serum tryptase

Markers of anaphylaxis can be measured. Unfortunately, tryptase can be an unreliable marker as it does not reliably increase in all episodes of anaphylaxis. This is particularly true of food-related anaphylaxis, the most frequent type in children. The 2011 NICE guideline on anaphylaxis mentions consideration of blood sampling for mast cell tryptase as soon as possible after initiation of treatment for anaphylaxis and a second sample 1–2 hours and no later than 4 hours from the onset of symptoms in children younger than 16 years of age if the cause is thought to be venom, drug-related or idiopathic.

A rise in serum tryptase levels (over 10 ng/ml) within 1–5 hours after suspected anaphylaxis indicates that the reaction was probably anaphylaxis. A persistently elevated serum tryptase after the cessation of an anaphylactic reaction, or in a well patient, suggests the possibility of systemic mastocytosis.

Biphasic anaphylaxis

In children who have recovered from anaphylaxis the major concern is the possibility of a biphasic reaction. Biphasic reactions are defined as a second reaction occurring 1–72 hours after the first. The frequency of biphasic reactions remains unclear, with estimates ranging from 1% to 23% of anaphylaxis cases.

Typically, biphasic reactions occur at 8 to 10 hours after the resolution of the acute phase and for this reason children should be monitored in hospital. The 2011 NICE guidelines on anaphylaxis recommend admitting children under 16 years who have required emergency treatment to hospital under the care of a paediatric team.

Admission to hospital should be arranged for any child who has had a particularly severe reaction and any of the following risk factors:

- severe initial phase
- delayed or suboptimal doses of adrenaline
- laryngeal oedema
- hypotension during the initial phase
- delayed symptomatic onset after allergen exposure
- previous history of biphasic anaphylaxis.

Follow-up

All children with anaphylaxis require follow-up by an allergy specialist even where there is an obvious cause. In a previously undiagnosed child, the onus to refer to a specialist clinic lies with the admitting physician. Allergy specialists will then consider the need for further investigations such as skin prick tests or blood tests for specific IgE (RAST) both to the likely trigger and to other commonly associated allergens.

The children and families will be given advice on avoidance (often in conjunction with a dietician) and provided with an anaphylaxis management plan. Where necessary the child and family will be supplied with an adrenaline auto-injector such as the EpiPen and trained in its use.

Children are then followed up in allergy clinic and monitored for signs that they have developed tolerance to an allergen. At this point a supervised in-hospital food challenge might take place.

Summary

The principles of managing a child with anaphylaxis are similar to those in adults. The follow-up of a child with anaphylaxis is essential in order to identify an allergen where possible. Avoidance of triggers and ensuring optimal asthma management, and carrying an adrenaline auto-injector form the mainstay of ongoing management.

Golden rules

- Anaphylaxis can occur without a rash or hypotension
- In life-threatening conditions IM adrenaline should be given if there is any doubt about the cause
- Biphasic reactions mean that children should be monitored closely and the 2011 NICE guideline on anaphylaxis recommends admitting children under 16 who have required emergency treatment to hospital
- Follow-up in an allergy clinic must be arranged by the admitting physician

Further reading

Advanced Paediatric Life Support: The Practical Approach, 5th edn. BMJ Books, 2011.

Ben-Shoshan M, Clarke AE. Anaphylaxis: past, present and future. *Allergy* 2011;**66**(1):1–14.

Braganza SC, *et al.* Paediatric emergency department anaphylaxis: different patterns from adults. *Arch Dis Child* 2006;**91**(2): 159–163.

Du Toit G. Food-dependent exercise-induced anaphylaxis in childhood. *Pediatr Allergy Immunol* 2007;**18**(5):455–463.

Gupta R, Sheik A, Strachan DP, Anderson HR. Time trends in allergic disorders in the UK. *Thorax* 2007;**62**(1):91–96.

Kemp SF. The post-anaphylaxis dilemma: how long is long enough to observe a patient after resolution of symptoms? *Curr Allergy Asthma Rep* 2008;**8**(1):45–48.

Lieberman P, Camargo CA, Bohlke K, *et al.* Epidemiology of anaphylaxis: findings of the American College of Allergy, Asthma and Immunology Epidemiology of Anaphylaxis Working Group. *Ann Allergy Asthma Immunol* 2006;**97**(5):596–602.

National Institute for Health and Clinical Excellence. *Anaphylaxis: assessment to confirm an anaphylactic episode and the decision to refer after emergency treatment for a suspected anaphylactic episode.* (Clinical guideline 134.) 2011.http://guidance.nice.org.uk/CG134.

Pumphrey RS. Lessons for management of anaphylaxis from a study of fatal reactions. *Clin Exp Allergy* 2000;**30** (8):1144–1150.

Sampson HA, Muñoz-Furlong A, Campbell RL, *et al.* Second symposium on the definition and management of anaphylaxis: summary report – Second National Institute of Allergy and Infectious Disease/Food Allergy and Anaphylaxis Network symposium. *J Allergy Clin Immunol* 2006;**117**(2): 391–397.

Sampson HA, Mendelson L, Rosen JP. Fatal and near-fatal anaphylactic reactions to food in children and adolescents. *N Engl J Med* 1992;**327**(6):380–384.

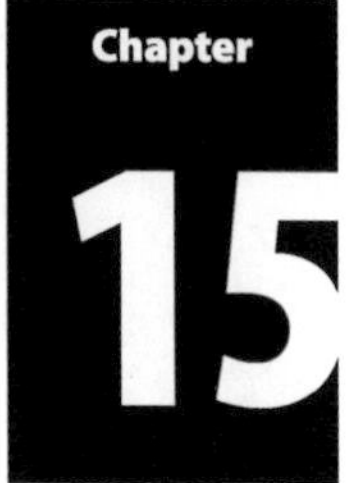

The child with stridor

Ed Carver and Tim Day-Thompson

Introduction

Stridor may be a sign of emergency or non-emergency airway pathology. Its presence, especially in the acute setting, may herald critical airway obstruction and respiratory collapse, demanding timely and effective management.

This chapter focusses on assessment, management and preparation for transfer for definitive care of the acutely stridulous infant or child.

Definition and features

Stridor is a vibratory, often high-pitched sound produced by abnormal airflow through a partially obstructed airway at the level of the supraglottis, glottis, subglottis or proximal trachea. It is a pathological sign rather than a diagnosis. It should be differentiated from breath sounds caused by abnormal airflow elsewhere in the respiratory tree such as stertor (snoring) or wheeze.

The relationship of stridor to phase of breathing varies with location and severity of the underlying pathology:

- biphasic stridor suggests critical narrowing or fixed obstruction at or below the glottis
- inspiratory stridor suggests partial obstruction of the extrathoracic large airways as these are usually narrowest during inspiration
- expiratory stridor (or wheeze with more distal narrowing) suggests partial obstruction of the intrathoracic upper airways as these are usually narrowest during expiration.

The volume and pitch of stridor correlate poorly with severity of airway obstruction.

How does stridor differ in children?

Important differences in paediatric anatomy and physiology increase susceptibility to stridor and its effects.

Size

The paediatric airway is small. During laminar airflow resistance is inversely proportional to the fourth power of its radius. Therefore significant reductions in airflow result from modest reductions in diameter. When a child is distressed airflow may become turbulent leading to further increases in flow resistance and increased work of breathing.

Managing the Critically Ill Child, ed. Richard Skone *et al.* Published by Cambridge University Press.

Immaturity

Immature cartilaginous structures support the airway and chest wall. These are relatively compliant and prone to collapsing inwards with excessive negative airway pressure or extrinsic compression. This compounds the inefficiency of laboured breathing and may cause gas trapping.

Infants are more reliant on diaphragmatic breathing due to immaturity of the rib cage and accessory muscles. Their diaphragm also has fewer fatigue-resistant muscle fibres.

Other factors

Respiratory reserve is further reduced by the high metabolic rate and small functional residual capacity, particularly in infants.

Causes of acute paediatric stridor

Causes of stridor can be congenital or acquired, with acquired forms further divided into infective or non-infective causes.

Infective

Viral croup (laryngotracheobronchitis)

This is the most common cause of acute stridor in children. It is most frequently caused by parainfluenza virus, and commonly occurs between 6 months and 3 years of age.

An upper respiratory tract coryzal prodrome is followed by inflammation and oedema of the subglottis, resulting in a characteristic barking cough. There may be a low-grade fever, hoarse cry, stridor and increased respiratory effort. These symptoms are often worse at night.

Most patients experience a mild, self-limiting illness; however, stridor may prompt an emergency department visit. Of those patients admitted, only around 1% require intubation and ventilation, the rest being managed with humidified oxygen and steroids. A high temperature in any child with the symptoms of croup should prompt consideration of the pathologies below.

Epiglottitis

This is a medical emergency with potential for rapidly progressive, life-threatening airway obstruction. It is caused by bacterial infection of the epiglottic/supraglottic tissues. It usually occurs between 2 and 7 years of age.

Typical clinical presentation involves rapidly progressive high fever, sore throat, dysphagia, drooling and stridor leading to respiratory failure and shock. Spontaneous cough is usually absent; the patient appears toxic and prefers sitting forwards if able.

The UK introduction of the *Haemophilus influenzae* type B (HiB) vaccine (given to children during the first year of their life) in 1992 dramatically reduced the incidence of childhood epiglottitis. Despite this, HiB-related epiglottitis has occurred in HiB-immunized individuals. Epiglottitis may also be caused by other organisms. It therefore remains an important differential diagnosis in acute stridor. An immunization history should be sought in all children, as over 4% of the UK population are partially immunized or unimmunized.

Most children will require intubation and ventilation to secure the airway and antibiotic treatment.

Bacterial tracheitis

This is a super-added tracheal bacterial infection following a viral respiratory tract infection. The most common causative organism is *Staphylococcus aureus*.

Bacterial tracheitis is usually preceded by upper respiratory tract coryza with subsequent rapid onset of high fever, stridor, respiratory distress and painful cough with copious mucopurulent tracheal secretions (Table 15.1).

Table 15.1. Differentiating features of viral croup, tracheitis and epiglottitis.

	Viral croup	Bacterial tracheitis	Epiglottitis
Commonest age	6 months–3 years	Wide range, average 3 years	2–7 years
Progression	Gradual	Follows a viral prodrome, then rapid deterioration	Very rapid
Febrile?	Usually mild fever	High fever	High fever
Swallow	Normal	Normal	Very difficult/drooling
Cough	Frequent, barking	Barking, painful, productive	None /muffled
Toxaemic appearance?	No	Yes	Yes
Vocalizations	Hoarse	Possibly hoarse	Unable to speak
Other features	Worse at night		Agitated and distressed

Abscess

Metastatic abscess formation in the space between the posterior pharyngeal wall and the prevertebral fascia (retropharyngeal abscess) usually occurs before 6 years of age. Similar seeding in the space between the tonsils and the superior constrictor muscles (peritonsillar abscess) is commoner in older children and adolescents. Staphylococcal and streptococcal infections are the most common causes.

Typical presentation involves high fever, dysphagia and trismus with swelling and limited movement of the neck. Stridor and respiratory distress are uncommon.

Non-infective

Foreign-body aspiration

Inhaled small food items are the commonest cause of foreign-body aspiration. Peak incidence is at 1 to 2 years of age. There is often a history of choking or coughing, but this may be absent. Depending on the location, degree and time course of airway obstruction, there may be a change in voice, stridor, cough, wheeze, dyspnoea or signs of complete obstruction.

Eighty per cent of inhaled foreign bodies lodge in the lower airways and therefore stridor is less common as a presenting feature.

External airway compression

Neoplasm, enlarged lymph nodes, haematoma and vascular structures may all cause extrinsic compression of the airway.

Spasmodic croup

This mimics viral croup but is not related to upper respiratory tract infection. It often occurs with sudden onset at night, can be recurrent and may be related to gastric reflux or atopic triggers. Clinical management is the same as for viral croup.

Other

Non-infective acute causes of stridor include severe allergic/angioneurotic reaction and thermal airway injury. Both require careful assessment as airway inflammation may worsen rapidly. Early intubation is therefore advised.

Chronic causes of stridor

It is important to be aware of a number of structural, often congenital, abnormalities that can cause chronic stridor. Although they may be incidental and stable, these patients are susceptible to acute exacerbations and may respond less well to treatment.

Parents may present late with these children, and seem disproportionately calm. It is useful to get a history of the usual respiratory pattern for these children as they may normally have a tracheal tug or subcostal recession. The stridor in children with chronic airway problems may also be a red herring in that it may worsen dramatically with increased effort of breathing, such as in chest infections.

The main causes of chronic stridor can be divided into either structurally weak airways (such as laryngomalacia or tracheomalacia) or stenotic airways. The former may present with acute life-threatening events secondary to airway collapse and difficulty in ventilation, while the latter may cause difficulty at the time of intubation in finding a small enough ET tube to pass through the obstruction.

Assessment of a child with stridor

Assessment

Where possible the child should be assessed undisturbed, in their own comfortable position with parents nearby, as distressing these children can exacerbate stridor.

A timely clinical assessment should be made of the effectiveness and work of breathing. Any available history will assist diagnosis and thus facilitate targeted treatment. Further examination involves assessment of the phase of breathing associated with the stridor. Loudness of stridor correlates poorly with severity and decreases in near complete obstruction or exhaustion. Cautious chest examination should be possible. The severity of airway stridor should not distract from other potential problems, e.g. cardiovascular compromise.

Pulse oximetry should be used where tolerated. Low saturations or a significant supplemental oxygen requirement are a sign that the child's work of breathing has become excessive.

Croup severity scoring systems can been used to guide management, but these are rarely used nowadays. More important is recognition of signs of severe croup, including:

- delayed inspiratory breath sounds
- biphasic stridor
- suprasternal and intercostal recession
- nasal flaring
- cyanosis in oxygen of 40% or more.

Intrusive interventions such as cannulation or direct airway examination should be avoided, unless judged to be low-risk or clinically indicated. This should not delay timely intervention when indicated. Assessment by the most experienced clinicians present and advice from ENT and PICU/retrieval teams should be sought, if in doubt.

If, after assessment, a decision is taken to watch the child and wait for further help, this opportunity should be taken to get as many things prepared as possible in anticipation of the child deteriorating before help arrives.

Signs of a really sick child

Signs of severe airway obstruction and increased work of breathing

These include:

- choking
- head bobbing and nasal flaring in the infant or 'seesaw' paradoxical chest and abdominal movements, subcostal, sternal or intercostal recession and tracheal tug; these signs occur earlier in infants
- adopting a specific posture to keep the airway open, e.g. tripod posture in children or arching in infants
- grunting in infants (an attempt to splint the airways open with auto-PEEP)
- biphasic stridor
- respiratory rate of > 50 in an infant or > 30 in a child.

Signs of respiratory decompensation

- Worsening oxygenation, especially with oxygen supplementation.
- Hypercarbia – this may produce sympathetic overdrive, altered consciousness or cardiovascular collapse.

Signs of exhaustion and impending respiratory arrest

It is vitally important to recognize these. They may mean that a child is too sick to move to a theatre to intubate.

Table 15.2. Signs of exhaustion.

Signs of exhaustion
Paradoxical reduction in minute ventilation (with/without decreased stridor intensity)
Paradoxical silent chest
Reduced conscious level
Apnoeas
Bradycardia
Cyanosis

Beware of severe cardiovascular compromise in addition to respiratory distress in certain conditions such as sepsis associated with bacterial tracheitis.

Targeted treatments

A variety of treatments to reduce the effects of airway obstruction are available. These may prevent the need for intubation, or simply buy time to seek help and arrange equipment. As in other chapters, these treatments follow on from basic medical management (see Chapter 4).

Reduction of mucosal inflammation

These are usually of greater value where potentially reversible mucosal inflammation is responsible for airway obstruction, e.g. croup or stridor post-intubation/bronchoscopy. They may have minimal effect in conditions such as bacterial tracheitis and epiglottitis. These conditions should therefore be considered early if presumed croup fails to respond to treatment.

Nebulized adrenaline

For moderate to severe croup, not controlled by steroids, 400 μg/kg of adrenaline (0.4 ml/kg of 1:1000, maximum 5 ml) delivered by a nebulizer may reduce mucosal inflammation quickly. It can be repeated at 30–60-minute intervals. Significant tachycardia and dysrhythmias are rare; nevertheless ECG monitoring should be performed with repeated doses.

Because of the short-term nature of the effects of nebulized adrenaline, the patient must continue to be closely observed as the stridor will return. The aim of adrenaline nebulizers is to provide time for the steroids to work. More than two doses of nebulized adrenaline suggests that the child may need to be monitored on PICU or intubated. Contact your local PICU retrieval team for advice at this point.

Corticosteroids

Corticosteroids reduce inflammation with a delayed effect of 6–24 hours. Their effectiveness in croup is well established. They can be given orally, parenterally or by nebulization. A single dose of dexamethasone (PO (per oral), IV or IM – equal efficacy) 0.15 mg/kg should be administered. Alternatively 2 mg of nebulized budesonide may be used.

Optimization of airway gas flow

Humidification

Where increased airway secretions are present, inspired gases should be humidified to avoid dried secretions exacerbating airway obstruction.

Heliox

This is a 70:30 helium:oxygen mixture with lower density than air or oxygen. Lack of availability and limitation of inspired oxygen concentration may limit its utility, but it may buy time for other targeted treatments to be effective.

Antibiotics

Bacterial infection of the airway requires early antibiotic treatment. First-line antibiotics should be broad-spectrum and parenteral.

A broad-spectrum cephalosporin, e.g. ceftriaxone 80 mg/kg/day (maximum 4 g/day) or cefotaxime 50 mg/kg 8 hourly (maximum 2 g/dose), would be an appropriate first-line therapy for most upper airway bacterial infections including epiglottitis and tracheitis. If MRSA infection is likely, vancomycin should be considered.

Foreign-body removal

An inhaled foreign body preventing cough or vocalization needs immediate basic life support manoeuvres for the choking child. Pneumothorax from 'ball-valve effect' gas trapping behind a foreign body must be considered and treated promptly if present.

Severe partial upper airway obstruction may be worsened by attempts to remove the foreign body in the emergency department. Supplemental oxygen and avoidance of further distress to the child are required while rapid transfer to theatre for rigid bronchoscopy is arranged.

The rigid bronchoscopy will require a spontaneously breathing patient, inhalational induction and maintenance of deep anaesthesia, and topical application of local anaesthetic to the airway.

Intubating a child with stridor

Intubation considerations

Pre-intubation

The three scenarios that must be anticipated in this situation are a difficult view for intubation, a narrowed airway (needing a smaller than predicted ET tube) and loss of airway on induction of anaesthesia.

Unless circumstances mandate a lifesaving attempt elsewhere, intubation should take place in a safe environment for inhalational induction with all necessary equipment ready and expertise available. If the child is being transferred to theatre an experienced anaesthetist should accompany them. An appropriately trained ENT surgeon may be required to perform emergency tracheostomy or bronchoscopy.

The presence of parents with the child up to induction of anaesthesia often helps to keep the child calm and should be encouraged where possible. The parents can be asked to step out (with a nurse) once the child is anaesthetized. This should be explained to the parent before induction.

Equipment that may be required includes:

- a selection of small ET tubes (down to a size 2.5mm in babies)
- stylet or pre-stiffened refrigerated ET tube
- difficult intubation equipment
- surgical equipment for bronchoscopy and tracheostomy
- fluids and IV access – in the severely obtunded child with cardiovascular instability, early IO access should be obtained where IV access has failed. Syringes (50 ml) preloaded with fluid boluses for rapid administration are helpful. Where there is relative cardiovascular stability in a non-obtunded child, IV access can be obtained under anaesthesia.

Depending on the clinical situation glycopyrrolate pre-treatment should be considered to reduce airway secretions and obtund vagally mediated bradycardia.

Intubation

A challenging and possibly failed intubation should be anticipated, especially in conditions associated with difficulty visualizing the vocal cords, such as epiglottitis, pharyngeal masses or craniofacial abnormalities.

Inhalational induction in oxygen with a volatile agent that causes least airway irritation is the usual technique. This needs to be carefully planned and performed by the most senior anaesthetist present. Monitoring for induction should include oxygen saturations and end-tidal carbon dioxide measurement. ECG monitoring should be attached as a saturation probe may fail if the child becomes bradycardic.

Gas induction

- The position adopted for induction should be the most comfortable for the patient, usually upright in most patients, irrespective of the pathology.
- Alveolar ventilation may be severely compromised by airway obstruction, slowing the uptake of volatile agents. Patience is crucial – it may take up to 10 minutes before the patient is ready for laryngoscopy and intubation.
- Application of CPAP during induction helps to maintain airway patency as muscle tone diminishes.
- Attempting to intubate too early can be disastrous. As a general rule, once the pupils are small and central wait for a further 30 breaths.
- Topical local anaesthetic applied to the airway (e.g. lignocaine spray) will assist in blunting unwanted responses to intubation in the spontaneously breathing patient.

Laryngoscopic view may be compromised by oedema, especially in epiglottitis. Compression of the chest may produce glottic bubbles to guide intubation. If attempts at intubation fail, advanced difficult airway rescue techniques, such as emergency cricothyrotomy or tracheostomy, may be required (see Chapter 16). All of the necessary equipment to undertake such procedures should be readily available. The ENT team should also be present when possible.

Post intubation

In the presence of pre-existing hypovolaemia, initiation of ventilation may lead to hypotension. This can usually be rectified by giving fluid boluses.

Muscle relaxation should be continued by infusion to prevent coughing and ET tube dislodgment. The ET tube position should be confirmed by CXR, and it should be well secured to minimize accidental extubation. Nasal reintubation for transfer of the child is not recommended when the intubation has been difficult, or the airway narrowed by disease or attempts at intubation.

A further reason why controlled ventilation is desirable in this situation is that spontaneous ventilation may be difficult because of the small diameter of the ET tube, lung disease and sustained hypoxia.

Should the child's ventilation deteriorate acutely it is essential to rule out the following:

- obstruction of the small ET tube by secretions or a foreign body
- pneumothorax from ball/valve effect of obstructing foreign body or secretions
- other underlying lung pathology, e.g. chest infection, pulmonary oedema
- inadequate sedation and paralysis.

Preparations for transfer

A record should be made describing:

- the state of airway pre-intubation
- method of induction of anaesthesia
- adjuncts required for airway maintenance and/or intubation
- description of view at laryngoscopy and grade of intubation, including manoeuvres undertaken to achieve it
- details of ET tube size, position and fixation
- any complications encountered.

Documentation should also include radiological and microbiological investigations, blood tests and specific treatments given. A CXR should be taken to assess ET tube position and any chest pathology. If an arterial line is present, blood gas analysis should be undertaken to determine the effectiveness of ventilation.

The major risk in transferring a child with stridor is accidental extubation. The ET tube should be fixed well and the child well sedated and paralysed prior to departure.

Summary

Children are particularly susceptible to stridor. They may tire quickly from the effort of breathing. Therefore, senior, experienced clinicians should be involved early in the management of these children. In most cases planning and ensuring that the right equipment and team are available will make the process calm and safe.

Golden rules

- The volume and pitch of stridor correlate poorly with severity of airway obstruction
- Stridor does not usually lead to low oxygen saturations unless airway obstruction is severe. Alternative reasons should be sought
- Timely interventions should not be delayed by efforts to minimize distress to the child
- If a child is being monitored at a distance, preparations should be made in anticipation of rapid deterioration
- Expect a difficult airway/intubation
- Once the child is intubated, secure ET tube fixation is paramount

Further reading

Handler SD. Stridor. In Fleisher GR, Ludwig S. (eds.), *Textbook of Pediatric Emergency Medicine*. Baltimore: Williams & Wilkins, 1993.

Maloney E, Meakin GH. Acute stridor in children. *Contin Educ Anaesth Crit Care Pain* 2007;7(6):183–186.

Robinson D. Airway management. In Morton N. (ed.), *Paediatric Intensive Care*. Oxford: Oxford University Press, 1997.

Samuels M, Wieteska S. *Advanced Paediatric Life Support: the practical approach/Advanced Life Support Group*, 5th edn. Chichester: Wiley-Blackwell, 2011.

Chapter 16

The difficult paediatric airway

Oliver Masters and Alistair Cranston

Introduction

The combination of a critically ill child and a difficult airway might be considered to be one of the most challenging situations for an anaesthetist, intensivist or ED specialist. Fortunately, the difficult airway in the paediatric population is rare and generally easier to identify prior to laryngoscopy than in adults.

For those unfamiliar with the paediatric airway, adult skills are transferrable to the paediatric population. The same basic principles apply. The overall goal is to ensure adequate oxygenation and ventilation and always to have a back-up plan in the event of difficulty.

There comes a point when one has to weigh up the urgency of the situation and ask yourself the following questions.

- Am I the right person to be managing the airway?
- If not, how long will it take for the right person to arrive?
- In the meantime, how do I manage the airway?

The aims of this chapter are to provide some of the tools necessary to make this decision, as well as giving the confidence and knowledge to successfully apply your adult skills to the paediatric setting.

How do children differ from adults?

It is beyond the scope of this book to go into an extensive list of anatomical and physiological differences between the paediatric and adult airways – this information can be found in any standard textbook. Instead, we will look at the differences that result in a need for changes in management between the two.

Head position

The correct head position is the first step in effective airway management. Neck flexion and head extension (sniffing the morning air) is a position that is suitable for most children over 2 years of age. In younger children, the head must be kept in a neutral position. The relatively large head of an infant means that it is sometimes necessary to place a roll under the shoulders, to prevent over-flexion of the head.

Managing the Critically Ill Child, ed. Richard Skone *et al.* Published by Cambridge University Press.

Bag and mask ventilation

Most of the principles that apply to effective bag and mask ventilation in adult practice can be applied to children. These are:

- select a mask of appropriate size
- ensure an airtight seal around the nose and mouth
- ensure that the fingers do not compress the area under the chin – this can easily cause airway obstruction
- pull the jaw forward by placing a finger behind the angle of the mandible
- hold the mouth open with the face mask itself.

Difficulties in bag–mask ventilation can be brought about by an obstruction to gas flow at the laryngeal, supralaryngeal or infralaryngeal levels. Algorithm 16.1 highlights the basic manoeuvres that should be used to aid ventilation.

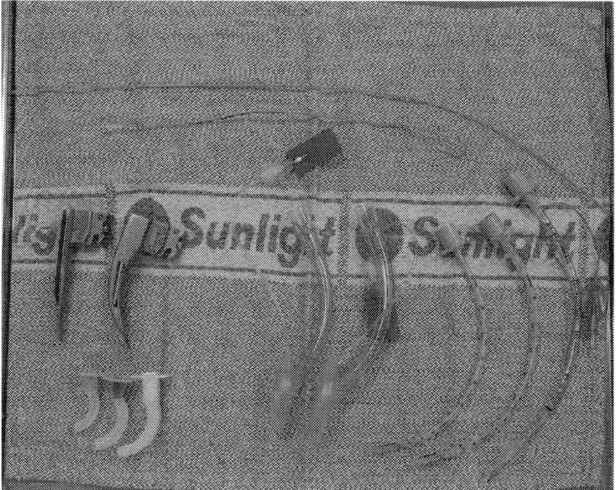

Figure 16.1. Basic airway equipment needed to manage a paediatric airway.

Airway adjuncts

In the unconscious patient, a Guedel airway may improve airway patency, especially if there is some degree of functional supralaryngeal obstruction. Nasopharyngeal airways (NPA) are much better tolerated in semiconscious patients. An endotracheal tube (ET tube) one size smaller than that for intubation may be used, though care must be taken not to insert it too far, as this may precipitate laryngospasm. There are no hard and fast rules for ascertaining the length, but the following guides may be used:

- insert the NPA until audible breath sounds and movement of gas is felt at the external opening
- measure from the tip of the nose to the tragus of the ear

- as a rough guide, in the first year of life insert about 8 ± 0.5 cm and 8.5 ± 0.5 cm in the second year.

Nasogastric tubes

Children are much more susceptible to a reduction in pulmonary compliance secondary to insufflation of the stomach during bag-mask ventilation. Fortunately gastric tubes are much easier to pass blind in children than in adults. Any degree of gastric distension is worth reducing with a gastric tube.

Intubation

As in adult practice, in the emergency situation pre-oxygenation is mandatory. The combination of relatively high metabolic rate, closing capacity encroaching on FRC and underlying disease processes means that desaturation is likely to occur more quickly in small children.

There are a few anatomical differences in the paediatric airway with which the experienced adult operator may not be familiar. These include:

- high larynx (located at C2 in neonates descending to C5/6 by 4 years)
- relatively large tongue
- small mandible
- large, floppy, tubular epiglottis.

A straight-bladed laryngoscope may be preferred in babies. The epiglottis is picked up with the tip of the laryngoscope. This is more likely to precipitate a bradycardia than placement in the vallecula, so attempt the conventional approach first and only if the epiglottis is obscuring the view should the epiglottis be picked up.

It may be necessary to perform a 'backwards, upwards, rightwards pressure' (BURP) manoeuvre to facilitate proper visualization of the larynx. Although this manoeuvre can be performed by an experienced assistant in infants, in babies it is often easiest to perform this with the little finger of the hand holding the laryngoscope.

Cuffed ET tube

Until about 10 years of age the narrowest point of the paediatric airway is the cricoid ring. A tube that passes with relative ease through the cords may not necessarily be the right size and care should be taken not to force it through the cricoid ring, as this may precipitate airway oedema.

Traditionally uncuffed ET tubes have been used in children under the age of 10 years, as it was thought that a cuffed ET tube was more likely to cause trauma. It is now considered acceptable to use a cuffed tube in any paediatric airway. In many circumstances, particularly if the airway is expected to be difficult, it is preferable to use a smaller, cuffed ET tube. This reduces the likelihood of repeated intubations, in an attempt to gain a snug fit. In certain circumstances such as the child who has sustained a burn to the airway, it is considered mandatory to use an uncut, cuffed ET tube to avoid the need for reintubation in the presence of evolving airway oedema.

Length of ET tube

Another significant difference in the paediatric airway is length. It is important to be meticulous regarding ET tube length to ensure endobronchial intubation does not occur. Use the following principles:

- the formula (age/2)+12 cm is a useful guide
- most full-term neonates require the 10 cm mark to be located at the lips
- it is essential to listen in both axillae for equal and bilateral breath sounds.

Predicting the difficult paediatric airway

Predicting that an airway is likely to be difficult prior to attempted laryngoscopy gives a significantly greater chance of being able to deal with ensuing problems. As mentioned, the difficult paediatric airway is often easier to predict than the adult one. In older children, characteristics of a difficult adult airway, such as obesity, become more applicable. Predictors applicable to paediatrics are detailed below.

History

The main points to elicit in the history are:

- history of snoring or sleep apnoea
- previous facial surgery, e.g. cleft lip or palate
- presence of any syndrome, particularly involving the face or airway.

Examination

Any degree of facial deformity should be noted. Particular reference should be paid to:

- facial asymmetry
- small jaw (micrognathia)
- low-riding ears
- difficulty with mouth opening.

What do I need when faced with a difficult paediatric airway?

Three things are required once you suspect a difficult paediatric airway:

- appropriate equipment
- appropriate help
- a plan.

Equipment

There is a whole host of equipment and airway adjuncts that are designed to be of assistance when dealing with a difficult airway. However, the most important equipment is the basic airway equipment you are already familiar with. Some of the most useful basic equipment is shown in Figure 16.1.

Consider the following things before starting:

- make sure you have equipment in a range of sizes rather than just the one that you're expecting to use
- check that the bougie you have will pass through the ET tube you have selected (note – the smaller bougies may be very flimsy and difficult to use)
- for very small ET tubes it may be preferable to pre-insert a stylet, so it can be shaped in a specific manner (often with an anterior bend) to facilitate passage through the larynx. Ensure the stiff wire does not protrude from the end of the tube, as this may cause airway trauma.

A significant proportion of airway problems come via the ED. Although this area should be fully equipped to deal with difficult airways, if the child is stable enough it may be preferable to transfer the child to the operating theatre. It is a more familiar environment, with a comprehensive range of airway equipment.

Help

When faced with a potentially difficult airway in an emergency setting, the more help you have, the more likely the outcome will be successful. Help falls into two main categories:

- on-site help – readily available in a short time-frame, e.g. ODPs or anaesthetic assistants, other anaesthetists, paediatricians, neonatologists, critical care and ED personnel
- off-site help – you may have to wait for this, e.g. specialist paediatric anaesthetist, ENT surgeon, and retrieval service personnel.

Even in the urgent setting, it is usually possible to wait for the arrival of additional personnel in the first category. Paediatricians and neonatologists are likely to have experience of intubating children and neonates, so are worth having around – especially for younger children and babies.

The decision on whether to proceed without help from the second category depends on a risk:benefit assessment. However, when faced with a potentially difficult paediatric airway, it would be sensible to concentrate on oxygenation and wait for this level of help to come, unless immediate intervention is necessary.

Plan

Irrespective of the airway difficulty, it is crucial to have a plan for what to do when things go wrong. The Association of Paediatric Anaesthetists and the Difficult Airway Society have produced a guideline for the management of the difficult airway in children between 1 and 8 years (see algorithms). It is split into three sections and deals with:

- difficulty in bag–mask ventilation
- unanticipated difficulty with tracheal intubation
- failure to intubate and ventilate.

Although primarily aimed at difficulties encountered during routine induction of anaesthesia, the basic principles can equally be applied to the emergency setting.

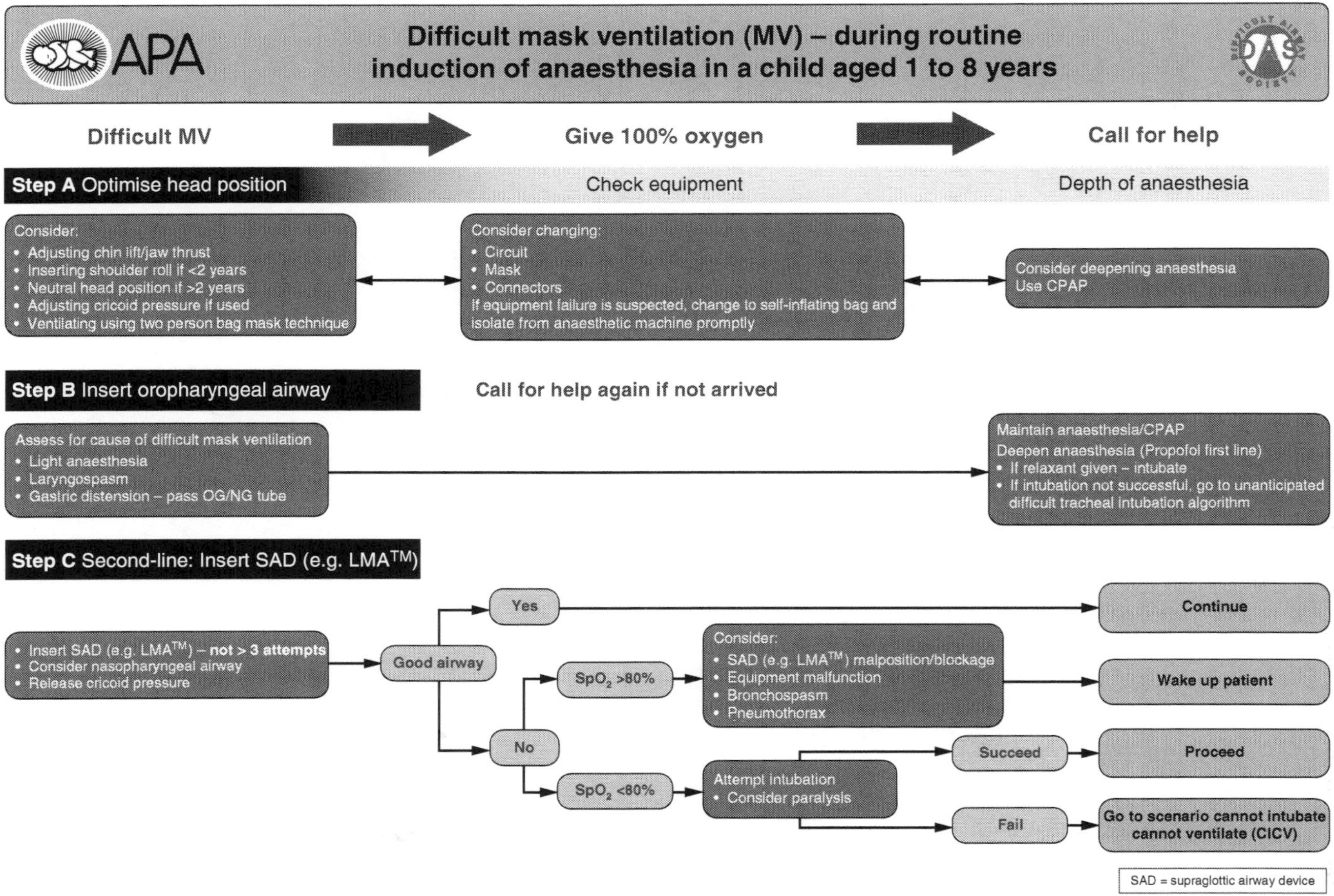

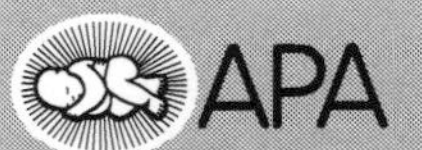
APA

Difficult mask ventilation (MV) – during routine induction of anaesthesia in a child aged 1 to 8 years

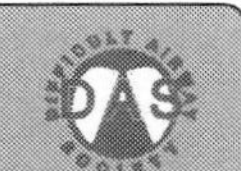

Difficult MV → Give 100% oxygen → Call for help

Step A Optimise head position — Check equipment — Depth of anaesthesia

Consider:
- Adjusting chin lift/jaw thrust
- Inserting shoulder roll if <2 years
- Neutral head position if >2 years
- Adjusting cricoid pressure if used
- Ventilating using two person bag mask technique

Consider changing:
- Circuit
- Mask
- Connectors

If equipment failure is suspected, change to self-inflating bag and isolate from anaesthetic machine promptly

Consider deepening anaesthesia
Use CPAP

Step B Insert oropharyngeal airway

Call for help again if not arrived

Assess for cause of difficult mask ventilation
- Light anaesthesia
- Laryngospasm
- Gastric distension – pass OG/NG tube

Maintain anaesthesia/CPAP
Deepen anaesthesia (Propofol first line)
- If relaxant given – intubate
- If intubation not successful, go to unanticipated difficult tracheal intubation algorithm

Step C Second-line: Insert SAD (e.g. LMA™)

- Insert SAD (e.g. LMA™) – **not > 3 attempts**
- Consider nasopharyngeal airway
- Release cricoid pressure

Good airway
- Yes → **Continue**
- No
  - SpO_2 >80% → Consider:
    - SAD (e.g. LMA™) malposition/blockage
    - Equipment malfunction
    - Bronchospasm
    - Pneumothorax

    → **Wake up patient**
  - SpO_2 <80% → Attempt intubation
    - Consider paralysis

    → Succeed → **Proceed**
    → Fail → **Go to scenario cannot intubate cannot ventilate (CICV)**

SAD = supraglottic airway device

Algorithm 16.1.

Difficulty with bag-mask ventilation

Algorithm 16.1 is self-explanatory and involves working through the issues in a step-wise fashion. It moves through checking basic technique and equipment, through to insertion of an oropharyngeal airway, attempted intubation (if muscle relaxant is administered) and use of a laryngeal mask airway (LMA).

If the LMA provides adequate ventilation and the child has a full stomach, consideration needs to be given towards intubation. This may be possible via conventional means, or by using the LMA as a conduit for a fibreoptic scope (see below). If the LMA does not result in a good airway and the SpO_2 is below 80%, then intubation must be attempted. If the SpO_2 is over 80%, then consideration needs to be given towards addressing the reasons for this.

Difficult intubation

The most important aspect of dealing with any difficult intubation scenario, as highlighted in bold along the top of Algorithm 16.2, is to ensure adequate oxygenation with mask ventilation.

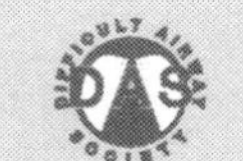

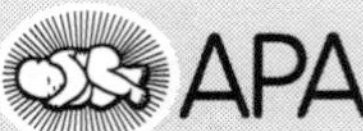

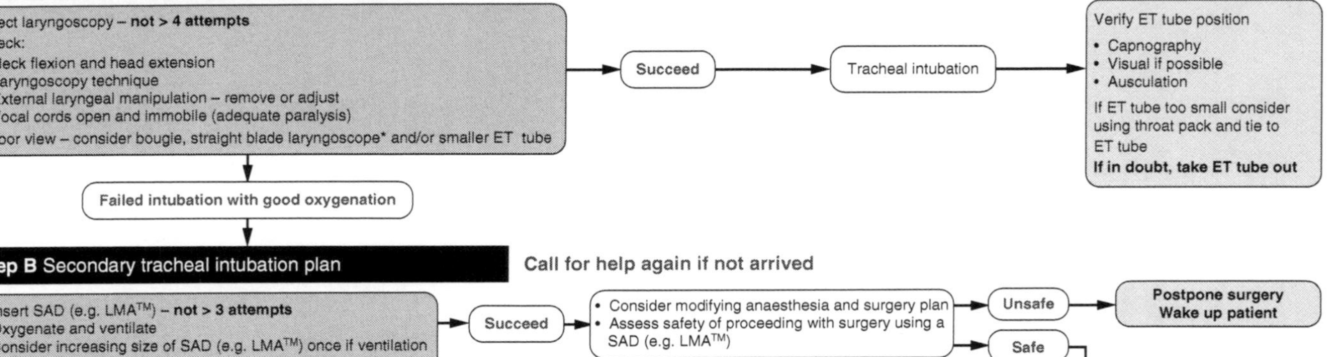

Algorithm 16.2.

Step A applies to the difficult intubation with satisfactory mask ventilation. It addresses simple manoeuvres that we have discussed earlier to try and improve the chances of successful intubation. No more than four attempts are recommended. It also highlights the importance of checking tube position. The old adage of 'If in doubt take it out' is also emphasized.

Step B moves onto more advanced techniques and what to do when oxygenation starts to fail. The use of the LMA to facilitate oxygenation is once again emphasized in addition to its role as a conduit for fibreoptic intubation. This is discussed in more detail below. If oxygenation is inadequate via the LMA, then bag–mask ventilation must be attempted. If still unsuccessful, move onto the next algorithm, 'cannot intubate and cannot ventilate'.

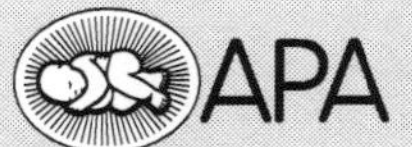

Cannot intubate and cannot ventilate (CICV) in a paralysed anaesthetised child aged 1 to 8 years

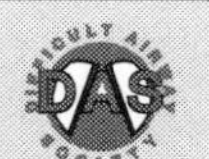

Failed intubation inadequate ventilation → Give 100% oxygen → Call for help

Step A Continue to attempt oxygenation and ventilation

- FiO_2 1.0
- Optimise head position and chin lift/jaw thrust
- Insert oropharyngeal airway or SAD (e.g. LMA™)
- Ventilate using two person bag mask technique
- Manage gastric distension with an OG/NG tube

Step B Attempt wake up if maintaining SpO_2 >80%

If rocuronium or vecuronium used, consider suggamadex (16mg/kg) for full reversal

Prepare for rescue techniques in case child deteriorates

Step C Airway rescue techniques for CICV (SpO_2 <80% and falling) and/or heart rate decreasing

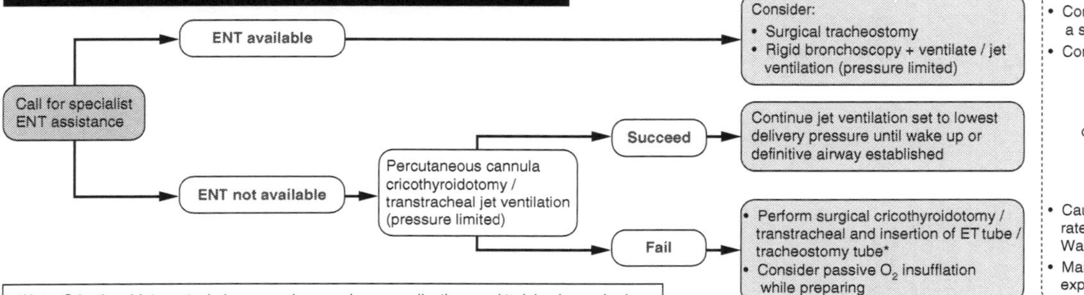

*Note: Cricothyroidotomy techniques can have serious complications and training is required – only use in life-threatening situations and convert to a definitive airway as soon as possible

Algorithm 16.3.

Failure to intubate and failure to adequately ventilate (Algorithm 16.3)

In this situation, continued attempts at oxygenation must be made while a more definitive solution is sought. The ongoing oxygenation attempts are listed in the Step A section. The points already discussed are re-emphasized.

If the child is maintaining SpO_2 over 80% then it may be possible to attempt to wake the child up. If an aminosteroid muscle relaxant such as rocuronium has been used, sugammadex in a dose of 16 mg/kg should reverse neuromuscular blockade.

If the child is desaturating below 80% and/or becoming bradycardic, Step C covers rescue techniques. The first plan is to have an ENT surgeon available to perform either a surgical tracheostomy or a rigid bronchoscopy. If an ENT surgeon is not immediately available, then percutaneous cannula cricothyroidotomy should be attempted. It is likely to be technically challenging in children and reinforces the importance of having planned properly so that you don't reach this stage.

The algorithm covers the technique for performing cannula cricothyroidotomy. Of note is the importance of using a pressure-limited transtracheal jet ventilator, if available. If unavailable, a 4 bar oxygen source connected via a Y connector or a three-way tap with an occludable orifice should be used.

As a starting point the oxygen flow-rate (in litres/minute) should be matched to patient age, but increased depending on the degree of chest expansion. Keeping an LMA in place to help upper airway patency is essential to prevent barotrauma and to facilitate adequate expiration.

Fibreoptic intubation via an LMA

As mentioned previously, the LMA can provide a useful conduit through which to pass a fibreoptic scope to facilitate intubation. There are a few problems with this:

- most adult fibreoptic scopes have an external diameter of 4 mm; consequently the smallest size ET tube that can be successfully railroaded over this is a 4.5 mm
- the internal diameter of a paediatric LMA may not be large enough to accommodate a fibreoptic scope and ET tube
- the ET tube may not be long enough to protrude far enough from the end of the LMA to pass through the vocal cords
- once in place there is no easy way of removing the LMA.

There are a few ways around these problems. One method is to use the suction port of the fibrescope to pass a J-shaped guide-wire through the larynx in the following sequence:

- pass fibreoptic scope through the LMA, and past the vocal cords
- insert J-shaped guide-wire through the suction port of the scope into the trachea
- remove fibreoptic scope and LMA, leaving guide-wire in place
- pass airway exchange catheter over guide-wire into larynx
- remove guide-wire and connect catheter up to breathing circuit, ensuring presence of end-tidal CO_2 and maintaining oxygenation with 100% oxygen
- railroad appropriate sized ET tube over catheter and remove catheter.

The process is one that is worth practising prior to being faced with this problem in an emergency setting.

Stabilization prior to transfer

Once the airway is secured there are a few issues to address. The main points are:

- ensure the tube position is correct
- ensure the tube doesn't come out
- ensure that the documentation is complete.

Ensure the tube position is correct

As soon as the tube is in, the end-tidal carbon dioxide ($ETCO_2$) trace should be checked, as should the presence of equal and bilateral air entry in both axillae. Absence of a CO_2 trace means that tube position must be confirmed visually.

ET tube length (especially in small babies) is crucial – too long and endobronchial intubation will occur, too short and there is a risk of accidental extubation. Prior to transfer a CXR should be requested and checked.

Neck flexion and extension significantly affect ET tube position in babies, with flexion pushing the ET tube closer to the carina. Make sure that the CXR is taken with the neck in a neutral position. If the ET tube length needs to be adjusted, make sure that it is well documented what the length was when the X-ray was taken and what the length is after repositioning. This avoids unnecessary confusion at the receiving unit.

Ensure the tube does not come out

The method used to secure the ET tube is not important as long as it is effective. The difficult airway is best secured using tapes rather than ties.

Ties are often able to work loose and don't hold the tube in as precise a position as well-placed tapes. It is important to ensure that the tapes are well stuck to the skin. It is reasonable to use elastoplast initially. If there is difficulty sticking the tapes to the skin a chlorhexidine wipe can be useful as long as the area is allowed to dry thoroughly. 'Sleek' may stick better than elastoplast and sometimes zinc oxide tape can be useful when other tapes do not stick to the skin.

Ensure the documentation is complete

It is important that other medical practitioners know what problems were encountered and how these were overcome. List the following information:

- a clear and concise summary of the indications for intubation
- the clinical assessment involved
- the names of all the practitioners present
- what was actually done.

This provides a useful template and allows others to make an informed decision as to how things might be done differently in the future. Any investigations relating to the airway must be commented upon and any actions clearly stated. You must ensure that all documentation is complete and photocopied for the receiving team prior to transfer.

Summary

The difficult paediatric airway is a rare phenomenon. When faced with one the key is to be well-prepared, seek help and use generic airway skills. Most importantly, as with any other situation in medicine, 'do no harm'.

Golden rules

- Try and maintain oxygenation and ventilation at all times
- Have a plan – including for when things go wrong
- Use all available help
- Keep things simple
- Don't make things worse – be prepared to bail out
- Don't forget the LMA

Further reading

Cook TM, Woodall N, Frerk C. Fourth National Audit Project. Major complications of airway management in the UK: results of the Fourth National Audit Project of the Royal College of Anaesthetists and the Difficult Airway Society. Part 1: anaesthesia. *Br J Anaesth* 2011;**106**:617–631.

Cook TM, Woodall N, Harper J, Benger J. Fourth National Audit Project. Major complications of airway management in the UK: results of the Fourth National Audit Project of the Royal College of Anaesthetists and the Difficult Airway Society. Part 2: intensive care and emergency departments. *Br J Anaesth* 2011;**106**:632–642.

Cote CJ, Hartnick CJ. Pediatric transtracheal and cricothyrotomy airway devices for emergency use: which are appropriate for infants and children? *Pediatr Anesth* 2009: **19**(Suppl.1):66–76.

Walker RWM, Ellwood J. The management of difficult intubation in children. *Pediatr Anesth* 2009;**19**(Suppl. 1): 77–87.

Weiss M, Engelhardt T. Proposal for the management of the unexpected difficult pediatric airway. *Pediatr Anesth* 2010;**20**:454–464.

Chapter 17

The surgical abdomen

Suren Arul

Introduction

Children differ from adults in both pathology and presentation when suffering from abdominal disease. The abdominal pathology seen in sick children admitted to the ICU can either be the cause of their deterioration or a consequence of the hypotension and sepsis that results from their main pathology.

This chapter aims to discuss common abdominal pathologies according to age in children. It will then discuss the management of acutely unwell children with abdominal pathology, which remains remarkably consistent regardless of cause.

How abdominal pathology differs in children

Pathology

Essentially there are a few basic patterns of primary abdominal emergencies. They include:

- bowel obstruction ultimately leading to bowel ischaemia, e.g. intussusception or incarcerated hernia
- intra-abdominal sepsis, e.g. appendicitis
- sudden increase in intra-abdominal pressure causing decreased venous return and splinting of the diaphragm, e.g. massive abdominal tumours
- haemorrhage.

The range of possible diagnoses varies with age in children. Table 17.1 gives a brief outline of common abdominal pathologies according to age. It is useful to bear in mind as it may help guide investigations and timing of interventions.

Managing the Critically Ill Child, ed. Richard Skone *et al.* Published by Cambridge University Press.

Table 17.1. Differential diagnosis of abdominal pathology in children according to age.

Age	Diagnoses
0–3 months	Congenital abnormalities of the GI tract, e.g. atresia, stenosis, duplication cysts Congenital abnormalities of the lower urinary tract (often complicated with UTI), e.g. pelvic or vesico-ureteric junction obstruction, postero-urethral valve disorder Malrotation or volvulus Incarcerated inguinal hernia Trauma/non-accidental injury (NAI)
3 months – 2 years	Intussusceptions Trauma/NAI Obstruction (e.g. Meckel's band, bezoar) Hirschsprung's enterocolitis
2–5 years	Appendicitis Trauma/NAI Obstruction (various causes) Massive abdominal tumours
5+	Appendicitis Trauma/NAI
Teenagers	Appendicitis Inflammatory bowel disease Pancreatititis

Presentation

The general adage of paediatric surgery is that the younger the child the more non-specific the presentation. The classic problems seen in paediatric patients are that:

- infants and older children may give little verbal history, or make misleading comments
- signs in children can be misleading, e.g. many abdominal signs occur in children who are severely unwell especially if associated with sepsis
- children with abdominal pathology will not have the classic history or signs that we associate with significant abdominal pathology in adults, e.g. pelvic appendicitis.

The key to management is therefore to have a high index of suspicion and to ask advice from the relevant specialist early. There are, however, certain pointers that act as 'red flags' for children with abdominal disease (Table 17.2).

Table 17.2. Red flags in abdominal pathology.

History of: • Abdominal pain as the very first symptom to develop • Refusing to even try food/bottle • Bilious green vomiting (rather than yellow) • Increasing lethargy and refusing to move
Symptoms or signs: • Pain on percussion and when child is asleep (often seen as facial grimaces or quiet crying rather than screaming) • Lying very still • Allowing painful procedures (e.g. cannulation) without moving away • Increasing abdominal distension

Specific conditions

Congenital anomalies

Most congenital anomalies will either be detected antenatally or present acutely at birth. However, occasionally conditions may be missed because they have developed late in pregnancy or cause only partial obstruction to the bowel. The cardinal signs of congenital bowel disease are:

- bilious dark green bile
- intestinal obstruction
- sepsis
- ischaemia
- shock.

Malrotation

This is a congenital condition in which the small and large bowels are abnormally attached to the retroperitoneum. The midgut (small bowel and colon) can then twist on the axis of the superior mesenteric artery, causing a volvulus. This initially leads to pain and vomiting and eventually midgut ischaemia followed by infarction, circulatory collapse and death. The majority of children will present within the first month of life while the remaining minority can potentially develop a volvulus at any age. Once again the red flag sign is bilious green vomiting; however, if this is missed it can progress to bloody stools and systemic collapse. In some patients there are few signs prior to the event, so malrotation should be considered as a diagnosis for any patient with sudden unexplained deterioration.

Hirschsprung disease

This is a rare condition with an incidence of 1 in 3000 in males and much lower incidence in females. In the classic form the neuro-enteric plexus fails to develop from the rectum to the sigmoid colon; however, it can extend proximally and potentially affect the entire bowel. The affected bowel tends to go into spasm, causing a functional intestinal obstruction. The presentation is by failure to pass meconium in the first 24 hours with increasing evidence of abdominal distension and bilious green vomiting.

Hirschsprung's enterocolitis

This is a life-threatening condition in which functional obstruction rapidly develops into systemic sepsis. It can occur both before a diagnosis has been made and also after the operation has been done to remove the aganglionic segment. The signs and symptoms of this condition include constipation, abdominal distension, evidence of systemic sepsis, and dilated loops of fluid-filled bowel on the plain X-ray.

Urinary tract pathology

Hydronephrosis secondary to pelvi-ureteric junction obstruction is one of the commonest antenatal ultrasound findings. It is usually managed conservatively. Other conditions which can cause hydronephrosis include vesico-ureteric obstruction, posterior-urethral valve disorder or severe vesico-ureteric reflux. Babies often tolerate significant hydronephrosis well. However, once an obstructed system becomes infected the baby can develop life-threatening septic shock within a matter of a few hours.

Acquired intestinal obstruction

Various pathologies can lead to intestinal obstruction, including incarcerated inguinal hernia, adhesive obstruction, intussusception and internal herniation around a band (such as a Meckel's band). In most cases the presentation is similar:

- pain
- abdominal distension
- bilious vomiting
- 'redcurrent jelly' stools
- hypotension and sepsis.

Finally the obstructed bowel can perforate, causing a significant deterioration in the patient's condition.

Intussusception

This is the commonest cause of obstructive symptoms in children between 3 months and 2 years of age. The usual pathology is of the ileum invaginating into the ileocaecal valve (although ileo-ileal intussusception can occur). Recurrent intussusceptions or a presentation outside the classic age group are all suggestive of a pathological lead point such as inflamed Peyer's patches or Meckel's diverticulum, which usually needs to be resected surgically to resolve the problem.

Symptoms are classic in that the child develops the following:

- bouts of severe, inconsolable crying
- drawing up of knees
- intense pallor that lasts approximately 5 to 15 minutes
- deep, unrousable sleep
- repetition of the cycle.

Non-bilious vomiting may occur in the early stages; however, significant vomiting is not an early feature. Late signs suggestive of established obstruction and bowel ischaemia include bilious green vomiting, systemic sepsis and the classic 'redcurrant jelly' stools.

Incarcerated inguinal hernia

Indirect inguinal hernia is very common in babies and children. The general rule is that the earlier the hernia presents the higher the likelihood of incarceration, hence babies and infants with a reducible inguinal hernia should be referred early for elective repair (i.e. within days). Reducible, unobstructed hernias do not usually cause significant pain. Warning signs that a hernia is incarcerated include:

- intense pain
- inconsolable crying
- tender, red fullness in the groin.

Bilious vomiting, systemic sepsis and bloody stools are late signs associated with bowel ischaemia. All babies or infants admitted with collapse should have their nappy removed and their groins carefully checked for signs of an inguinal hernia.

Intra-abdominal sepsis

Appendicitis

This is by far the commonest cause of an intra-abdominal catastrophe in children. The peak age of presentation is at 11 years old, although it can present at any age, including in infants. Younger children are more likely to have an atypical presentation. In particular pelvic appendicitis is relatively common in the under 5-year-olds and usually presents late with perforation or small bowel obstruction.

Although the child will have obvious signs of systemic sepsis the abdominal signs may still be relatively sparse, especially if the inflamed appendix is walled off within a pelvic mass. Radiological investigations frequently give false-negative results (especially to radiologists not specializing in paediatrics), therefore there is no substitute for an experienced clinician repeatedly examining the child.

Peritonitis

Other causes of peritonitis in children include primary peritonitis, perforation of the bowel from ingested foreign bodies, obstruction and trauma. Sometimes these children present *in extremis* with no history of abdominal symptoms, and little to find on examination. Unless there is another very obvious source, the abdomen should always be considered as a potential culprit in the list of suspects.

Trauma

Injury to the abdomen is covered in the chapter on trauma. Unexplained collapse can sometimes be explained by injuries sustained by non-accidental means.

Abdominal signs secondary to other conditions

Pathologies such as meningitis and urinary tract infections can cause vomiting and abdominal pain or distension, the probable cause being the paralytic ileus secondary to systemic sepsis. It is important not to get overly distracted by the abdominal signs in these patients, as it is not unheard of for patients to undergo an unnecessary laparotomy.

Children with chronic disease or being treated for other conditions

Most children who are treated for chronic or complex congenital bowel conditions, such as cancer, chronic liver disease or short gut requiring long-term intravenous parenteral nutrition, will be managed in the community at a considerable distance from their specialist paediatric centre. If these children become unwell they are likely to present to their local hospital.

Usually the families of these children will be well versed in their child's condition and will also have the contact details of the relevant specialist services. It is important to take advice from the relevant specialist before embarking on major investigation or treatments in these children, as otherwise significant delays in transfer or unnecessary duplication of investigations can occur.

Long-term central lines are often a feature of children with chronic or complex disease, such as short gut syndrome or cancer. Be aware that one of the commonest causes of collapse in these patients is central line infection.

Initial management

As with other conditions, a systematic approach (as seen in Chapter 4) is important. Regardless of the particular abdominal pathology, a thorough assessment of the child while administering oxygen, IV fluids and antibiotics is essential, followed by urgent referral for a specialist surgical opinion.

In any child where an abdominal pathology is suspected the principles of management are as follows:

- manage the child's physiology (goal-directed therapy)
- give broad-spectrum antibiotics
- get a prompt surgical opinion
- investigate the abdomen radiologically if there is any doubt (and it is safe)
- keep other pathologies in mind (and continue to treat them).

Table 17.3. Initial management of surgical child.

Phase of management	Assessment	Action
Initial phase • On presentation of the child (see Chapter 4 for detailed management)	Assess for need to intubate • Poorly responsive • Hypoxia refractory to oxygen • Rising CO_2 • Poor respiratory effort • Moribund	Give oxygen • Ventilate by hand if needed Gain IV access • IO if more than three IV attempts Give fluid bolus • 20 ml/kg of crystalloid Take blood including ABG, clotting and cross-match Give antibiotics
After initial assessment • Once imminently life-threatening risks have been addressed and abdominal source is suspected	Reassess need to intubate • Signs of persisting deterioration despite treatment • Need for interventions such as: CVC/surgery/transfer to PICU	Surgical review Repeat blood gases to assess ventilation • Hypoxia refractory to oxygen • Rising CO_2 • Worsening metabolic acidosis • Give analgesia Site NG tube and aspirate prior to intubation Assess response to fluid bolus • If BP and HR improve continue with boluses • Consider blood and inotropes at 60 ml/kg fluid replacement
Further stabilization • Not immediately life-saving procedures	Continue to reassess clinical condition and blood results Definitive plan (transfer vs. operate) Decide on further monitoring	Contact retrieval team Arterial line if: • Haemodynamic instability • Starting inotropes • Repeated blood gases CVC if: • More definitive access needed • Starting inotropes • Giving high concentration drugs • Need to measure CVP Correct coagulopathy

Decision to ventilate

Abdominal distension causes a significant challenge to a spontaneously breathing child. The high closing capacity of infants coupled to a relatively small functional residual capacity can lead to a large increase in work of breathing and hypoxia. Most children can cope well with the incursion on lung volume by increasing their respiratory rate. However, as with many other pathologies, it must be remembered that children can decompensate rapidly after initially appearing relatively well.

Should a child need intubation it must be remembered that induction of anaesthesia can lead to rapid desaturation, reflux, vomiting or cardiovascular collapse, especially if dehydration has been underestimated.

Cardiovascular support

As with adults it is quite easy to underestimate fluid loss in children with abdominal pathology. All sick patients with significant abdominal pathology will have a degree of shock and so early vascular access and appropriate resuscitation with fluid boluses are essential. The initial management is similar to that of sepsis in that aggressive use of fluid resuscitation and antibiotics is important. Blood cultures should be taken as soon as possible (without delaying other interventions).

The volume given in each fluid bolus is to a large degree irrelevant. What is important is to keep track of how much has been given and to track the child's response (as a reference value it is useful to remember that the circulating volume of a child is between 70 and 90 ml/kg).

Blood should be cross-matched early, and blood products requested, as these children may suffer from dilutional coagulopathy or disseminated intravascular coagulation. Once the child has received 60 ml/kg of fluid consider giving blood products (guided by blood gas haemoglobin or formal laboratory results).

Other supportive measures

Broad-spectrum antibiotics that include Gram-negative and anaerobic cover are essential for patients with suspected abdominal sepsis. They should be given early in the management but ideally after blood and urine cultures are taken. A urinary catheter should be used to gain a sample quickly. If no urine is forthcoming antibiotics need to be given without delay.

Nasogastric tube

A nasogastric (NG) tube is essential in the management of children with abdominal pathology (minimum size 10FG (French Gauge)). This can help confirm the diagnosis if thick green bile is aspirated. It may also decompress the stomach and help alleviate any impairment to ventilation (especially if there has been over-vigorous bagging of a child prior to intubation). Although conventional wisdom teaches to remove an NG tube prior to an RSI in order to minimize reflux, there are many conditions in children where it might be considered prudent to place one prior to induction. These include conditions such as congenital diaphragmatic hernia (CDH) or in a child where the X-rays show a large dilated stomach.

Urinary catheter

Urinary catheter insertion is important in any critically ill child. However, in this situation it fulfills a dual role. As well as monitoring urine output, it can be used to monitor intra-abdominal pressure. The relatively small size of the child's abdomen means that a small increase in intra-abdominal fluid or organ size can lead to a significant increase in abdominal pressure. This, in turn, can cause the child to be significantly compromised due to splinting of the diaphragm or reduced venous return from inferior vena cava obstruction.

Table 17.4 details further potential pitfalls in the management of children with abdominal pathology.

Central line/arterial line

Central lines may be very difficult to site in these children. The children are often hypovolaemic, may be coagulopathic, and their distended abdomen may make femoral access challenging. It is worth getting as many factors as possible in your favour before attempting a line, so give plenty of fluid and clotting products.

If the operator feels able, an internal jugular CVC using ultrasound guidance is best for these children. Remember that during the initial phase an IO cannula can be used for fluids and inotropes.

Investigations

If there is suspicion of abdominal pathology in a critically unwell child, the following investigations should be considered:

- abdominal X-ray
- ultrasound scan
- CT scan with double contrast.

If there is a suspicion of perforation or obstruction then a left lateral decubitus abdominal X-ray should be performed to look for free air or fluid levels.

Other considerations when considering investigations:

- do not send for radiological investigations until clinically stable
- investigations are dependent on the expertise of the person performing and reporting them
- negative investigations should not prevent further consideration of abdominal pathology if suspicion is high
- there is simply no substitute for repeated examination by an experienced clinician.

Surgery

Immediate surgery is almost never indicated in the management of children with significant intra-abdominal pathology and that includes trauma. One of the few indications for surgery in the seriously unwell child would be for the removal of an obviously infected Hickman line.

Resuscitation, stabilization and appropriate antibiotics are the essential mainstay of management. Surgery, whilst often needed relatively urgently, is dependent on the appropriate surgical, anaesthetic and intensive care specialists available. Postoperative care in these children is also very complicated. Hence, it is usually much better to attempt urgent transfer prior to embarking on surgery if all the appropriate facilities are not available.

Table 17.4. Potential pitfalls for general surgical patients.

System	Organ system specific problems	Consequence of these problems
Respiratory	Lung compression from abdominal distension Metabolic acidosis Developing lung injury	Shunting Tachypnoea to overcome smaller tidal volume Increased minute volume due to metabolic acidosis Increased work of breathing May tire from respiratory effort Rapid desaturation on induction of anaesthesia
Cardiovascular	Decreased fluid intake Vomiting Sepsis Third space loss Hypovolaemia	Child may be more hypovolaemic than anticipated Hypotension Poor perfusion of already compromised gut May 'crash' on induction of anaesthesia
Gastrointestinal	Pain Vomiting Ileus	Potential to aspirate is high Will be hypovolaemic Will have electrolyte imbalance Distended abdomen affecting breathing Pain affecting breathing
Other problems	May be in DIC Dilutional coagulopathy Dilutional anaemia 'Hidden' bleeding	Coagulopathy Anaemia Hypovolaemia

Summary

The management of children with abdominal pathology is remarkably consistent regardless of the exact diagnosis. As with much other pathology in children, early contact with a specialist centre can help speed up management by reducing the duplication of investigations. The abdomen should always be considered as a cause of illness in a critically ill child, but should not deter investigation and treatment of other potential disease processes.

Golden rules

- Bilious vomiting is a sign of significant pathology
- Repeated clinical examination by an experienced clinician is essential
- Initial management should include oxygen, fluid resuscitation and antibiotics
- Early intubation and ventilation is advisable if significant cardiorespiratory compromise is present
- Immediate surgery is rarely warranted

Chapter 18

Paediatric trauma

Karl Thies

Introduction

Trauma is the primary cause of death in children above the age of 1 year. Injury patterns in children are age-dependent. The majority of injuries are traumatic brain and limb injuries. Thoracic and abdominal injuries occur less frequently but carry a high mortality, especially if combined with other injuries.

In the UK, the structure of trauma management has changed towards children being managed in large tertiary centres. However, all hospitals with the capacity to receive children should be prepared to manage a sick child who is too unstable to move to another hospital. Given the low frequency of major trauma in children, trauma teams must receive regular training and should rehearse repeatedly to enable all team members to fulfil their roles.

This chapter cannot cover trauma management in detail; instead it aims to build on existing experience that anaesthetists and ED doctors already have from managing adult patients. It also aims to highlight the differences between trauma in adults and children.

Paediatric trauma resuscitation

Preparation

When information is received from ambulance control the paediatric trauma team should be assembled as early as possible. This will allow time to prepare the team and equipment. Designation of the trauma team leader (TTL) and allocation of roles must happen before the patient arrives.

When taking a call from ambulance control about an imminent arrival, the agreed national 'pre-alert' information delivered should consist of:

- age
- time of injury
- mechanism of injury
- injuries sustained
- signs (A–E)
- treatment received.

Managing the Critically Ill Child, ed. Richard Skone *et al.* Published by Cambridge University Press.

If a child is being brought to a non-major trauma centre then the pre-hospital system may have triaged them as too unstable to pass the nearest hospital. Therefore, receipt of a major trauma alert from the ambulance service should trigger a system that ensures senior doctors (consultants) are present at the time the child arrives.

Resuscitation and anaesthetic drugs should be prepared according to the age of the patient and an equipment check should be carried out. If immediate surgical intervention is likely (penetrating chest injuries, uncontrolled external haemorrhage) theatres should be informed immediately.

The primary survey

The purpose of the primary survey in trauma is to identify and treat injuries that pose an immediate threat to life using the established CABCDE system, where the first C stands for 'C-spine' and 'catastrophic haemorrhage control'.

The team should carry out the primary survey systematically and simultaneously under the supervision of the TTL. Although X-rays and, where indicated, abdominal sonography form part of the primary survey, many trauma centres now replace these by performing full-body CT scans in adults. This should be considered in children.

Table 18.1. The primary survey – timing of interventions.

Within 5 seconds
Initial assessment by TTL to identify
- Altered level of consciousness (final common pathway for all vital functions!)
- Complete airway obstruction
- Massive external haemorrhage
- Shock
- Cardiac arrest

Within 1 minute
Immediately life-saving interventions ('CABC')
- Establishing oxygenation and ventilation with basic airway manoeuvres
- Compression of massive external haemorrhage

Within 10 minutes
Very urgent interventions
- Immobilization of the cervical spine
- Chest decompression
- Pelvic compression splint
- Large-bore vascular access and bloods sent for laboratory examination
- Commence monitoring
- Analgesia, anaesthesia and definitive airway
- Fluid therapy, transfusion of blood products
- Sonography
- Undressing the patient
- Complete primary survey
- Chest and pelvic X-ray

Within 30 minutes
Urgent tests and interventions
- Urinary catheter
- CT scan
- Focussed X-rays

Within 3 hours
- Completion of diagnostics and therapy
- Special investigations and X-rays
- Operative care

Secondary survey is carried out after all immediate threats to life are resolved.

A standard 'trauma panel' of blood investigations usually include:

- FBC
- glucose
- group and save with/without cross-match
- clotting profile
- urea and electrolytes
- LFTs including amylase and lipase
- a pregnancy test in all female patients of childbearing age.

Airway management, anaesthesia and ventilation

During handover from the pre-hospital team the person responsible for managing the airway should:

- establish contact with the patient
- check airway patency
- check conscious level.

A quick check for any overt haemorrhage can be done at the same time. Untreated large scalp lacerations are notorious for causing significant blood loss in children. All findings then need to be reported to the TTL.

Initial airway management

All trauma patients should receive high-flow oxygen. If there is any sign of obstruction, the airway should be cleared with basic manoeuvres:

- suction the upper airway carefully with a soft catheter to avoid mucosal lacerations and reflex vomiting
- jaw thrust with/without oropharyngeal airway (Guedel)
- cervical collars should be loosened if they impair airway access
- if tolerated by the child the stomach should be decompressed with a large-bore orogastric tube
- immobilization of the spine should be maintained at all times until a spinal injury is ruled out.

In children who arrive with an ET tube in place, the correct position and size need to be confirmed immediately by auscultation and capnography.

Endotracheal intubation and general anaesthesia

Initial airway control can usually be achieved with basic measures, but the majority of severely traumatized children require endotracheal intubation (ETI) early on during resuscitation. The decision to intubate is made by the TTL and the anaesthetist but needs to be communicated to the whole team. Whilst the primary survey is proceeding, the anaesthetic team can prepare for ETI.

Anaesthetic drugs

The choice and dosage of the drugs used for induction and maintenance depends on the cardiovascular and neurological condition of the child.

Ketamine is the preferred induction agent in the compromised child because of its more favourable cardiovascular profile. Ketamine further reliably reduces raised intracranial pressure (ICP) without decreasing cerebral perfusion pressure (CPP), as long as normoventilation is maintained. Propofol and thiopentone are less suitable because of their cardiovascular side effects. Etomidate causes long-lasting suppression of the adrenal cortex, probably affecting the physiological endocrine response to trauma.

Anaesthesia in haemorrhagic shock

Most anaesthetic drugs, analgesics and sedatives attenuate the compensatory vasoconstriction in shock and may cause a dramatic fall in blood pressure in a hypovolaemic child.

Ketamine is a useful drug in haemorrhagic shock, because it produces analgesia and amnesia without affecting compensatory vasoconstriction. For induction of anaesthesia, ketamine 1 mg/kg can be given repeatedly until the patient becomes unresponsive.

High-dose rocuronium (1.5 mg/kg) provides fast-onset muscle relaxation and has, for many, replaced suxamethonium as first choice for rapid-sequence induction (RSI). Ensure sugammadex is available immediately to reverse muscle relaxation if airway control is lost and ETI is not possible.

A failed ETI protocol needs to be part of the regular paediatric trauma training (see Chapter 16).

Spinal immobilization

For trauma patients, spinal immobilization before, during and after intubation is essential. The cervical collar should be removed and manual in-line stabilization of the C-spine established. The operator should try to intubate with the head in the neutral position, which inevitably makes laryngoscopy more difficult. A bougie is often useful in this situation, as it may be easier to pass than the ET tube initially. Intubation of these patients therefore requires a minimum of four people to manage the process (in-line immobilization, cricoid pressure, intubator, assistant).

Cricoid pressure

There is no evidence that cricoid pressure is beneficial in paediatric RSI. A common-sense approach to cricoid pressure should be applied. If it impairs the operator's view of the glottis it should be lessened or removed. It should be used with care (or bimanually) if a C-spine injury is suspected. It should be avoided altogether if there is laryngeal trauma (swelling, local crepitus, hoarse voice). The endotracheal tube position must be confirmed by auscultation and capnography immediately after ETI.

Blood in the upper airway

Severe head injury or maxillofacial injury can result in ongoing haemorrhage into the upper airway, leading to airway obstruction and aspiration. In severe maxillo-facial trauma a soft nasopharyngeal airway can be life-saving if an oropharyngeal airway is ineffective.

Endotracheal intubation can be difficult or impossible in bleeding patients and constant oropharyngeal suction should be applied during ETI to obtain an acceptable view. If intubation is not possible, a supraglottic device (LMA or other device) can be inserted, which partially protects the lower airway from aspiration of blood. A surgical airway is required immediately if oxygenation cannot be maintained.

Provisional haemostasis can be achieved with two nasally inserted urinary catheters, which are inflated in the nasopharynx and fixed under traction. An anterior nasal tampon can complete haemostasis.

Management of shock

Circulatory shock after major trauma is in most cases due to haemorrhage, although a tension pneumothorax after ETI decreases venous return and can also cause circulatory shock.

Assessing blood loss

Unfortunately there is no single clinical measurement that can be consistently used for assessment of blood loss. Blood pressure and heart rate are unreliable because they depend on too many other factors, e.g. anxiety, pain and concomitant traumatic brain injury (TBI). They further depend on the type of injury. Penetrating injuries cause less tachycardia than blunt injuries with extensive tissue injury, for a similar degree of hypovolaemia. Systolic blood pressure and heart rate can remain normal in the awake patient until more than 30% of the blood volume is lost.

Other signs when assessing hypovolaemia are capillary refill time (CRT – normal < 2 seconds), skin colour and temperature. Loss of up to 25% blood volume will be associated with a slight increase in CRT, cool peripheries and mild agitation. As blood loss increases the peripheries will become cold and mottled and the child increasingly lethargic. Once more than 40% of the blood volume is lost, peripheral perfusion will be absent, often with no discernible CRT and cold, waxy-looking skin. Bradycardia in shock usually precedes cardiac arrest.

A metabolic acidosis can be used to help guide fluid resuscitation. Serum lactate is also valuable, but has a slower response time than a base deficit.

As with adults, transthoracic echocardiography (TTE) can be used to assess ventricular filling, and other causes of shock such as pericardial tamponade, myocardial contusion, valve rupture or haemothorax. TTE can help to optimize cardiac pre- and afterload in shock but clearly requires an experienced operator.

Fluids

Balanced electrolyte solutions are first-line treatment of hypovolaemia and should be administered in 10 ml/kg boluses IV or IO. Colloids are second-line treatment for hypovolaemia unless blood products are needed urgently. As with adults, the actual choice of fluid is a regular point of disagreement amongst physicians. The important factors that should be remembered are:

- the fluid should be warmed
- any fluid lost should be replaced.

Blood products, massive haemorrhage and trauma-induced coagulopathy (TIC)

Massive haemorrhage is defined as loss of 50% of the circulating blood volume within 3 hours, or ongoing blood loss of 2 ml/kg/min (150 ml/min in an adult).

In the treatment of uncontrolled haemorrhage, balanced electrolyte solutions and colloids both aggravate TIC, which increases mortality. Therefore early use of packed red blood cells (PRBC) in combination with fresh frozen plasma (FFP) is necessary. Long-standing European clinical practice and recent experience from the UK defence service show that early transfusion of FFP in haemorrhagic shock increases survival. If there is ongoing haemorrhage, PRBC, FFP and platelets should be transfused in a ratio of 1:1. Even this regimen cannot reliably prevent TIC.

Every hospital should have a massive haemorrhage guideline or protocol (see Chapter 21), which should be activated in such cases. Early recognition is important, as it can take significant time for the necessary blood products to be assembled and delivered to where they are needed.

Damage-control resuscitation

The combination of metabolic acidosis and hypothermia leads to severe coagulopathy and further blood loss. This in turn triggers a vicious circle of worsening hypothermia, intensifying acidosis, and coagulopathy and bleeding. Damage-control resuscitation aims to break this circle early, by addressing all three factors simultaneously:

- fluid resuscitation and early transfusion of blood products and clotting factors to re-establish tissue oxygenation and blood clotting
- haemorrhage control by hypotensive resuscitation and early surgical intervention, targeting haemostasis, but not necessarily definitive repair (damage-control surgery)
- hypothermia prevention and treatment.

The definitive surgical repair is carried out after retrieval, 12–24 hours later, once tissue oxygenation, blood clotting and normothermia have been re-established.

Hypotensive resuscitation

In adult patients with uncontrolled haemorrhagic shock it is common practice to maintain the systolic blood pressure at 80 mmHg until haemostasis is achieved. This approach increases survival by limiting blood loss and maintaining perfusion of the vital organs at the same time. Evidence in children is limited, but blood pressure should be maintained in the low-normal range (see Chapter 35), except where there is TBI, when blood pressure of at least normal levels must be maintained to ensure adequate cerebral perfusion. Blood pressure targets for isolated head injury are detailed in Chapter 19.

Endpoints of resuscitation

The endpoints of resuscitation in shock are not well defined. As a general recommendation in the anaesthetized patient one would aim for:

- normal blood pressure once the haemorrhage is under control
- haemoglobin of above 100 g/l
- platelet count of above 100×10^9/l
- CVP of 8–10 cmH_2O
- improving base excess and lactate levels
- normal clotting
- adequate urine output
- good ventricular filling and contractility as shown by transoesophageal echocardiography (TOE) or transthoracic echocardiography (TTE).

Tranexamic acid

The CRASH 2 trial revealed that administration of the antifibrinolytic tranexamic acid (TXA) in bleeding trauma patients decreases the relative risk of death by 30% if given no later than 3 hours after the injury. However, TXA should not be started later than 3 hours after the injury because the relative risk of death is then increased. Children should receive a loading dose of 20 mg/kg over 10 minutes (up to the adult dose of 1 g) and then 10 mg/kg over 8 hours.

Hypocalcaemia

Hypocalcaemia is a common problem in massive transfusion. It can worsen coagulopathy and cause ECG changes and myocardial dysfunction. Therefore the plasma calcium concentration should be monitored frequently and corrected as necessary.

Hypothermia

Hypothermia is a common finding in severe trauma. It is associated with a significantly increased incidence of multiple organ dysfunction in severely injured patients. There is also evidence that hypothermia is an independent predictor of mortality in major trauma. This is due to the following factors:

- decreased platelet function
- decreased clotting factor activity
- increased oxygen demand (in awake, hypothermic patients the oxygen demand can be increased five-fold).

Treatment of hypothermia must start as soon as the patient arrives in hospital, as children will become cold faster than adults. Forced air-warming devices, overhead heaters, warmed IV solutions and blood products and high room temperature are used to prevent and treat hypothermia.

Traumatic brain injury (TBI)

Sixty per cent of all severely injured children suffer isolated TBI. The outcome after TBI depends on the initial rapid access to definitive care and minimizing 'secondary injury', which is aggravated by:

- hypoxaemia
- hypotension
- hypo- or hypercapnia
- hypo- or hyperglycaemia.

Anaesthesia for TBI

Patients with major TBI (GCS < 10) require early intubation to secure the airway and to restore oxygenation of the brain whilst maintaining an adequate cerebral perfusion pressure (see Chapter 19).

Management of acutely raised intracranial pressure

A decreased GCS, dilated pupils, bradycardia and hypertension despite adequate analgesia are late signs of increased ICP. Deepening of the sedation and administration of IV mannitol (0.5 g/kg) or hypertonic saline (5 ml/kg initial dose of 3% saline, followed by 2 ml/kg boluses) can be used to decrease the ICP (see Chapter 19 for the emergency management of raised ICP).

Chest injury

Serious chest injuries in children are rare, but can present without visible external signs. They are associated with significant morbidity and mortality.

Blunt chest injury

Rib fractures only occur if exceptional force is involved and should raise suspicion regarding further underlying serious injuries. These patients are at risk of developing a tension pneumothorax on initiation of mechanical ventilation and consideration should be given to elective chest drain insertion. Lung contusions can be identified on plain X-ray. Patients with severe lung contusions require early intubation and mechanical ventilation (MV), with high PEEP often being required to maintain oxygenation.

If a traumatic broncho-pleural fistula is suspected (pneumothorax, increasing mediastinal size and surgical emphysema) it may be necessary to ventilate a child on one lung. Older children can be managed as adults; i.e. lung separation with a bronchus blocker or double-lumen tube can be tried to minimize the air leak. For younger children, simply advancing the ET tube with manipulation into a bronchus can isolate a lung. Because the angles at which the bronchi come off the trachea are similar, it is possible to isolate either lung with this technique. Urgent thoracotomy is then necessary to repair the fistula.

Aortic rupture in children is seen much less frequently than in adults. A widened mediastinum on the chest X-ray after deceleration trauma could indicate such an injury. The diagnosis is confirmed by CT scan or CT angiography.

Penetrating chest injury

Penetrating chest injuries in children are very rare but do occur, mainly as stab wounds in the adolescent population. These injuries can present as haemopneumothorax, haemopericardium, or transdiaphragmatic injuries. Management is the same as for adults. Some patients need immediate thoracotomy for haemorrhage control.

Abdominal injury and pelvic fracture

Abdominal injuries are the primary cause of circulatory shock. The abdomen is also the most common site of initially unrecognized, fatal injury in traumatized children. Focussed assessment with sonography in trauma (FAST) will identify free fluid in the peritoneal cavity. CT scanning is necessary to detect solid organ or retroperitoneal injuries. Fortunately, solid organ injuries rarely require laparotomy, current treatment being primarily conservative or the use of radiological embolization.

Fractures of the elastic immature pelvis are relatively rare, and generally have a good prognosis. In adolescents, fractures of the pelvic ring can lead to severe life-threatening retroperitoneal haemorrhage, which requires external splinting in the emergency department. A range of pelvic splints of different sizes should be available in all EDs for children. Sources of bleeding in pelvic fractures can be arterial, venous or from bones and ligaments. To control an arterial bleed, immediate radiological embolization should be considered. If the haemorrhage is primarily venous or if there is no immediate access to interventional radiology, temporary retroperitoneal packing can be carried out in theatres or the ED.

Anaesthesia for emergency laparotomy

Patients requiring emergency laparotomy usually present hypothermic and in circulatory shock. In blunt abdominal trauma the blood loss is limited by the amount of blood that can be accommodated in the abdominal cavity or retroperitoneal space; eventually the haemorrhage tamponades itself. When opening the peritoneum, the tamponading effect is lost, causing severe hypotension and sometimes exsanguination if the surgeon cannot control the haemorrhage immediately. These patients should be stabilized by transfusion of blood products before the peritoneum is opened. Good communication between surgeon and anaesthetist is necessary to prevent this from happening.

Complex abdominal injuries often require damage-control resuscitation before definitive repair can be carried out safely. The goal is to achieve haemostasis and prevent contamination of the peritoneal cavity in cases of intestinal perforation.

Preparation for transfer

If a child does need to come to a DGH for management, it is likely to be because they were too sick to transfer safely to a major trauma centre (MTC). The aim of stopping in the nearest hospital is to rectify the immediately life-threatening problems before swift transfer on to the MTC.

The primary survey should be completed swiftly, and any immediate life-threatening problems rectified. The decision as to whether to operate in a DGH will be decided based on the child's need, advice from the MTC and the expertise of the surgeons and anaesthetists. It should also involve discussion with the local PICU retrieval team. Ideally, the child should be operated on in the MTC wherever possible.

This means that the transfer process often needs to be swift, but safe. Details on conducting a local team-led transfer are covered in Chapter 24. If the child is to be transferred, then careful planning needs to take place. The team should not leave without the following:

- written history of what has happened to date – including what aspects of the secondary survey have been performed
- drug chart detailing what has been given (including fluids)
- blood products
- adequate monitoring (this does not necessarily mean a central line – discuss with PICU)
- radiological images in a format that can be viewed
- a plan of where to take the child (e.g. PICU or theatre at the receiving hospital).

Summary

Current management strategies for major trauma mean that a child should not be managed outside an MTC unless necessary. However, each department should be ready to treat those children who are too unstable to reach an MTC safely by ambulance.

Golden rules

- The principles of the team approach to trauma are the same in children as they are in adults
- Do not underestimate blood loss in children
- The patterns of injury are different, but the aims of management are similar to adults
- Aim to avoid the triad of:
  - Hypothermia
  - Acidosis
  - Coagulopathy

Chapter 19

The child with raised intracranial pressure

Phil Hyde

Introduction

Raised intracranial pressure (ICP) is a serious consequence of a variety of pathologies in children. Without prompt treatment a raised ICP results in morbidity and mortality. The key components of the management of raised ICP in children are:

- recognition of the presence or potential for raised ICP
- emergency management of raised ICP
- urgent computed tomography of the brain
- transfer of the child to a neurosurgical and paediatric intensive care facility.

The aim of this chapter is to cover the management of acutely raised ICP.

Intracranial pressure and cerebral perfusion in children

Pressure

Intracranial pressure is determined by the force exerted on the inner surface of the skull by:

- brain
- blood volume
- cerebrospinal fluid (CSF).

Intracranial pressure may rise if any one of the normal tissues increases in volume or if an additional mass is present within the skull (Figure 19.1). Normal values for ICP in infants and children are from 8 to 15 mmHg.

Managing the Critically Ill Child, ed. Richard Skone *et al.* Published by Cambridge University Press.

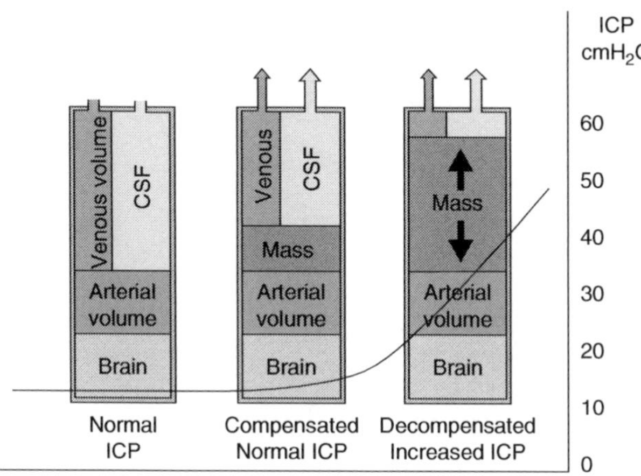

Figure 19.1. Intracranial pressure increases with additional mass within the skull or an increase in the volume of brain, CSF or blood.

Perfusion

With normal levels of ICP and normal systemic blood pressure, arterial blood is able to enter the skull and perfuse the brain. If the ICP is greater than the arterial pressure, blood will not flow through the brain.

Cerebral perfusion pressure is defined as follows:

$$\text{cerebral perfusion pressure} = \text{mean arterial pressure} - \text{intracranial pressure}$$

As can be seen from this equation, an increase in ICP will cause a decrease in cerebral perfusion pressure unless a corresponding rise in mean arterial pressure occurs. When cerebral perfusion pressure falls below a critical value, the corresponding reduction in cerebral blood flow results in brain ischaemia.

Autoregulation of arterial pressure

In healthy individuals the cerebral blood flow supplying the brain is maintained at a constant value over a range of blood pressure values. This 'autoregulation' is demonstrated in Figure 19.2 (using adult values). Autoregulation is lost in the following situations:

- at extremes of systemic blood pressure
- following traumatic brain injury (perfusion becomes completely pressure-dependent).

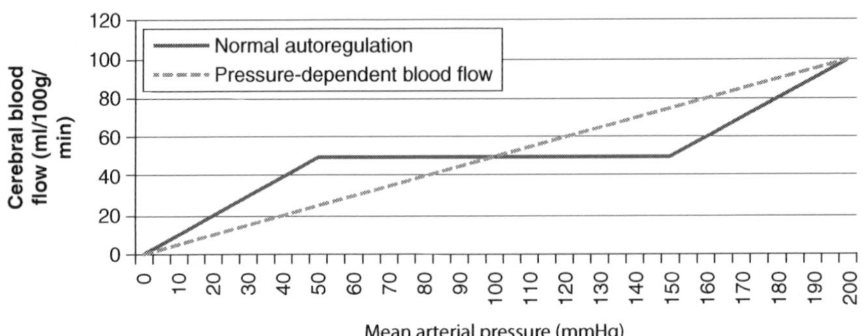

Figure 19.2. Autoregulation of cerebral blood flow with pressure. Values shown in this graph are adult values. Corresponding pressure values will be lower in children.

The consequence of the loss of autoregulation, e.g. after head injury, is that maintaining an adequate blood pressure becomes essential in order to maintain appropriate cerebral blood flow. It also highlights that surges in blood pressure should also be avoided.

Raised intracranial pressure in children

The age of the child and the rate of change of the volume of intracranial constituents are the primary determinants of the clinical presentation of raised ICP.

The younger child

The sutures of the skull are able to expand until about 18 months of age. Before this time, a slowly increasing intracranial volume will result in a rise in ICP and expansion of the cranial vault with the clinical features of:

- widely separated sutures
- full fontanelle
- enlarged head circumference
- setting-sun eyes
- vomiting
- developmental regression (see Table 19.1 for other signs).

Setting-sun eyes, where the sclera is visible between the upper eyelid and the iris, is an ophthalmological sign in small children resulting from an upward gaze paresis secondary to raised ICP.

The compensatory expansion mechanisms seen in young children initially prevent the ICP from rising to critical values, but have a limited capacity. When a critical volume is reached, or if the change in volume is rapid, ICP can rise quickly. Signs of raised ICP are seen in Table 19.1.

The older child

Children older than 18 months have a more limited capacity to accommodate rises in ICP and more rapidly present with the signs in Table 19.1.

Table 19.1. Historical features, symptoms and signs of raised intracranial pressure.

	Acute change in ICP	Chronic change in ICP
History prompting consideration of raised ICP	History of trauma	Previous ventricular shunt surgery Developmental regression
Symptoms of raised ICP	Headache Vomiting Diplopia	Headache Vomiting Diplopia
Signs of raised ICP	Decreased conscious level Tense cranial fontanelle Pupillary asymmetry Seizures	Widely separated cranial sutures Tense cranial fontanelle Enlarged head circumference Setting-sun eyes Ataxia
Signs of brain herniation (preterminal signs)	Pupillary dilatation Reduced conscious level Hypertension Bradycardia Respiratory depression	Pupillary dilatation Reduced conscious level Hypertension Bradycardia Respiratory depression

Conditions causing raised intracranial pressure in children

Table 19.2 categorizes the common causes of raised ICP in children.

Traumatic brain injury (TBI) is the commonest cause of raised ICP in children. It is also the leading cause of death in injured children. In the UK each year there are 2500 brain-injured children admitted to paediatric intensive care units, 500 of whom have severe injuries.

The three leading causes of brain injury in children over 1 year old are pedestrian versus car, pedal cyclist versus car and falling from height. In children younger than 1 year old, non-accidental injury is the leading cause of brain injury and must always be considered when examining the child (see Chapter 30).

Table 19.2. Causes of raised intracranial pressure in children.

Category	Examples
Traumatic	Intracerebral haemorrhage, diffuse axonal injury
Metabolic	Diabetic ketoacidosis, hepatic encephalopathy, hyperammonaemia, carbon monoxide poisoning
Hypoxic ischaemic injury	Drowning, seizures, post-cardiac-arrest
Infection	Meningitis, encephalitis, cerebral abscess
Vascular	Arterio-venous malformation, haemorrhagic or ischaemic stroke, venous thrombosis, malignant hypertension, eclampsia
Hydrocephalus	Communicating or non-communicating, blocked artificial shunt
Neoplastic	Malignant or non-malignant tumour

Treatment of acutely raised ICP in children

Treatment of raised ICP is focussed on:

- initial emergency treatment
- prevention of secondary brain injury
- treatment of the underlying cause.

Determining the nature and/or the extent of the underlying cause requires CT imaging of the head.

Often the child will need neurosurgical intervention and will need admission to a paediatric ICU. Therefore, early discussion with the regional paediatric intensive care retrieval consultant and neurosurgeon is vital.

Emergency management

A primary assessment of airway, breathing, and circulation (as detailed in Chapter 4) must be completed for all patients presenting with raised ICP. Prompt treatment of the major causes of secondary brain injury, particularly hypotension and hypoxaemia, must then be targeted.

Airway

All children with a GCS < 9 must be intubated and ventilated. Once intubated all patients must be adequately sedated with morphine and midazolam, and muscle relaxation maintained.

For trauma patients, spinal immobilization before, during and after intubation is essential. Intubation of these patients therefore requires a minimum of four people to manage the process (in-line immobilization, cricoid pressure, intubator, assistant). The choice of anaesthetic agent is up to the individual (e.g. thiopentone, ketamine). Ketamine is no longer considered contraindicated in head injuries and provides a favourable cardiovascular profile in trauma.

Ventilation

All patients must have end-tidal carbon dioxide (CO_2) monitoring. They can then be ventilated to an end-tidal carbon dioxide level that correlates to a blood carbon dioxide level ($PaCO_2$) of 4.5–5 kPa. All patients should be ventilated with a positive end-expiratory pressure (PEEP) of at least 5 cmH_2O and enough oxygen to maintain saturations $\geq 98\%$ or arterial $PaO_2 > 13$ kPa.

Circulation in trauma patients

Treat hypotension aggressively as it is the biggest cause of secondary ischaemic injury. Every patient should have a minimum of two large-bore peripheral cannulae or IO needles.

The systolic blood pressure should be maintained above the 95th centile for age, in order to ensure adequate cerebral perfusion pressure (see Table 19.3), accepting the risk of increased traumatic bleeding. After a maximum of 40 ml/kg of resuscitation fluid, packed red cells and fresh frozen plasma should be used for further resuscitation. All patients should have a urinary catheter placed (after the CT scan if it will delay imaging).

Table 19.3. Ninety-fifth centile systolic blood pressures by age.

Age of child	Target systolic blood pressure
< 1 year	> 80 mmHg
1–5 years	> 90 mmHg
5–14 years	> 100 mmHg
> 14 years	> 110 mmHg

If an injured child remains cardiovascularly unstable despite fluid resuscitation, it is vital to reconsider sites of bleeding. These are the same as in adults (external, chest, abdomen, pelvis or femur). In infants with an open fontanelle, intracranial haemorrhage can be significant. If there is ongoing bleeding in an injured child, the patient should not be transferred to CT until the bleeding has been controlled. This might mean that the patient goes directly to theatre to stop the bleeding, before a CT scan.

Circulation in non-trauma patients

Good intravenous access is still essential in these children in order to administer drugs and fluids.

In cardiovascularly stable head-injured children additional vasoactive drug support may be needed to maintain the high target blood pressures. If the patient only has peripheral access, then use dopamine to maintain their target systolic blood pressure. If the patient has central access, then use noradrenaline to maintain target systolic blood pressure. In patients with myocardial dysfunction, an inotrope, e.g. adrenaline, should be used in addition to noradrenaline.

For both sets of patients it is important not to delay computed tomography of the head for insertion of central and arterial access. Remember that an IO needle can be used for inotropes if necessary.

Immediate tests

Blood should be taken for:

- cross-match
- blood sugar
- blood gas
- urea and electrolytes
- full blood count
- coagulation
- blood culture
- liver function tests
- ammonia (if metabolic encephalopathy considered).

Carry out a bedside pregnancy test in all post-pubertal girls. Send urine for toxicology in all possible poisonings.

Neuroprotection

Regardless of the cause of raised ICP, once initial stabilization has occurred, focus moves to interventions that can minimize the ICP or prevent secondary injury. These are detailed in Table 19.4.

Refractory or progressive rise in ICP

Following optimization of the management described in Table 19.4, the continued presence of pupillary dilatation, hypertension and bradycardia should stimulate the use of temporary hyperventilation and a hyperosmolar agent (mannitol or hypertonic saline – see Table 19.4 and see Figure 19.3).

Temporary hyperventilation

Reduce the end-tidal carbon dioxide level to correlate with a $PaCO_2$ of 4 to 4.5 kPa. This is an effective method of reducing ICP acutely. It should be used as a temporizing measure whilst awaiting the effect of osmotic agents.

Hyperosmolar fluids

Give a dose of either:

- 2.5–5.0 ml/kg of 20% mannitol (1.25 ml/kg if cardiovascular instability)
- 5 ml/kg of 3% saline (2–3 ml/kg for subsequent doses – up to a maximum plasma sodium of 150 mmol/l).

These therapies act to reduce cerebral oedema by drawing water into the blood. Hypertonic saline is preferred in cardiovascularly unstable trauma patients, as the diuresis associated with mannitol is not well tolerated in these patients.

Further management with the regional paediatric intensive care consultant and neurosurgeon should occur while these interventions are ongoing (if not before).

Table 19.4. Neuroprotective manoeuvres.

Minimizing ICP

- Ensure adequate analgesia and sedation (often requires large amounts of morphine and midazolam)
- Give muscle relaxants (preferably by infusion)
- Ensure the patient's head is in the mid-line position
- Ensure the bed is tilted to 30 degrees head up
- Treat seizures if present
  In traumatic head injury, load with phenytoin as seizure prophylaxis (20 mg/kg over 20 min)
- Maintain $PaCO_2$ at 4.5–5.0 kPa (this can be measured on blood gases from venous, capillary or arterial sources)

Intravenous maintenance fluids should be given at 2/3 maintenance. If the patient weighs more than 10 kg, use 0.9% saline as maintenance fluid. If the patient weighs less than 10 kg, use 0.9% saline with 5% dextrose

Keep serum sodium more than 135 mmol/l. Boluses of 3 ml/kg of 3% hypertonic saline are safe and effective and will raise serum sodium by about 3 mmol/l

Preventing further injury

- Ensure blood sugar is >3 mmol/l
- Maintain blood pressure targets as already mentioned
- Give a broad-spectrum antibiotic (cefotaxime 50 mg/kg) and intravenous acyclovir if infection is a possible cause of the raised ICP
- Maintain good oxygenation (saturations ≥ 98% or arterial PaO_2 > 13 kPa)
- Maintain normothermia (core temperature 36–37°C)

Cross-sectional imaging

A CT scan of the head is required to assess the nature and extent of an underlying cause of raised ICP. This should be done in liaison with a consultant radiologist. A plain CT brain is useful for identifying surgically treatable lesions, to assess the size of the CSF spaces, including the basal cisterns, to detect herniation and shift and to show the presence of oedema, haematoma, contusions and fractures. A normal CT brain does not exclude raised ICP.

CT brain with contrast is advised if a cerebral abscess or venous sinus thrombosis is part of the differential. In trauma patients cervical spine CT should also be considered. Other imaging of the chest, abdomen and pelvis should be discussed with a consultant radiologist.

Lumbar puncture

Lumbar puncture is not required in the acute management of children with decreased conscious level and suspected or confirmed raised ICP. Relevant information gained from a lumbar puncture can be obtained after life-threatening physiology has been treated and the child stabilized.

Specific treatment of the underlying cause

Further management based on an intracranial diagnosis is often dependent on the results of CT of the brain. In the absence of CT scanning within a hospital (e.g. because of mechanical breakdown) the child should be treated as if time-critical.

Tumours with mass effect and surrounding oedema and raised ICP

CT scans of intracranial tumours require specialist interpretation from neuroradiologists and paediatric oncologists. The use of steroids to reduce the mass effect of the tumour should be discussed with an oncologist. Such advice may be available to you through your regional paediatric transport service's conference call facility.

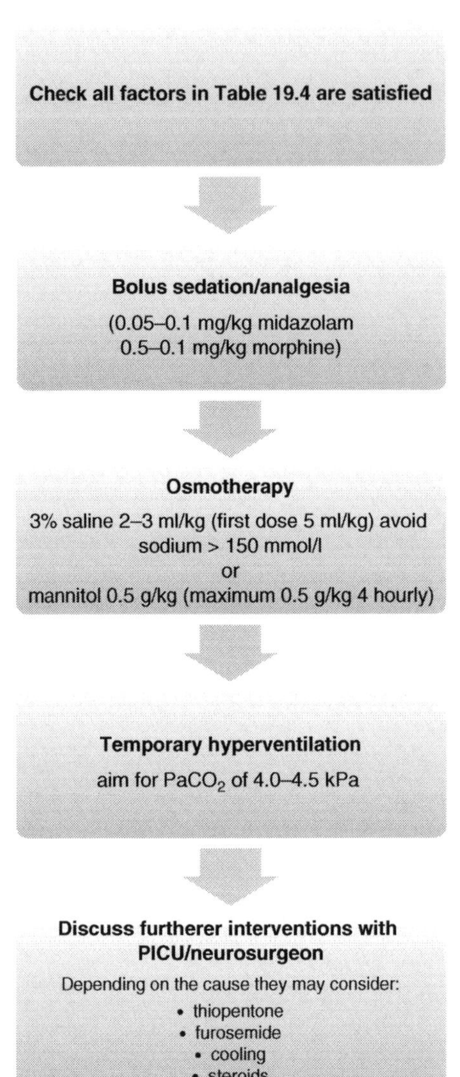

Figure 19.3. Management of acute rise in ICP with signs of herniation in a ventilated patient.

Blocked ventricular shunts and raised ICP

One group of children with raised ICP in whom immediate treatment is possible is those with a previously placed ventricular drain with reservoir bulb. Palpation of the ventricular drain as it passes subcutaneously along the skull and into the neck will enable recognition of the reservoir bulb. These have a depressible synthetic bulb. Physical depression of the bulb should result in downward flow of CSF. An inability to depress a rigid bulb can indicate a malfunction of the shunt system.

In a child who has a non-depressible reservoir bulb and signs of raised ICP it is possible to provide an immediate life-saving intervention prior to CT scan. First clean the skin overlying the reservoir bulb with 2% chlorhexidine and 70% alcohol solution. Pierce the child's skin overlying the bulb with an 18-gauge needle attached to a 20 ml syringe. Advance the needle into the centre of the bulb. Withdraw on the syringe and remove 20 ml of CSF (Figure 19.4).

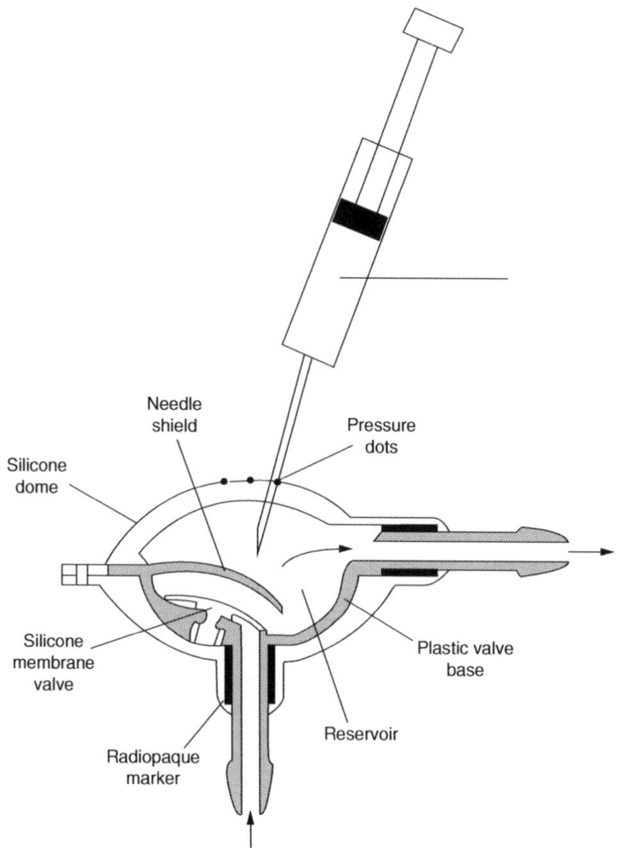

Figure 19.4. Ventricular drain reservoir. In a child with features of brain herniation from raised intracranial pressure, a needle and syringe can be used percutaneously to withdraw CSF.

Diabetic ketoacidosis and raised ICP

Patients with diabetic ketoacidosis and features of raised ICP need rapid institution of intensive care and neuroprotection. The most common cause of their deterioration is cerebral oedema. CT imaging of the head enables confirmation of cerebral oedema and exclusion of venous thrombosis, infarction or haemorrhage. Prior to being intubated and ventilated the patient will often have been maintaining their $PaCO_2$ very low with Kussmaul respirations. There are differences of opinion as to how hard you should try to replicate the low $PaCO_2$ once the patient is intubated. Some advocate aiming for a low $PaCO_2$ in order to keep the ICP at a minimum. Others advocate a more lung-friendly, conservative approach to ventilation.

Volume resuscitation should be strictly restricted and replacement of estimated fluid deficit should be stopped and when restarted will be spread over 72 hours (see Chapter 11).

Infectious causes of raised ICP

Suspected infectious causes of raised ICP should be treated with cefotaxime and acyclovir. A history of foreign travel within malaria zones should trigger appropriate investigations, a discussion with a consultant microbiologist and treatment with anti-malarial drugs.

Trauma

A pathway for the initial management of severe traumatic brain injury in children (GCS < 9) can be seen in Figure 19.5 (see also Chapter 18).

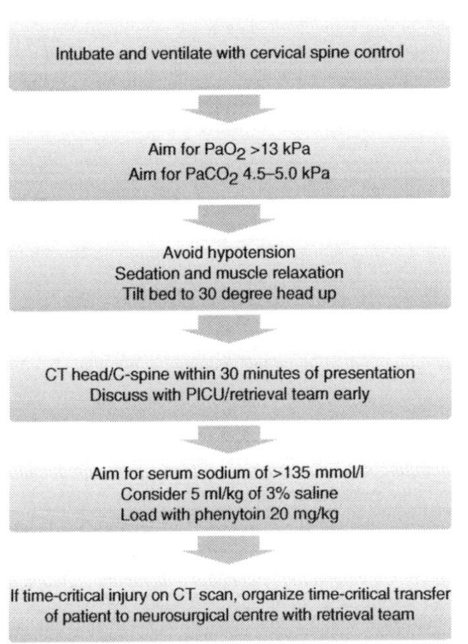

Figure 19.5. Initial basic management of a head injured patient with GCS < 9.

Hypertensive encephalopathy and raised ICP

Children with malignant hypertension should receive the standard neuroprotection described above. Antihypertensives should only be used with PICU advice. The aim is to reduce the child's blood pressure slowly with invasive monitoring. Always check a pregnancy test in post-pubertal females. The CT features of posterior subcortical oedema seen in eclampsia are identical to those observed in malignant hypertension.

Transport of children to the regional care centre

The recognition of a life-threatening abnormality on CT brain amenable to surgical intervention directs further management towards the safe and rapid transport of the child by the local team to a neurosurgical centre; this is known as neurosurgical time-critical transfer. A checklist of key interventions to enable time-critical transfer is found in Chapter 24. Neuroprotective measures, as already described, should be maintained throughout transfer.

Children without time-critical lesions, whose features of raised intracranial pressure have resolved, should receive continued neuroprotection and retrieval by the regional paediatric intensive care transport service. Discussion with the regional paediatric intensive care transport coordinator is essential in both cases.

Summary

ICP can be raised for many different reasons in children. The aims of management are to minimize the resulting injuries by maintaining adequate brain perfusion. Careful attention to detail is essential in order to have every chance of keeping the ICP low.

Golden rules

- Early recognition and rapid intervention are critical
- Attention to detail for all factors in Table 19.4 is important
- Make sure the patient is well sedated
- Consider seizures in an intubated child with autonomic disturbance and signs of raised ICP

Further reading

Curry R, Hollingworth W, Ellenbogen R, *et al.* Incidence of hypo-hypercarbia in severe traumatic brain injury before and after 2003 pediatric guidelines. *Pediatr Crit Care Med* 2008;**9**:141–146.

Kirkham FJ. Non-traumatic coma in children. *Arch Dis Child* 2001;**85**(4):303–312.

Kochanek PM, *et al.* Guidelines for the acute medical management of severe traumatic brain injury in infants, children, and adolescents – second edition. *Pediatr Crit Care Med* 2012;**13** Suppl 1:S1–82.

Tasker RC, Lutman D, Peters MJ. Hyperventilation in severe diabetic ketoacidosis. *Pediatr Crit Care Med* 2005;**6**(4):405–411.

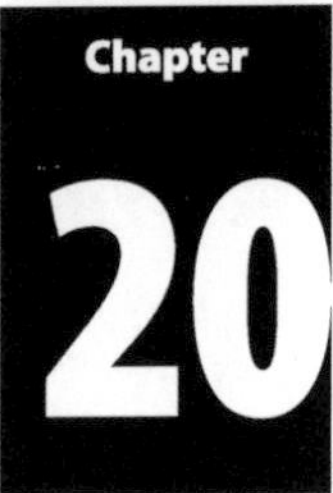

The child with burns

Sapna Verma and Manu Sundaram

Introduction

Children sustain burns in many different ways and this may be associated with other injuries. This chapter aims to cover the pertinent management for burns only. Other co-morbidities such as head or spine injuries should be managed alongside the burns in order of severity.

How do burns differ in children?

Pathophysiology

Although the assessment and management of a burn may at first glance appear the same for children and adults, there are significant differences.

Skin thickness

Children's skin is significantly thinner than adults'. The depth of the burn may therefore be much greater for the equivalent heat source, with burns occurring with temperatures as low as 40°C.

Airway

Children have narrower airways than adults; oedema can therefore rapidly lead to airway obstruction.

Surface area to volume ratio

Children will lose proportionately more fluid and rapidly become hypothermic.

Extent of burn

The 'rule of nines' cannot be universally applied to children. It must be modified to take into account their varying body proportions. See Figure 20.1.

The vast majority of burns occur within the home environment, especially in the kitchen or bathroom. The aetiology of burns varies with the age of the child; for example, scalds are more common in children under the age of 4, whereas flame burns are more common in children over 10 years of age.

Managing the Critically Ill Child, ed. Richard Skone *et al.* Published by Cambridge University Press.

Cause of burn

Consideration should always be given to the possibility of a non-accidental cause for burn injuries in children, particularly if the history is inconsistent with the injury and it involves scalds with a glove and stocking distribution.

Assessment of a child with burns

The child with burns should be managed as any critically ill patient (see Chapter 4). However, there are additional factors which should be considered for every burns patient.

Initial assessment

Initial assessment should follow the same principles as detailed in Chapter 4. The main aim, as always, is to treat immediately life-threatening problems and prevent further harm. Hence a thorough initial approach is essential, being aware of the potential for additional injuries.

Airway and facial burns

Facial and upper airway burns may cause oedema and airway compromise. A very low threshold for intubation should be set for burns patients. Oedema of the burned airway will worsen over the first 24–48 hours especially following fluid administration. Intubation with a cuffed and uncut endotracheal tube should be considered early on if there are signs listed in Table 20.1.

Table 20.1. Signs of potential impending airway compromise in burns.

Signs
Stridor
Hoarseness
Circumferential burns to the neck
Carbonaceous sputum
Singeing of the nasal hairs
Facial oedema

A cuffed endotracheal tube should be used (even in prepubescent children) when available. They are preferred in this situation for the following reasons:

- airway security
- no need to change tube if size too small
- when the oedema starts to improve there is no need to upsize.

Inhalational injury

The products of combustion cause irritation to the lower airways, resulting in bronchospasm and ciliary dysfunction. Similarly, burns to the lower airways or explosions may cause lung injury, pneumothoraces or pulmonary contusions. These may manifest themselves as respiratory distress, which can be assessed clinically (see Chapters 4 and 7) as well as with blood gases and radiological imaging.

Once ventilated, high airway pressures or FiO_2 may be required, and a lung-protective strategy of ventilation is recommended. Full-thickness burns or circumferential burns to the chest may hamper ventilation and rarely escharotomies may need to be performed in the emergency department, if this occurs.

Pulse oximetry must be continuously monitored in burns patients; however, in carbon monoxide poisoning the oxygen saturations may appear falsely normal. Blood gases should therefore be obtained and analysed with a co-oximeter to assess gas transfer (using PaO_2) and carboxyhaemoglobin levels. CO levels in excess of 25% should prompt consideration of ventilation.

If bronchospasm is present administration of β_2-agonists may be of benefit. Treatments such as bicarbonate lavage, nebulized heparin and nebulized *N*-acetylcysteine should generally only be undertaken in a tertiary centre.

Depth of burn

Accurate assessment of the burn depth is an essential component of burn management. The true depth may not be immediately obvious and is rarely uniform.

Superficial burns

These affect the epidermis of the skin only. The skin looks red and is mildly painful. The top layer of skin may peel a day or so after the burn, but the underlying skin is healthy. It does not require any treatment.

Partial thickness burns

These cause deeper damage and extend to the dermis. The skin forms blisters and is painful. As some of the dermis is unharmed these burns usually heal well within 10 days.

Full-thickness burns

These damage all layers of skin, resulting in a white, leathery appearance to the burn. There may be little or no pain as the nerve endings are destroyed. Skin grafting is usually required.

Deeper burns

These affect underlying structures, e.g. bone and muscle in electrical burns where there may be minimal damage to the overlying skin.

Exposure and extent of burns

The child must be exposed and examined to enable accurate estimation of both the depth and extent of the burn. This is essential to calculate the fluid requirements accurately. It also allows careful removal of wet clothing to minimize temperature loss. Adherent clothing can be left in place to minimize further damage to underlying tissues. It is important to document the child's temperature. Active rewarming with a Bair hugger should be used where appropriate. All jewellery must be removed immediately before tissue swelling occurs.

Assessing the extent of burns is important as it affects both management and outcome. The use of the 'Lund and Browder' charts (Figure 20.1), which detail these varying body proportions in relation to the age of the child, is essential in order to manage a child appropriately. Alternatively the child's palm with adducted fingers equates to 1% of their total body surface area. This method is particularly useful in the estimation of smaller burns.

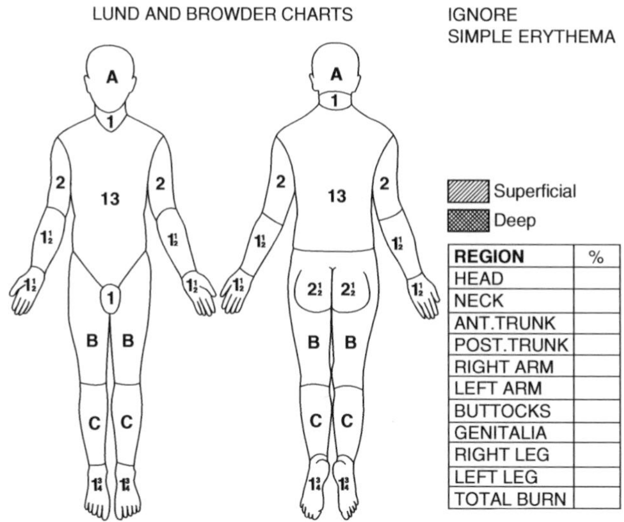

REGION	%
HEAD	
NECK	
ANT.TRUNK	
POST.TRUNK	
RIGHT ARM	
LEFT ARM	
BUTTOCKS	
GENITALIA	
RIGHT LEG	
LEFT LEG	
TOTAL BURN	

RELATIVE PERCENTAGE OF BODY SURFACE AREA AFFECTED BY GROWTH

AREA	AGE 0	1	5	10	15	ADULT
A = ½ OF HEAD	9½	8½	6½	5½	4½	3½
B = ½ OF ONE THIGH	2¾	3¼	4	4½	4½	4¾
C = ½ OF ONE LEG	2½	2½	2¾	3	3¼	3½

Figure 20.1. Lund and Browder chart.

Treatment of a child with burns

Immediate management should involve removal of smouldering clothing and removal from the heat source. Cooling of the burn is beneficial when performed within 20 minutes of injury. Thereafter a structured approach to the management of burns should always be followed to ensure that other associated life-threatening injuries are not missed.

Securing a definitive airway

There are specific issues relating to intubation of a child with a burn. The combination of facial swelling, possibility of a cervical spine injury and evolving oedema of the airway means that early intubation by an experienced anaesthetist with a cuffed uncut ET tube is recommended. In-line cervical immobilization should always be considered. When intubating a patient suffering from airway burns, it is important to:

- make sure that there is a selection of small ET tubes
- use a cuffed ET tube, even in prepubescent children
- note the position of the ET tube relative to fixed structures such as teeth or gums
- use ET tube ties rather than tapes.

Despite the problems with hyperkalaemia that may occur after 24 hours, suxamethonium 2 mg/kg can be used as a muscle relaxant in the immediate management of the acute phase.

Table 20.2. Initial management of a child with burns.

Phase of management	Assessment	Action
Initial phase On presentation of the child	Assess need to intubate: • GCS • Hypoxia refractory to oxygen • Inhalation injury • Airway compromise from oedema • Carbon monoxide levels • > 40% burns • Need for surgical intervention	Give oxygen Ventilate by hand if needed Remove burnt clothing Gain IV access preferably through unburnt skin IO if more than three IV attempts, or if difficulty is anticipated Give fluid bolus if indicated • 20 ml/kg of crystalloid • 10 ml/kg if trauma suspected
	Assess cardiovascular system	Take blood including ABG, clotting and cross-match
After initial assessment Once imminently life-threatening risks have been addressed	Reassess need to intubate in the presence of: • Stridor • Hoarseness • Circumferential burns (neck/chest) • Carbonaceous sputum • Singeing of the nasal hairs • Facial oedema	Repeat blood gases to assess ventilation • Hypoxia refractory to oxygen • Rising CO_2 • Carbon monoxide levels If intubating • Contact senior anaesthetist • Anticipate a difficult airway
	Assess extent of burn and calculate fluid deficit Examine and expose the whole body Measure temperature and start warming	Use cuffed, uncut ET tube Give analgesia Start fluid therapy immediately: • Start point is from time of burn • Give boluses if indicated • Catheterize bladder • Keep urine output > 1 ml/kg/h
Further stabilization Not immediately life-saving procedures	Continue to reassess clinical condition and blood results Decide on further monitoring	Contact retrieval team Definitive plan (transfer vs. operate) Arterial line if: • Haemodynamic instability • Starting inotropes • Repeated blood gases CVC if: • More definitive access needed • Starting inotropes • Giving high concentration drugs Correct coagulopathy

Fluid therapy

The largest amount of fluid loss occurs in the first 24 hours after the burn, while fluid leaks from the intravascular space into the interstitial space in the first 8 to 12 hours.

In children intravenous fluids must be commenced when the percentage body surface area affected is 10% or greater to maintain organ perfusion, ensure perfusion to the burnt area and therefore minimize the burn injury. Erythema of the skin on its own should not be included in the calculation of per cent body surface area affected.

Fluids are calculated using the Parkland formula as follows:

$$3-4\ \text{ml} \times \text{weight (kg)} \times \%\ \text{body surface area} = \text{volume in ml over 24 h}$$

Half of the calculated volume (as Hartmann's) should be infused over the first 8 hours from the time of the burn and the second half over the next 16 hours.

Although the fluid therapy is 'replacing' lost circulating volume, it is worth cross-matching large burns for blood and fresh frozen plasma early as it may often be needed prior to transfer.

In addition, the usual maintenance fluids should be given as 0.45% saline/5% dextrose (see Chapter 32).

Adjusting fluid replacement

Once fluids have been commenced the child's urine output will be used to adjust ongoing fluid therapy. The optimum urine output in children is 1 ml/kg/h or greater. Early urinary catheterization in burns to the genitalia is prudent to avoid subsequent problems with swelling. It is also a requirement in all burns greater than 20% of body surface area.

Shock and fluid boluses

Two reasonable-sized IV cannulae should be inserted peripherally, preferably into unburnt tissue. If this proves difficult insertion of an IO needle should be attempted and fluid boluses given.

Fluid boluses

Shock does not usually result directly from a burn unless there is a delay in presentation or concurrent pathology. If it is present, an alternative reason should be sought. Fluid boluses should be given when clinically indicated. The fluid boluses will usually not form part of the formula.

Analgesia

Anyone who has sustained even a very small burn will understand the pain that is associated with it. Covering a burn with cling film will cover exposed nerve endings and reduce pain. Analgesia in the form of morphine 0.1–0.2 mg/kg boluses and a morphine infusion may be required for severe burns. Alternatively, other opioids such as fentanyl may be administered, depending on individual preference and familiarity.

Dressings

Photographing burns before dressing will often obviate the need for repeated examination and hence reduce disruption to burnt tissue. Large blisters should be deroofed. Burns affecting more than 20% of the child's body surface area will almost certainly require debridement in theatre.

The burns should be covered with cling film to protect the underlying skin, reduce evaporative losses and allow visualization of the affected area if the patient is transferred to a burns centre. For burns less than 5% of body surface area a non-adherent dressing, for example silver urgotul, can be applied. Polyfax is the treatment of choice for facial burns.

Additional considerations

Antibiotics are not routinely administered for burns and should only be used where there is a high index of suspicion for infection. An immunization history should be obtained to ensure that the child is up to date with tetanus.

Suspicious burns

The incidence of intentional injury is very difficult to quantify, with quoted figures varying between 1% and 25%. Suspicion should be raised if there are:

- immersion burns, i.e. a scald with glove and stocking distribution or sacral sparing
- intentional contact burns, e.g. from cigarettes, iron or other hot implements
- delays in presentation
- burns that cannot be explained by the history provided
- unusual history for developmental stage of the child
- burns in areas that are not readily accessible, for example buttocks.

It is essential that a detailed history is obtained to determine the following:

- Who was present at the time of the burn?
- How did the burn occur?
- Where did the burn occur?
- What was the heat source?
- Was it an enclosed space?
- What first aid was carried out and for how long?
- When did the burn occur?

It is imperative that the circumstances surrounding the burn are clearly documented in the medical notes (see Chapter 30) and local safeguarding practice is followed.

Signs of a really sick child

Many of the other signs and symptoms used to assess children who are critically unwell, such as tachycardia, tachypnoea and pain, may be difficult to assess in severe burns patients. It is important to involve your local PICU/retrieval team early when managing severely burned children. Problems to look out for are detailed in Table 20.3. The indications for referral to a burns centre are as follows:

- partial thickness burns involving greater than 5% of the total body surface area
- full-thickness burns
- smoke inhalation
- circumferential burns
- electrical burns
- chemical burns

- burns to hands, feet, face and genitalia
- intentional burn.

Table 20.3. Potential problems for children with burns.

System	Specific problems	Consequence of these problems
Respiratory	Airway compromise Immediate Delayed (needs to be anticipated)	Need for clear management plan as a straightforward intubation at presentation may become very difficult with time. ET tube must be: • Cuffed • Uncut
	May develop acute lung injury from inhalation injury or trauma	May need higher airway pressures than anticipated
	Pulse oximeter probe unreliable	Falsely reassuring reading. Will need repeated blood gases and carbon monoxide reading (consider arterial line)
Cardiovascular	Hypovolaemia	Consider associated injuries as a cause (rarely the burn)
	Massive insensible losses	Will need carefully calculated fluid replacement Also likely to need fluid boluses prior to/during induction
	Very difficult IV access	IV access should be attempted through unburnt skin first Central venous access may be needed in large surface burns
	Difficult to assess cardiovascular system as Pain causes tachycardia Capillary refill unreliable	The most useful guide to fluid balance becomes the urine output Should be more than 1 ml/kg/h
	Fluid replacement regime may seem massive	Care is needed in calculating fluid replacement.
Gastrointestinal	Gastric stasis	Potential for regurgitation and aspiration is high
Other problems	May develop coagulopathy Dramatic nature of burn may distract from other life-threatening injuries	Care must be taken to assess the whole patient, not just the burn!
	Hypothermia may develop quickly	Make sure that active warming occurs in hypothermic patients, and that heat loss is minimized
	Rule of nines does not apply	Lund-Bower chart must be used to assess extent of burn

Pre-transfer management

As with any transfer, documentation and investigations should be prepared before departure. For burns patients this must include details of:

- extent of burn
- circumstances surrounding the injury
- fluids given up until the point of departure
- details of the airway management (size and length of ET tube)
- investigations performed.

If there are safeguarding concerns, for example the burn is thought to be intentional, to have arisen through significant neglect or there are other injuries that could be non-accidental in nature, then:

- all blood tests should be taken and sent to the laboratories with a chain of evidence form (see Chapter 30)
- clotting samples should be taken
- contact with social care services should be documented (including the name of the social worker, time of the call and a summary of the conversation).

Summary

Burns in children are distressing for all involved. Early intervention and aggressive fluid resuscitation are essential. Analgesia should not be forgotten. If there is any doubt about the management of a child with burns, contact the local PICU and burns team for advice.

Golden rules

- Start the fluid resuscitation calculation from the time of burn – not admission
- Early assessment and intervention for airway burns is important
- Do not trust the oxygen saturation reading if there is likely to be significant carbon monoxide inhalation
- Children will become hypothermic quickly unless warmed (including fluids)
- Always use a cuffed, uncut ET tube where available
- Hypovolaemia is usually associated with other injuries

Further reading

Advanced Paediatric Life Support: The Practical Approach, 5th edn. London: BMJ Books, 2011.

British Burn Association. *Emergency management of severe burns course manual*, UK version.

Fenlon S, Nene S. Burns in children. *CEACCP* 2007;7(3):76–80.

Hettiaratchy S. *ABC of Burns*. London: BMJ Publishing, 2004.

Young A. The management of severe burns in children. *Curr Paediatr* 2004;**14**:202–207.

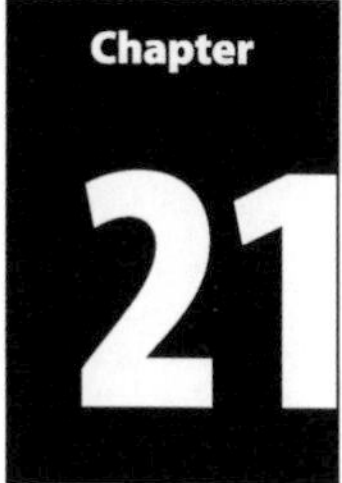

Blood product administration in children

Oliver Bagshaw

Introduction

Critically ill or injured children may need transfusion of blood or other blood products for a number of different reasons. These include:

- disseminated intravascular coagulation, e.g. secondary to systemic sepsis
- acute haemorrhage, e.g. trauma or reversal of anticoagulants
- acute anaemia secondary to an underlying condition such as haemolytic uraemic syndrome or sickle-cell disease
- plasma exchange for conditions such as thrombotic thrombocytopenic purpura.

This chapter assumes a degree of understanding of the principles of blood transfusion. The main considerations and basic rules that apply in children are similar to those in adults, but with a few key differences. The latter part of the chapter will give guidance for the management of a massive transfusion.

Considerations in children

Blood or blood products should only be administered if it is deemed essential for the child's wellbeing. Blood product transfusions can carry significant morbidity (see below) and this must always be borne in mind when the decision to transfuse is being made.

Cross-matching products for children

Red cells

Alloantibodies (antibodies produced against antigens from members of the same species) are very rare in infants younger than 4 months of age, unless the baby has already received repeated, massive transfusions. Formal cross-matching is therefore usually not necessary. A maternal sample for antibody screening and a sample from the baby for a direct antiglobulin test (DAT) are sufficient. If both are negative, blood can be issued according

Managing the Critically Ill Child, ed. Richard Skone *et al.* Published by Cambridge University Press.

to the blood group of the baby. If either is positive, serological investigation and formal cross-matching must be undertaken.

For older children, if antibodies are absent on screening it is possible to issue type-specific blood electronically for any patient. This makes the process much quicker and easier in situations where repeated transfusions are necessary as part of the child's acute management.

Ideally, donor exposure in children should be limited as much as possible. This can be achieved by avoiding transfusion altogether, or dividing a single unit into smaller satellite packs (pedipacks). These only have a volume of about 40 ml. They are ideal for top-up transfusion, but are not suitable if significant, ongoing haemorrhage is present. Local availability may be a problem.

Fresh frozen plasma (FFP)

FFP administered to children in the UK must be treated with methylene blue and have come from a donor pool that is free of possible CJD infection. Currently no FFP administered to children is sourced from the UK. An alternative is Octaplas, a pooled donor product that has some advantages in terms of consistency of clotting factor levels and a reduced risk of transmitting infection. Small volume packs of 60–70 ml are produced, but availability will depend on local sourcing.

Platelets

In patients who have frequent platelet transfusions, antibodies can become a problem. In these cases HLA-matched platelets need to be administered, otherwise a rise in platelet count may not occur.

Special circumstances

Irradiated blood products

In patients with impaired immune function there is a risk of precipitating graft-versus-host disease (GVHD), when transfused donor T cells (within blood products) proliferate and engraft in the recipient's bone marrow, then attack other organ systems. High-risk patients are given irradiated blood to try to minimize the risk of T cell transfusion. Examples of cases in which irradiated blood should be used are:

- congenital immune deficiencies
- DiGeorge syndrome (common in congenital heart disease)
- bone marrow transplantation
- lymphoma and leukaemia
- chemotherapy patients receiving purine antagonists (e.g. 6-mercaptopurine).

Only red cells and platelets need irradiation, FFP and cryoprecipitate do not. It is important to note that irradiated blood has a higher potassium concentration than normal blood, which increases with the age of the unit. Therefore, irradiated blood is not stored beyond 14 days. Rapid transfusion of irradiated blood has led to symptomatic hyperkalaemia in some patients.

If irradiated products are not immediately available and the clinical urgency of the situation dictates it, non-irradiated blood products can be administered, as the risks of not transfusing the patient may outweigh the small risk of GVHD.

CMV-negative blood products

In the UK a recent position statement by the Advisory Committee on the Safety of Blood Tissues and Organs (SaBTO) has recommended that cytomegalovirus-negative blood products need only be administered to neonates and pregnant women. Leucodepletion of blood products in the UK (with the exception of granulocyte) has significantly reduced the risk of CMV transmission in other patient groups such as immune deficiency or organ transplantation. If the urgency of the situation demands it then blood products may need to be administered, irrespective of the CMV status of the product or the patient.

Giving blood products

Packed red cell transfusion

Blood transfusion in stable children can be avoided if the haemoglobin concentration ([Hb]) is above 70 g/l and not dropping. Above a [Hb] of 70 g/l oxygen delivery to the tissues is likely to be sufficient and further blood administration does not improve outcome. Different [Hb] targets are aimed for in the following situations:

- $>$ 90 g/l patients with symptomatic sickle-cell disease (or [Hb]S $<$ 30%)
- $>$ 100 g/l patients with active haemorrhage
- $>$ 100 g/l neonates or ex-prems with apnoeic episodes requiring intervention
- $>$ 120 g/l patients with cyanotic congenital heart disease.

Calculation of packed red cell volume to be given

The circulating blood volume of the child is greater (per kg) than that of adults and varies with age. Newborn babies have a circulating blood volume of about 90 ml/kg, whilst in infants and older children it is closer to 80 ml/kg.

The formula below can be used (if active haemorrhage has ceased) to calculate the volume of packed red cells needed to achieve a desired increment in [Hb] (in g/l).

$$\text{Wt (kg)} \times \text{desired increase in [Hb] g/l} \times 0.5 = \text{ml needed to transfuse}$$

Thus for a 12 kg child with a [Hb] g/l of 70 g/l, in whom you would like to raise the concentration to 120 g/l, the equation would be

$$12 \times (120 - 70) \times 0.5 = 300 \text{ ml of packed red cells}$$

This only gives an approximation, due to the variation in circulating blood volume and the haematocrit of the blood being transfused. A formal haemoglobin or Hemocue estimation should always be checked following transfusion. Care should be taken in larger children, as the calculated volumes may be considerable. As a rule, it should never be necessary to administer more than one unit of blood (about 275 ml) to raise the [Hb] by 1 g/dl.

FFP

FFP is usually given to children in boluses of 10–15 ml/kg. In major trauma it should be given in a 1:1 ratio with packed red cells. For DIC or other coagulopathies it can be given as a source of fibrinogen and other clotting factors. This can be titrated to effect (through repeated boluses).

Platelets

Thresholds for platelet transfusion vary depending on the susceptibility to bleeding and the nature of the lesion or surgery. Suggested platelet counts that should trigger a transfusion are detailed below, although discussion with a haematologist is recommended:

- 10×10^9/l in individuals not susceptible to bleeding
- 20×10^9/l if bleeding is more likely (infection or pyrexia)
- 50×10^9/l for surgical procedures
- 100×10^9/l in cases of massive haemorrhage with ongoing bleeding.

If transfusion is necessary, do not worry about making complicated calculations to determine the desired rise in count. As a rule, children less than 15 kg should receive 10–15 ml/kg, whilst those over 15 kg can receive an adult unit (usually about 200 ml).

Massive haemorrhage

Massive haemorrhage is defined as loss of greater than 40 ml/kg of blood in less than 3 hours, ongoing losses in excess of 2 ml/kg/min or total blood volume loss in 24 hours. It is very rare in children, and is usually a consequence of a traumatic mechanism of injury or intraoperative bleeding during high-risk surgery. The sort of injury that causes haemorrhage in adults, e.g. high-speed motor vehicle accidents, penetrating injuries and abdominal and thoracic trauma, is unusual in children. However, if a child with a history of traumatic injury is admitted shocked, then active haemorrhage should be suspected and the cause sought. Concealed haemorrhage may occur in the:

- chest
- abdomen
- pelvis
- long bones
- brain and scalp (in babies).

When the blood group of a child who is actively haemorrhaging is not known, it may be necessary to administer O-negative blood. If active haemorrhage is significant and persists, a massive haemorrhage protocol (MHP) should be initiated (Figures 21.1 and 21.2). It is also important that steps to undertake any necessary damage-limitation surgery are initiated.

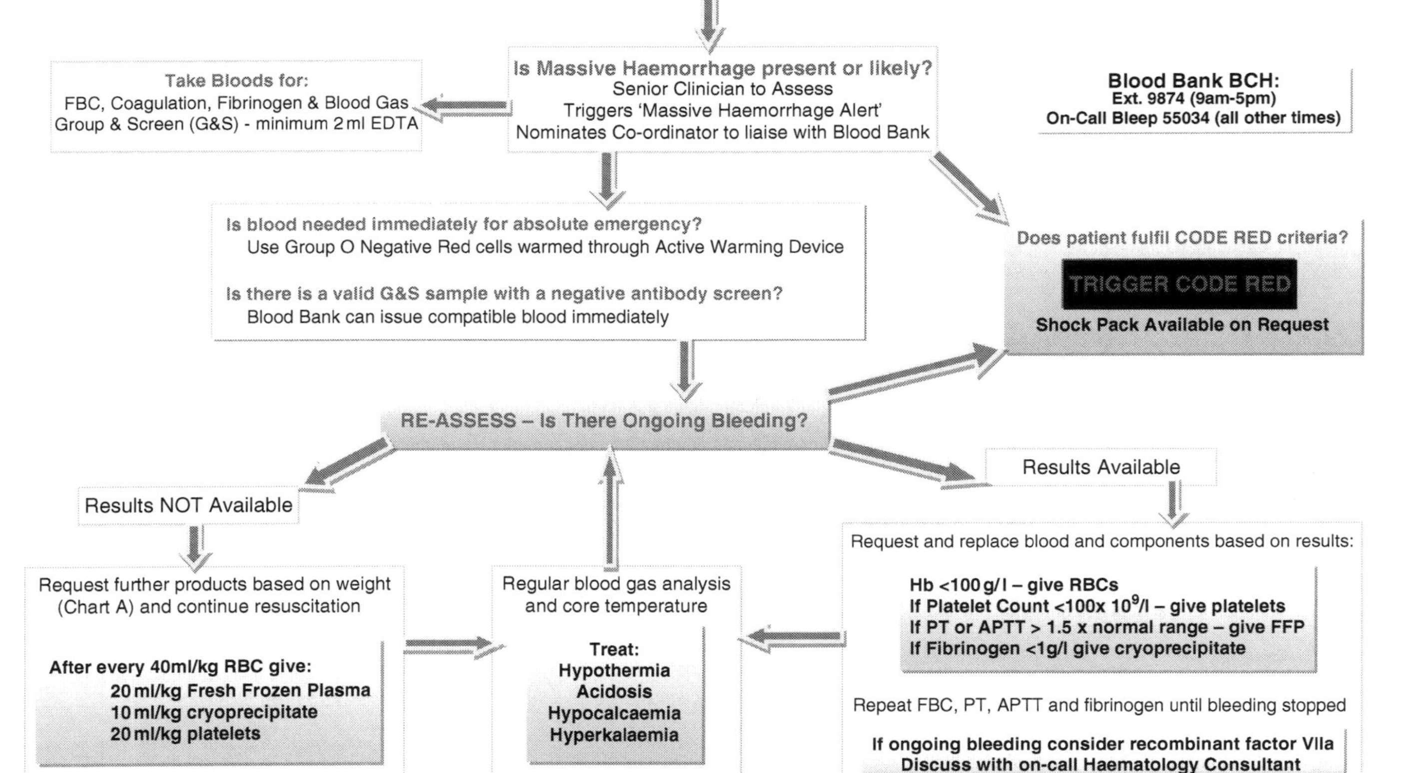

Figure 21.1. Management of suspected or likely massive haemorrhage in children. Reproduced with permission of Birmingham Children's Hospital Transfusion Committee.

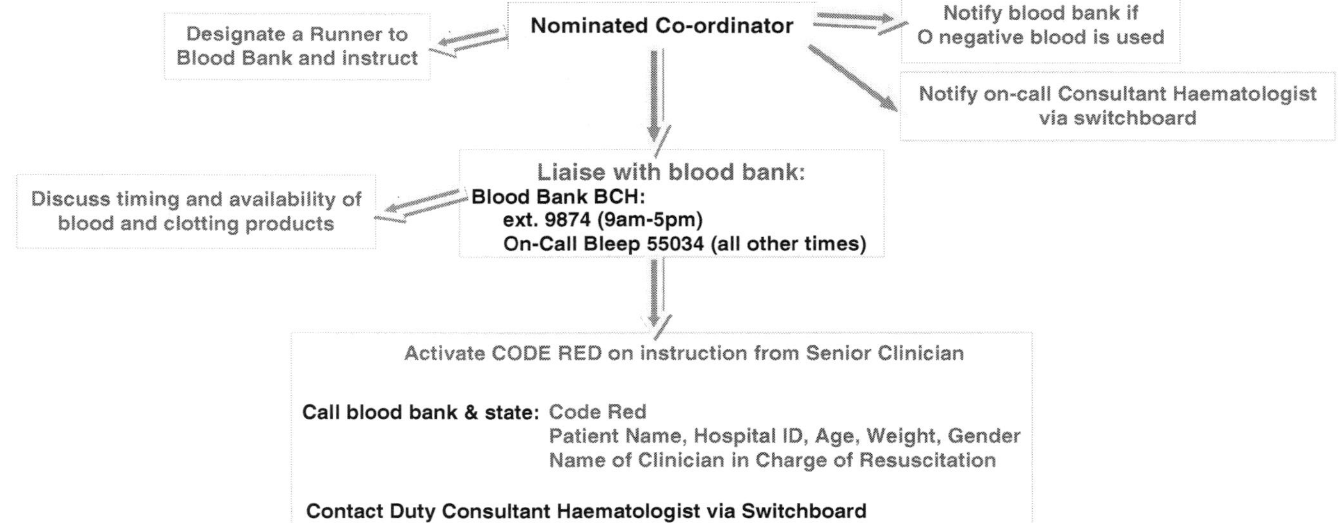

CODE RED **Definition**

Consider if:

ACTIVE HAEMORRHAGE SUSPECTED AND

>20 ml/kg Red Cells given in 1 hr

>40 ml/kg fluid given in 3 hr

>2 ml/kg/min blood loss

Code red activation enables release of 'shock pack' blood products i.e. red cells and FFP in 1:1 ratio with platelets and cryoprecipitate if available

Blue light delivery of platelets can be requested if they are unavailable.

In severe trauma red cells, FFP and platelets can be given in 1:1:1 ratio

Chart A

Blood Products to request by weight

	up to 10 kg	10–20 kg	20–50 kg	over 50 kg
Packed Cells	One Unit	Two Units	Three Units	Four Units
FFP	One Unit	Two Units	Three Units	Four Units
Platelets	One Unit	Two Units	Three Units	Four Units
Cryoprecipitate	Five Units	Eight Units	Twelve Units	Fifteen Units

HTC/NB 2011 Review November 2012

Figure 21.2. Management when 'Code Red' triggered. Reproduced with permission of Birmingham Children's Hospital Transfusion Committee.

Table 21.1. Key features of a massive haemorrhage protocol.

1. When to declare Code Red (see Figure 21.1)
2. Someone to coordinate with blood bank
3. Blood bank/consultant haematologist informed at earliest opportunity
4. Identification of the source of haemorrhage
5. Haemorrhage control – surgical opinion, tourniquets, Celox, tranexamic acid
6. Rapid availability and administration of blood products – shock packs
7. Ongoing assessment
8. Damage-limitation surgery

Airway management in massive haemorrhage

Ideally, the child should be resuscitated prior to induction of anaesthesia, but this is not always possible if haemorrhage is ongoing. Most children are able to mount a very effective sympathetic response to hypovolaemia which can make it easy to underestimate the degree of shock. Senior help should be sought urgently if a haemodynamically compromised child needs intubation.

Rapid-sequence induction is the method of choice. Children are generally much more robust than adults when it comes to tolerating induction of anaesthesia, but in the presence of hypovolaemia a significant fall in blood pressure may occur. Ketamine is usually the induction agent of choice, because of its sympathomimetic properties and greater haemodynamic stability. However, even ketamine is likely to cause a drop in blood pressure if hypovolaemia is present. It may be necessary to administer blood products and vasopressors to counteract this effect. Concerns about using ketamine in head injury patients are probably unjustified and the benefits of relative haemodynamic stability outweigh the risks of increasing ICP.

Circulation management in massive haemorrhage

Assessment of volaemic status is crucial prior to the induction of anaesthesia. The following clinical features are used:

- colour
- heart rate
- peripheral perfusion
- presence or absence of peripheral pulses
- respiratory rate
- conscious level.

Capillary refill is also used, but too much emphasis has been placed on this sign in the past, as it can be affected by other factors, such as cold and anxiety.

Two wide-bore peripheral cannulae should be inserted and blood taken for blood grouping and cross-match. If peripheral access proves difficult, IO access should be sought. The main aims of circulation management in this situation are:

- haemorrhage control
- rapid restoration of circulating volume
- avoidance of over-transfusion and the risks of clot displacement

- balancing associated pathology that may influence resuscitation targets, e.g. head injury
- avoidance of the deadly triad (see below and Chapter 18).

The deadly triad

The deadly triad within the context of trauma are:

- hypothermia
- coagulopathy
- acidosis.

Efforts to avoid these three factors should be made at all times by ensuring that any blood given is warmed, in adequate volume and in a 1:1 ratio with FFP (with sufficient platelet cover). Efforts should be made to warm the child by other methods also.

Tranexamic acid

Currently, no firm recommendations exist in children on the use of tranexamic acid in major haemorrhage. However, the results of adult studies suggest there may be some benefit in situations where fibrinolysis is likely to be ongoing, particularly if given early (within 1 hour). The dose in children is 20 mg/kg, although much higher doses have been used in cardiac surgery (50–100 mg/kg). It should be administered under haematological advice.

Imaging and transfer within the hospital

The patient should not be transferred for CT scan until haemodynamic stability has been achieved, unless it is co-located with the ED and scanning can take place as resuscitation continues. If haemodynamic stability cannot be achieved, it may be necessary to take the child straight to the operating theatre for haemorrhage control first.

By establishing a team approach to these patients and utilizing the available expertise, it should be possible for the initial assessment, resuscitation and stabilization to be successfully undertaken by the admitting hospital, prior to the arrival of a retrieval team or transfer to definitive care.

What do I need to consider before transfer to another centre?

If a child is actively haemorrhaging at the time transfer is anticipated, the transfer should be delayed until haemorrhage control has been established, even if this means undertaking haemorrhage control surgery at the referring hospital. An ambulance is not a safe environment for a child with ongoing haemorrhage. Transfer of the stable child should then be undertaken only by an expert retrieval team. If blood products have been commenced prior to transfer, it is perfectly reasonable to continue these during the journey, with the proviso that any blood product transfusions are completed within the 4 hour time-frame allowed.

Transfer of blood products may be necessary if the child is still actively bleeding or they are likely to go for immediate surgery on arrival. Under these circumstances, products should be issued by the blood bank in the referring hospital. They should liaise with the blood bank at the receiving hospital; products should be transferred in appropriate, sealed containers, with the necessary paperwork. The products should then be reissued at the receiving hospital if the blood bank is satisfied that the transfer has been undertaken appropriately. Failure to do this is likely to result in the products being wasted and may compromise the child's safety at the receiving hospital.

Problems with blood product administration in children

Blood administration

Always administer blood products manually by syringe or by infusion pump in smaller children (< 10 kg), due to the risks of over-transfusion if a free-running giving set is used. Even with massive haemorrhage it is usually possible to keep up with losses in this way. Care must always be taken to ensure that the three-way tap and giving set are not left open between boluses.

Complications

The main complications of transfusion are related to either the products being administered or the process of administration itself. Table 21.2 gives a list of the early and late complications that may occur as a consequence of administration of blood products. The main life-threatening complications of transfusion are transfusion-related circulatory overload (TRACO) and transfusion-related acute lung injury (TRALI).

Table 21.2. Early and late complications of blood product transfusion.

Timing	Complications
Early	Febrile reaction Allergic reaction (urticarial and anaphylactic) Incompatibility reaction (ABO and non-ABO) Transfusion-related circulatory overload (TRACO) Complications related to massive transfusion (hypothermia, hypocalcaemia, hyperkalaemia, acid–base disturbance) Bacterial contamination
Late	Transfusion-related acute lung injury (TRALI) Graft-versus-host disease (GVHD) Transmission of infection Post-transfusion purpura

Transfusion-associated circulatory overload (TRACO)

This is a pathological condition related to rapid or massive transfusion, characterized by:

- respiratory distress
- tachycardia
- hypertension
- evidence of pulmonary oedema on CXR occurring within a few hours of blood product administration.

Children most at risk are those under 3 years of age. Management involves stopping the transfusion, and administration of oxygen and diuretics. In severe cases, positive-pressure ventilation and inotropic support may be necessary.

Transfusion-related acute lung injury (TRALI)

TRALI produces many of the clinical symptoms of TRACO, but is a distinct entity. The pathological changes are caused by neutrophil activation within the pulmonary microvasculature. The lung injury leads to high-permeability pulmonary oedema, with respiratory distress and hypoxaemia, but no evidence of circulatory overload. Treatment is supportive, with positive airway pressure or mechanical ventilation, depending on the degree of respiratory compromise.

Summary

Administration of blood products to children is likely in many of the commonly encountered critical illness or injury scenarios, so the attending clinicians should have a good understanding of the main considerations specific to the child. Good lines of communication need to be established with blood bank and haematology staff early on in the child's admission.

Golden rules

- Blood product administration carries significant morbidity
- When indicated blood transfusion needs to be organized and timely
- Every hospital should have a massive transfusion protocol to speed up administration of blood products where needed
- Irradiated blood is needed for children with immunodeficiency syndromes

Further reading

Association of Anaesthetists of Great Britain and Ireland. Blood transfusion and the anaesthetist: management of massive haemorrhage. *Anaesthesia* 2010;**65**:1153–1161.

British Committee for Standards in Haematology. Transfusion guidelines for neonates and older children. *Brit J Haematol* 2004;**124**:433–453 (amended in 2005 and 2007). http://www.bcshguidelines.com/4_HAEMATOLOGY_GUIDELINES.html.

McLelland DBL (ed.). *Handbook of Transfusion Medicine*, 4th edn. NHS Blood and Transplant. London: The Stationery Office, 2007. http://www.transfusionguidelines.org.uk/.

The sick neonate presenting with shock

Fiona Reynolds

Introduction

The sick neonate may present to the emergency department with a range of symptoms from poor feeding through to collapse with shock. The differential diagnosis of the sick, shocked neonate is different from that in other stages of life.

The difficulties in diagnosis should not detract from the basic steps of ensuring oxygen delivery to tissues. The immediate management of a neonate who presents in shock follows the principles set out in Chapter 4.

Most of the conditions mentioned below are discussed in greater detail within their respective chapters. This chapter aims to give a brief overview of the main pathologies that affect neonates as well as giving advice about management.

Initial management

Airway and breathing

The management of the airway in neonates follows the same principles as that in older children. The decision to intubate a neonate is a clinical decision based on:

- paediatric GCS score
- airway obstruction
- respiratory failure
- persistent apnoeas.

Glasgow Coma Scale

Although difficult to assess, an attempt should be made to assess the consciousness level of the neonate using an appropriate Glasgow Coma Scale (GCS) scoring system (see Chapter 35).

Airway obstruction

The airway may be obstructed as a consequence of shock or decreased consciousness or due to pathologies such as inflammation or infection. Additionally, congenital conditions such as laryngomalacia may affect the neonate. The child may present with sterterous breathing or stridor (as discussed in Chapter 15) depending on the condition.

If the airway is compromised to the point of compromising ventilation then intubation is likely to be indicated. If there is concern about airway calibre, a careful, planned gas induction is warranted (as in Chapter 15).

Managing the Critically Ill Child, ed. Richard Skone *et al.* Published by Cambridge University Press.

Respiratory failure

It is important to identify respiratory failure rapidly and intervene promptly. Delaying intubation in severe respiratory failure may turn a difficult procedure into a high-risk one in many instances.

Apnoeas

Sick neonates suffering from respiratory failure may suffer apnoeas. They should not be ignored, as they are a sign of severe disease. The apnoeas themselves are often easy to manage by stimulating the child or by bagging them.

If the child is stable and the apnoeas are short then a child with bronchiolitis may be observed, or treated with CPAP. However, if a child comes in with signs of shock and apnoeas, or the apnoeas are increasing in frequency and duration, then intubation is indicated.

Never forget, apnoeas may be a symptom of hypoglycaemia in the neonate.

Circulation

The management of the paediatric circulation, again, follows the same principle as that in older children. That is:

- give fluid boluses of 10–20 ml/kg
- watch for a response in heart rate, capillary refill and blood pressure
- gain intravenous (IV) access early
- move to intraosseous (IO) access if IV access is not possible within 90 seconds
- if in doubt about choice of inotropes, start with adrenaline or dopamine.

The main differences in neonates, when managing the circulation, are that:

- it is important to correct calcium levels
- it doesn't take much fluid loss to become hypovolaemic (circulating volume is only 80–90 ml/kg)
- neonates should be cross-matched early.

Attention to detail

This is perhaps the area that causes the most problems to doctors who manage children. Small derangements in physiology can have a disproportionate effect on the child. Factors that need to be actively managed include:

- temperature (hypothermia and hyperthermia)
- blood glucose
- sodium and calcium levels
- ET tube size and position (length).

Conditions that affect neonates

Septic shock (Chapter 5)

Septic shock is the most common reason for cardiovascular collapse in the neonate. The most common pathogens include:

- group B *Streptococci*
- *Escherichia coli*
- herpes simplex virus
- enterovirus.

The presentation of the septic neonate is often non-specific, with poor feeding, crying and listlessness, or an unusually quiet baby. Pyrexia or hypothermia may be present. Tachypnoea may reflect pyrexia or an attempt to compensate for metabolic acidosis. Tachycardia with poor perfusion and cold hands and feet may be present along with hypotension.

The stabilization of the neonate with septic shock follows the principles outlined in Chapters 4 and 5:

- optimize oxygen delivery
- fluid balance
- electrolytes and glucose correction
- temperature control.

Neonates with shock should receive antibiotics early according to local policy, e.g. amoxicillin and cefotaxime. Aciclovir should also be considered. The administration of antibiotics is time-critical as delay increases mortality.

Congenital heart disease (Chapter 6)

Many neonates with congenital heart disease (CHD) are identified by antenatal ultrasound scans. However, some neonates may present to the ED with cyanosis or shock secondary to a previously unsuspected CHD. The deterioration usually coincides with the physiological closure of the ductus arteriosus (DA). Re-opening of the DA with prostaglandin E1 or E2 (PgE) will improve the circulation in most cases (see Chapter 6).

In the shocked state opening of the ductus arteriosus is only one part of the treatment required. Some thought should be given to what the primary problem associated with the child's CHD is. The circulatory problem may relate to:

- reduced pulmonary blood flow
- reduced systemic blood flow
- globally impaired ventricular function.

Reduced pulmonary blood flow

The neonate with reduced pulmonary blood flow to the lungs from a right-sided obstruction, e.g. tricuspid atresia, will present with cyanosis, which will increase as the DA closes. The increasing hypoxaemia may lead to tissue hypoxia, hypoperfusion and shock. It may be impossible to differentiate from the neonate with septic shock.

The resuscitation should aim to increase oxygen delivery with artificial ventilation, optimizing preload and cardiac contractility. The induction agent should be chosen to minimize the effect on cardiac output. Ketamine is often chosen for this reason.

If cardiac disease cannot be confidently excluded PgE should be commenced by intravenous infusion. The re-opening of the DA allows increased pulmonary blood flow and improvement in saturations. PgE may cause apnoea if ventilation is not controlled.

Reduced systemic blood flow

Poor femoral pulses may give a clue to an obstructive left-sided heart lesion but may also reflect poor perfusion in a neonate with a structurally normal heart. A difference in saturations between the right hand and the lower limbs is also suggestive of congenital heart disease.

The resuscitation aims are to restore oxygenation and cardiac output. Restoration of cardiac output is dependent on re-opening of the DA as well as the optimization of preload, myocardial contractility and afterload.

Globally impaired ventricular function

Impaired ventricular function may occur as a primary condition in:

- cardiomyopathy
- myocarditis
- myocardial ischaemia from congenital abnormalities of coronary arteries.

Secondary impairment of cardiac function may occur in conditions such as critical aortic stenosis and coarctation of the aorta.

Neonates with impairment of cardiac function may have respiratory distress, hepatomegaly and enlarged heart with pulmonary oedema on CXR. Emergency treatment aims to optimize oxygen delivery. This may require intubation and ventilation to reduce oxygen consumption by reducing the work of breathing. As in adults, a high-risk induction of anaesthesia would need to be undertaken, allowing extra time for circulation of drugs.

Arrhythmia

Abnormalities of heart rhythm may be either slow or fast arrhythmias. These may present before birth with fetal distress and hydrops or after birth with poor feeding, respiratory distress or shock.

Supraventricular arrhythmias are often well tolerated. An unremitting supraventricular arrhythmia or a ventricular arrhythmia will result in impaired ventricular function and potentially shock. ECG monitoring is sometimes omitted in infants thought to have simple respiratory distress. This can lead to a delayed diagnosis of a supraventricular tachycardia. A 12-lead ECG is required if an arrhythmia cannot be excluded on the standard ECG. If interpretation is difficult it can be faxed to the local paediatric cardiologist.

The management of arrhythmias is dealt with in Chapter 6.

Metabolic disease (Chapter 12)

Metabolic disease in the neonatal period may present with:

- encephalopathy
- cardiomyopathy
- severe metabolic acidosis
- hyperventilation
- hypoglycaemia
- shock
- hyperammonaemia.

Hyperventilation may be secondary to metabolic acidosis. It may also be secondary to hyperammonaemia, which stimulates the respiratory centre and drives a respiratory alkalosis.

Initially the cardiovascular system tolerates the metabolic derangement but the progressive acidosis will adversely affect myocardial contractility and tissue hypoxia will compound the primary metabolic derangement.

Metabolic disease should be suspected in any infant presenting with shock. Measurement of plasma ammonia levels is important in any shocked infant in whom the diagnosis is not clear. Treatment to reduce ammonia levels is time-critical in order to optimize neurological outcome. The emergency treatment of hyperammonaemia is described in Chapter 12.

Glucose delivery in intravenous fluids is important to provide substrate and promote anabolism, which may help reverse the metabolic derangement.

The key steps in management of inherited metabolic disease in a neonate are:

- treatment of shock
- delivery of glucose
- emergency treatment of hyperammonaemia (if present).

Non-accidental injury (Chapter 30)

Non-accidental injury may present with shock. Injury may cause occult bleeding leading to cardiovascular compromise. The most common form of non-accidental injury is abusive head trauma. Intracranial blood loss may be of sufficient volume to cause cardiovascular compromise or anaemia in the small infant.

Endocrine disease

A deficiency of adrenal steroids may present with cardiovascular compromise. Steroid deficiency is suggested by:

- hyponatraemia
- hyperkalaemia
- hypoglycaemia.

Steroid deficiency in the neonatal period is most commonly secondary to congenital adrenal hyperplasia, which results in virilization of female infants. This may be evident at birth, although presentation may be delayed in male infants.

Treatment requires rehydration with saline, glucose infusion and steroid replacement.

Technical details (size of equipment)

Most of the sizes and tips for accomplishing technical procedures are found in Chapter 37. However, this is a brief summary of the immediate life-saving equipment that needs to be at hand.

Airway and breathing

Bagging patients

It is vitally important to use the correct-size facemask for neonates. The appropriate-size oropharyngeal airway should be used early in order to improve airway management and minimize gastric insufflation. A nasogastric tube should also be inserted early in order to minimize the impact of air passing into the stomach.

Make sure that the bag attached to the ventilation circuit, such as a T-piece, is the right size. Too large a bag encourages hyperinflation with each breath.

Intubation

Start with a size 3.5 mm endotracheal tube (ET tube) for a full-term neonate who weighs about 3 kg. It is important to have smaller and larger ET tube available and ready. A bougie that passes down a small ET tube should also be readily available. Make sure that the head is in the neutral position when intubating.

If the ET tube inserted is the wrong size, i.e. the leak is too large, change to a larger ET tube over a bougie once the child has been preoxygenated.

Circulation

Intravenous access

If a neonate presents in cardiac arrest, the first line for access is the intraosseous route. If there is time, most of the drugs needed during the resuscitation of a sick neonate can be given through a 24G cannula. However, if large volumes of fluid are needed, e.g. sepsis or trauma, a 22G cannula will be needed, usually sited in the long saphenous or femoral vein.

Central venous access

Central venous access should be gained if the operator feels able. Ultrasound-guided insertion of a 4.5 or 5FG central venous catheter (CVC) is the usual means of access.

Arterial line

A 24G cannula is usually used to site an arterial line in the radial or posterior tibial artery in neonates. If these are not palpable, then a 22G cannula (or Seldinger arterial line) in the femoral artery (preferably under ultrasound guidance) will often be more straightforward.

Capillary gases

Capillary gas analyses will be performed by paediatricians as a surrogate for arterial blood gases. They can provide important information, but are prone to certain errors. For example:

- blood glucose can be unreliable if the child has any sugary substance on their hand/foot
- lactate and potassium can be falsely elevated if the sample has been difficult to obtain
- it usually does not reflect the arterial oxygen tension
- if peripheral perfusion is very poor all figures are likely to be inaccurate.

The information that can be gleaned from a capillary sample includes:

- a normal potassium or lactate is probably normal
- a high lactate, base deficit or potassium from a good flowing sample is probably high
- a high $PaCO_2$ from a good sample is probably high.

As a result all capillary samples should be interpreted in the context of the clinical assessment of the child. Abnormal results that do not fit the clinical picture should be rechecked, or confirmed with an arterial sample, if possible.

Summary

The management of specific conditions in neonates is detailed in individual chapters within this book. However, when managing a small baby the main differences are the wider differential diagnosis, immature physiology and paying scrupulous attention to detail.

Golden rules

- Attention to detail is the key to managing neonates
- Always consider cardiac and metabolic conditions
- If in doubt about whether the pathology is cardiac start PgE
- Check all of the blood gas parameters – especially glucose and electrolytes
- Seek expert advice early

Ongoing management of the successful arrest

Barney Scholefield

Introduction

The return of a pulse during paediatric resuscitation is often seen as a triumph for the resuscitation team, the child and their family. However, for the critical care physician the hard part is to yet come in managing the post-resuscitation phase.

The four phases of resuscitation (Table 23.1) need to be expertly managed to minimize further injury to the child and maximize the chance of a permanent return of spontaneous circulation (ROSC) with successful short- and long-term outcomes.

Table 23.1. The four phases of cardiac arrest.

Phase	Interventions
1. Pre-arrest phase (prevention)	Child safety and injury prevention strategies Early recognition of patient deterioration through adequate patient monitoring and early-warning systems
2. No-flow 'arrest' (period of cardiac arrest prior to starting CPR)	Minimize delay to basic and advanced life support Rapid cardiac arrest team activation Minimize delay to defibrillation
3. Low-flow 'resuscitation' (CPR in progress)	'Excellent' CPR to optimize coronary and cerebral perfusion Avoidance of over-ventilation whilst maintaining adequate ventilation and oxygenation Treat reversible causes of cardiac arrest
4. Post-resuscitation phase (post-ROSC)	Optimize coronary and cerebral perfusion Treat arrhythmias Manage 'post-cardiac-arrest syndrome' (see Table 23.2) Rehabilitation

This chapter aims to highlight the epidemiology of paediatric cardiac arrest, emphasizing the differences between adults and children. It will also highlight the current recommendations for post-resuscitation management, in particular those targeting the post-cardiac-arrest syndrome during the 'immediate' and 'early post-arrest' stages. Interventions during these stages, prior to the safe transfer to a tertiary paediatric intensive care unit, may improve the patient's overall outcome.

Managing the Critically Ill Child, ed. Richard Skone *et al.* Published by Cambridge University Press.

Why are paediatric arrests different from adult?

The overall incidence of out-of-hospital cardiac arrests in children younger than 16 years old is low (8–20/100 000/year). It is much more frequent in infants less than 1 year old, reaching an incidence comparable to adult levels of 70/100 000/year. The in-hospital cardiac arrest incidence in children is nearly 100 times higher than out-of-hospital. Unfortunately, the survival and neurological outcome from cardiac arrest remains poor. Out-of-hospital survival rates are reported to be as low as 5–12%, with only 0.3–4% being neurologically intact.

Paediatric cardiac arrests are usually secondary to severe respiratory compromise or circulatory shock. These lead to a respiratory arrest with subsequent hypoxia-induced cardiac arrest, usually presenting as a non-shockable rhythm. This contrasts with the much higher incidence of ischaemic heart disease in adults, where cardiac arrest is often secondary to a myocardial infarction-induced shockable rhythm.

Nearly 50% of children who suffer a cardiac arrest will also have a chronic underlying condition such as:

- congenital cardiac disorders
- chronic respiratory conditions (e.g. asthma)
- neurological and developmental impairment.

Awareness of the differences in aetiology is important. Early reversal of the cause of the respiratory arrest can quickly convert a weakly perfusing or impalpable pulse into an adequate one. The existence of preceding severe illness with resultant acidosis and hypoxia can lead to significant neurological and systemic damage before the true cardiac arrest occurs. However, this cannot be ascertained until later, after stabilization and further neurological assessment.

The currently recommended compression to ventilation ratio of 15:2 for all infants and children is a compromise. It aims to provide enough ventilation for oxygenation, and sufficient cardiac compressions to provide adequate coronary and cerebral perfusion.

In studies of adult patients suffering from ventricular fibrillation the success of compression-only resuscitation is due to the retained aortic blood oxygen concentration and pulmonary oxygen reservoir. Only 14% of paediatric cardiac arrests present with a sudden-onset shockable rhythm, hence there is a need for both ventilation and compressions in the vast majority of cases.

Post-cardiac-arrest syndrome

The post-resuscitation stage after ROSC is the period of highest risk of developing ventricular arrhythmias and reperfusion injuries. The International Liaison Committee on Resuscitation consensus statement and current paediatric resuscitation guidelines now emphasize the existence of the 'post-cardiac-arrest syndrome' (PCAS). This syndrome is the consequence of prolonged whole-body ischaemia and reperfusion affecting the brain and myocardium. It also has systemic effects similar to those seen in severe sepsis.

PCAS can be divided into four phases with specific treatment goals:

- immediate post-arrest (first 20 min)
- early post-arrest (20 min to 6–12 h)
- intermediate (6–12 to 72 h)
- recovery phase (3 days onwards).

Post-cardiac-arrest therapeutic hypothermia applied during the intermediate phase after adult ventricular fibrillation has produced positive results in some studies. This has renewed focus on specific therapies that could further improve survival and neurological outcome after cardiac arrest (Table 23.2).

Table 23.2. Monitoring and treatment targets for the post-cardiac-arrest syndrome.

Post-cardiac-arrest syndrome	Monitoring strategy	Potential therapy	Physiological target	Pitfalls
Pyrexia	Core (rectal, oesophageal and bladder) temperature monitoring	Therapeutic hypothermia or strict normothermia	Initially target temperature 33–37°C	Avoidance of temperature <32°C or >38°C
Seizures	Clinical signs CFAM or EEG monitoring	Benzodiazepines, phenytoin, phenobarbitone	Cessation of clinical and sub-clinical seizures	Hypotension, over-treatment
Hyperoxia, hypoxia	Saturation monitoring, arterial PaO_2	'Normoxia'	100% O_2 during arrest Titrate O_2 to achieve sats of 94–96% post arrest	New diagnosis of congenital heart disease
Hypercapnia, hypocapnia	Arterial $PaCO_2$, $ETCO_2$	'Normo'ventilation	Aim $PaCO_2$ 4.5–5.5 kPa (normocapnia)	
Cerebral perfusion	Haemodynamic monitoring	Fluid therapy Inotropic support, vasopressors Head-up 45-degree position	Physiological age-specific normal parameters for blood pressure (see Chapter 19)	Consider need for neuroradiology (e.g. cranial CT scan)
Myocardial dysfunction	Clinical signs, heart rate, blood pressure, liver size, capillary refill, central venous pressure	Fluid therapy. colloid, crystalloid or blood products as required Inotropic support: dobutamine or adrenaline	Physiological age specific normal parameters Urine output >1 ml/kg Improving lactic acidosis	Potential acquired heart disease (e.g. myocarditis or cardiomyopathy)

CFAM, continuous functional amplitude integrated electroencephalography monitoring; EEG, electroencephalography; sats, saturation; $ETCO_2$, end-tidal carbon dioxide; BP, blood pressure.

The brain

The brain is the most vulnerable organ in the body when subjected to hypoxia and ischaemia during cardiac arrest. Even the best, closed-chest standard CPR can only achieve

50% of normal cerebral blood flow. The cascade of neurologically damaging processes that occur during cardiac arrest and over the following hours to days leads to neurodegeneration by a number of mechanisms:

- impaired cerebrovascular reactivity
- cerebral oedema
- cerebral hyperaemia
- post-ischaemic biochemical cascades.

The extent of damage is dependent on numerous factors, including the duration of cardiac arrest and the area of the brain affected. The subsequent brain injury can manifest as:

- seizures
- cognitive dysfunction
- myoclonus
- stroke
- coma or persistent vegetative state
- brain death.

Neurological assessment

Assessment and recording of the patient's neurological status, both before cardiac arrest and after ROSC, can aid prognostication. A short period of assessment prior to administering intravenous sedation and neuromuscular blockade can help to ascertain the neurological status. If possible, the following should be assessed:

- formal recording of when the patient starts to gasp or make spontaneous respiratory effort
- the components of the GCS
- pupillary size and pupillary reactivity.

Timing of sedation or anaesthesia and the use of neuromuscular blockade will depend on the patient's neurological status and haemodynamic stability after ROSC. Rarely, the patient will wake up, demonstrate intact recovery and be rapidly extubated. Usually, the patient will remain comatose, and require continued ventilatory and haemodynamic support. Sedation will need to be adequate to manage the patient on the ventilator and aid additional interventions, such as central venous access and targeted temperature management.

The heart

The paediatric myocardium is remarkably resilient following cardiac arrest and in cases where the underlying problem is not related to the heart, such as asphyxial arrests, the heart can recover function within 12–24 hours.

In the immediate and early post-arrest phase, function is impaired due to profound systemic vasoconstriction and cellular acidosis. Initial support for the myocardium involves the following:

- adequate fluid resuscitation
- targeting normal blood pressure for age
- monitoring of perfusion and central venous pressure to avoid circulatory overload
- inotropic support of the myocardium to achieve these goals.

The choice of inotrope follows the same rationale as in adults, and depends on the balance between inotropy and vasoconstriction. The former favours the use of adrenaline or dobutamine, whilst the latter is best achieved with noradrenaline.

Specific interventions

Hyperthermia and hypothermia

Hyperthermia after cardiac arrest is common and there is strong evidence linking core temperature above 38°C with worse neurological outcome. Hyperthermia should trigger targeted temperature management to reduce the core temperature.

Targeted temperature management to produce mild hypothermia (32–34°C) has been used with success after adult ventricular fibrillation cardiac arrest. It has also been shown to be safe and effective in neonates suffering hypoxic–ischaemic encephalopathy soon after birth. Mild hypothermia after paediatric cardiac arrest is utilized by some paediatric critical care units. Patients are cooled to a temperature of 33–34°C for 24 to 48 hours, followed by gradual, controlled rewarming. Avoidance of temperatures below 32°C is essential, as this is associated with the following:

- worse survival
- arrhythmias
- immune suppression
- coagulopathy
- infections.

Shivering should be prevented by the use of adequate sedation and neuromuscular blockade.

During the discussion for tertiary transfer of the post-cardiac-arrest patient, a decision on the target temperature should be made, whilst undertaking accurate and continuous core temperature monitoring.

Various methods for targeted temperature management are available including:

- surface cooling with wet blankets
- servo-controlled air or fluid cooling blankets
- boluses of cold intravenous fluids (10 ml/kg at 4°C over 10 minutes)
- intravenous cooling catheters (unsuitable in smaller children).

Anticonvulsants

The incidence of seizures after paediatric cardiac arrest has been reported to be as high as 47%, with 35% of patients in refractory SE. Seizures can produce further secondary neurological damage by increasing metabolic demand. They should be identified quickly and treated.

In post-cardiac-arrest patients who remain comatose, sedated and receiving neuromuscular blocking drugs, identification of seizures will require a high level of clinical suspicion, unless continuous neurophysiological monitoring is undertaken. Clues include unexpected changes in pupillary size and abrupt changes in heart rate or blood pressure.

Treatment of identified or suspected seizures will follow standard guidelines (see Chapter 10).

Oxygen: hypoxia and hyperoxia

Maintaining adequate ventilation and oxygenation is essential during resuscitation and post-resuscitation care. Hypoxia will cause continued secondary brain injury and must be avoided. Hyperoxia (defined as $PaO_2 > 40$ kPa) may also be associated with worse survival. In children, the commonly occurring respiratory compromise preceding cardiac arrest necessitates high-concentration oxygen therapy during the low-flow resuscitation and in the early post-resuscitation phase. Targeting oxygen saturations between 94 and 96%, with a reduction in FiO_2, would appear appropriate whilst avoiding hypoxia.

If anaemia or carbon monoxide poisoning is suspected, then the highest concentration of oxygen should be administered.

Cardiac arrest in the infant may be secondary to unidentified congenital cardiac disease. Initial resuscitation of these infants with a high FiO_2 is appropriate; however, introduction of alprostadil (Prostin) and reduction of FiO_2 to 0.5 is necessary in a suspected or confirmed duct-dependent circulation and should be discussed with a paediatric intensivist or cardiologist (see Chapter 6).

Ventilation: hypocapnia, hypercapnia

During and after cardiac arrest cerebral autoreactivity is often lost; however, cerebrovasular reactivity can be preserved. Therefore targeting normocapnia ($PaCO_2$ 4.5–5.5 kPa) through controlled age-appropriate ventilatory rates is recommended. Hypoventilation may cause hypoxia and raise intracranial pressure due to hyperaemia. Hyperventilation may cause further cerebral ischaemia and risks raising intrathoracic pressure and impairing cardiac venous return to an already stunned myocardium.

Metabolic control

Hypoglycaemia and hyperglycaemia

Post-cardiac-arrest paediatric patients are at high risk of developing hypoglycaemia (plasma glucose < 3.0 mmol/l). Early glucose monitoring and correction with 2 ml/kg of 10% dextrose followed by a continuous infusion of a glucose-containing solution is essential to avoid neurological damage and seizures. Hyperglycaemia (plasma glucose > 13 mmol/l) can also occur as a physiological stress response and is associated with worse outcome. However, aggressive glucose control with insulin in the non-diabetic patient has not been proven to be beneficial in the paediatric population and hyperglycaemia will usually correct itself within a few hours.

Metabolic acidosis

Profound metabolic acidosis is common during cardiac arrest and after ROSC. However, the routine use of sodium bicarbonate solution is not recommended. Evidence in other critically ill states (e.g. adults with septic shock) has failed to show improvements in haemodynamics when metabolic acidosis is treated with sodium bicarbonate. However, acidosis may depress the action of catecholamine, so treatment may be considered in the following situations:

- acidosis with resistance to catecholamine therapy
- cardiac arrest secondary to tricyclic antidepressant overdose
- hyperkalaemia
- hypermagnesaemia.

Sodium bicarbonate administration will need adequate ventilation, due to the production of carbon dioxide.

Further investigations and child protection

During the stabilization and management of the post-cardiac-arrest syndrome further investigations and clinical history will be required to guide ongoing therapy. Table 23.3 outlines, with reasons, useful investigations for use after all cardiac arrests in infants and children, with suggestions for additional investigation in certain circumstances.

Blood tests

Routine blood sampling for haematological and biochemical blood tests, blood glucose analysis and arterial blood gas analysis will allow rapid correction of physiological derangement and allow manipulation of the post-cardiac-arrest syndrome treatment strategies. Additional blood testing is indicated for specific conditions such as:

- toxicology for poisoning
- carbon monoxide assessment post-burns or fires
- metabolic investigations (especially plasma ammonia and lactate where inborn error of metabolism is suspected).

Other investigations

A chest radiograph will be helpful to assess ET and NG tube placement. If there is any suspicion of head trauma, an acute intracranial bleed or raised intracranial pressure, urgent cranial computed tomography scans should be arranged.

Child protection considerations

In all out-of-hospital cardiac arrest situations involving infants and children, consideration should be given to the initiation of full child protection investigation proceedings (see Chapter 30). Any infant or child who dies unexpectedly in the UK is subject to a sudden unexpected death in infancy (SUDI) investigation by a trained team of clinicians, social workers and police. A 'near-miss' unexpected death, as is the case in most resuscitated cardiac arrests, should undergo the same level of investigation to ensure non-accidental injury is not missed as a cause of cardiac arrest. Accurate history-taking and recording of information during and after resuscitation will be invaluable, not just in the cases of non-accidental injury, but also in helping families during the aftermath of the cardiac arrest if the child dies.

Table 23.3. Post-resuscitation investigations.

	Post-resuscitation investigation	Reason
For all cardiac arrests	Full blood count and clotting screen and group and save for cross-match	Baseline haematology
	Sodium, potassium, urea and creatinine	Baseline biochemistry Risk of hyperkalaemia and renal failure
	Arterial blood gas analysis	Targeting oxygenation and carbon dioxide level Assess acid–base status Rule out carbon monoxide exposure (if required)
	Glucose	Hypoglycaemia, hyperglycaemia
	Chest radiograph (CXR)	Post-intubation tube check, Assess underlying lung pathology
	Electrocardiograph (ECG)	Evidence of myocardial ischaemia/ infarction Underlying arrhythmias (prolonged QT interval)
	Microbiology cultures: blood and/ or urine cultures	Investigation of sepsis with prompt, appropriate antibiotic treatment
Additional investigations if indicated	Computed tomography (CT)	Rule out acute intraventricular bleed or hydrocephalus. Also consider chest or abdominal pathology
	Child protection investigation	Involving local child protection team, social services and police should be considered promptly in ALL out-of-hospital cardiac arrests in children
	Further investigations for unknown cause of cardiac arrest	Toxicology screen (urine and blood) Inborn error of metabolism screen

Retrieval and transportation considerations

Post-cardiac-arrest patients with sustained ROSC will require transportation to a paediatric critical care unit for a number of reasons:

- continued management of their post-cardiac-arrest syndrome
- ongoing investigation and treatment of the underlying cause for the cardiac arrest
- sufficient time to allow accurate prognostication of the likely survival outcome.

Stabilization and preparation for transportation of the critically ill child are covered in greater detail in Chapter 24.

In the post-cardiac-arrest scenario, early discussion with the destination intensive care unit regarding appropriate physiological targets can be helpful. During transportation the parameters detailed in Table 23.4 should be maintained:

Table 23.4. Targets for physiological parameters.

Ventilation to achieve normocapnia ($PaCO_2$ 4.5–5.5 kPa)
Oxygenation to target arterial saturations of 94–96%
Myocardial and circulatory support to maintain age-appropriate normal haemodynamic values
ECG monitoring for arrhythmias
Neurological assessment of seizures and GCS
Continued core temperature monitoring to target temperature range (33–37°C)

Summary

The successful resuscitation of an infant or child is just the start of an important phase in post-cardiac-arrest care. During the period of stabilization prior to transportation to a paediatric intensive care unit, monitoring and early management of the post-cardiac-arrest syndrome can potentially limit further damage to the brain and other vital organs. The historically poor survival and neurological outcome seen after paediatric cardiac arrest can be improved by applying the increasing body of evidence-based practice outlined in this chapter.

Golden rules

- Monitor temperature continuously
- Pay close attention to electrolytes and glucose
- Be aware of potential for seizures
- Once things have settled, consider further investigations and child protection issues
- Contact PICU early and set targets for temperature and ventilation

Further reading

Berg R, Zaristky A, Nadkarni V. Paediatric cardiopulmonary resuscitation. In Fuhrman BP, Zimmerman JJ (eds.), *Paediatric Critical Care*, 3rd edn. St Louis: Mosby, 2006.

Samuels M, Wieteska S (eds.). *Advanced Paediatric Life Support*, 5th edn. Oxford: Blackwell, 2011.

The Royal College of Pathologists and The Royal College of Paediatrics and Child Health. Sudden unexpected death in infancy. A multiagency protocol for care and investigation. http://www.rcpch.ac.uk/sites/default/files/SUDI_report_for_web.pdf.

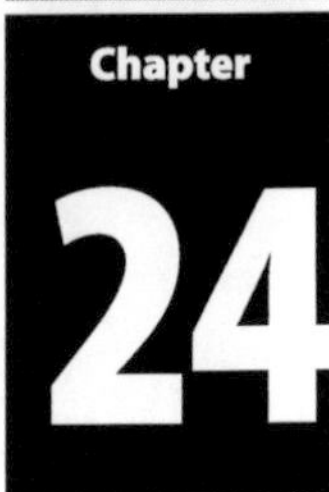

Referring-team-led transfers

Andrew J. Baldock and Gareth D. Jones

Introduction

Transfers conducted by referring teams are usually performed for neurosurgical emergencies. Occasionally clinicians from a referring hospital may also be asked to perform transfers to PICU for non-neurosurgical patients.

This chapter aims to provide a reference point for those individuals tasked with fulfilling these obligations. The emphasis is on neurosurgical transfers, but the same principles apply to other pathologies. Further details on the management of specific conditions can be found in the relevant chapters.

Planning for transfers

Children who need to be transferred to a tertiary centre must be identified early and referred to the regional specialists, e.g. neurosurgeons and paediatric intensive care teams, at the first available opportunity.

The decision to transfer a child must be taken by senior clinicians in each hospital, and only after appropriate resuscitation and stabilization have taken place. Once the child has been stabilized, and the decision taken to transfer, management is focussed on the prevention of secondary injury and on the safety of the child in transit to the definitive centre.

In anticipation of the above scenario local guidelines should be written for paediatric transfers. They should contain:

- clear contact information for the regional referral teams
- defined management goals
- named personnel who will undertake the transfer (e.g. senior anaesthetist and trained assistant)
- details on how these staff will be freed from other duties
- details of the equipment to be used during transfer for children of all ages.

In the case of neurosurgical emergencies, they should be written as a collaboration between local hospitals and the regional neurosurgical and critical care services. The local ambulance service should also contribute to such guidelines, in order to respond appropriately to requests that the neurosurgical team have defined as time-critical.

Managing the Critically Ill Child, ed. Richard Skone *et al.* Published by Cambridge University Press.

Preparing the patient for transfer

Anticipating problems can make them a lot easier to manage. Table 24.1 addresses common questions that face the clinician when preparing a patient for transfer.

Table 24.1. Likely management questions when preparing for transfer.

Management questions for transfer	Answers
Should I intubate?	Consider intubation if: • There is an obvious clinical indication at presentation • The patient is deteriorating despite treatment • There is any chance that the patient will need intubation during the transfer • It is being used as a treatment modality; e.g. control of CO_2 in head injury or oxygen delivery in carbon monoxide poisoning
Do I need a nasal ET tube?	No. A well secured oral ET tube will usually suffice and a nasal tube may be contraindicated
What sedation should I use?	Whatever the transfer team is happy to use, as long as it is age-appropriate. Morphine and midazolam are commonly used in paediatrics. Propofol is controversial in children, but can be used in the short term
Should I paralyse the patient?	Most retrieval teams will routinely paralyse patients for transfer (with an infusion of muscle relaxant)
Do I need an arterial line?	Consider if: • Cardiovascularly unstable • Non-invasive readings are unreliable • Accurate blood pressure readings are essential Arterial line should not delay a timely transfer in time-critical conditions, but can be hugely beneficial
Do I need a central line?	Consider if: • IV access is difficult/inadequate • Inotropes are being administered • CVP monitoring is necessary to guide treatment Central line should not delay a timely transfer as IO needles can be used for most access/drugs
How much of everything do I need?	Make certain that you have enough oxygen/infusion drugs to last at least twice the expected duration of transfer, and anticipate traffic or ambulance breakdown

Table 24.1. *(cont.)*

Management questions for transfer	Answers
When should I contact the destination hospital	Contact: • As soon as the need for tertiary intervention is recognized • Immediately prior to leaving your hospital 10 minutes before arrival
What problems can occur specific to transfers?	Hypothermia • Measure temperature throughout Lack of assistance • Make sure that a mobile phone is at hand throughout Limited supplies (see above) Difficult to get to patient • The ambulance should stop where safe if any intervention is being carried out

Intubation and spinal protection

A controlled intubation pre-departure is likely to be safer than attempting to secure an airway en route. As a result, any patient with a GCS < 9 or a fall in GCS of more than 3 should be intubated for transfer. Similarly a low threshold should be applied to any patient whose respiratory or cardiovascular function is likely to deteriorate en route.

Triple immobilization with a hard collar, blocks and tape should be instigated for head injuries, and maintained throughout the transfer. A NG tube should be considered for all patients prior to transfer.

Ventilation

All patients requiring ventilation for transfer should be adequately sedated and paralysed. This is standard practice for many paediatric retrieval teams because of the risk of accidental extubation. End-tidal CO_2 monitoring should be used throughout transfer to confirm ET tube placement and to monitor the efficacy of ventilation.

The patient should be placed on the transport ventilator for long enough to highlight any difficulties prior to departure. Before leaving, blood gases should be checked and the difference between $ETCO_2$ and $PaCO_2$ measured (to guide ventilator management during the transfer). Although the difference between the two is unlikely to remain constant, it helps to establish a relationship prior to departure.

During transfer, if gas exchange deteriorates, the management remains similar to that in hospital:

- ventilate the patient manually
- ensure that they are adequately sedated and paralysed
- check that the ET tube has not moved or kinked
  - use an appropriately sized catheter to suction the ET tube (see Chapter 3)
  - the slope on the upward phase of the $ETCO_2$ may be the first obvious sign of airway obstruction
- assess for evolving lung pathology (e.g. pneumothorax).

Circulation

The occurrence of hypotension should be anticipated during the course of a transfer and prepared for. Again the management follows the same principle as in hospital events.

In cases where it is uncertain whether inotropes/vasopressors are needed they should be made up and attached to the patient prior to departure. Running these drugs at low rates, e.g. 0.1 ml/h, will help to overcome the dead space in lines and infusion pumps and reduce the time lag once started.

Access

Where possible at least one cannula should be reserved for fluid boluses and intermittent drug administration during transfer, e.g. 3% saline to manage intracranial hypertension. This should be attached to an extension line with a three-way tap at the doctor/nurse end, so that boluses can be given without having to stop and get out of the ambulance seat.

Central lines may be considered for transfers, but should not be considered essential. For time-critical transfers it is important that attempts to establish central venous or arterial access do not slow down the process of transferring the patient for definitive management, unless the benefits are seen to outweigh the risks. Remember that inotropes and vasopressors may be administered by the intraosseous route.

Adrenaline and inodilators can be administered in weak concentrations peripherally (e.g. at a quarter of the strength delivered centrally – see Chapter 36), although the access must be good and monitored regularly throughout transfer due to the risk of extravasation. If there is any doubt about the quality of the cannula, insert an IO needle or central line for inotrope delivery. The regional paediatric retrieval team can be contacted for advice.

Indications for an arterial line are the same as for any sick child. Consideration should be given to the fact that automatic non-invasive blood pressure cuffs can use a lot of energy (battery power) on portable monitors and can become unreliable on bumpy roads. However, as with central lines, siting an arterial line should not be allowed to slow down a time-critical transfer.

Sedation

Midazolam and morphine infusions are commonly used in paediatrics for all children over 3 months. Younger children are usually managed on morphine as a sole agent. The doses and infusion are detailed in Chapter 36. As with adult patients, sedation should be titrated to effect as sedative drugs may contribute to hypotension. This is especially true for midazolam in small children. Whichever drugs are used, it is helpful to prepare infusions using the same drugs and concentrations that are used in the regional PICU to facilitate handover.

Maintenance fluids

Maintenance intravenous fluid should be started if the child is not already receiving too much fluid (see Chapter 32). The choice of fluid will be dictated by the pathology, e.g. head-injured patients should receive isotonic fluid (0.9% saline is preferred). Patients over 10 kg are unlikely to require the addition of dextrose to maintenance fluid. Both hyperglycaemia and hypoglycaemia may worsen the outcome of neurological insults.

Temperature control

Hypothermia is another serious issue for children during transfer. They should be well covered and kept warm throughout (with the obvious exception of therapeutic hypothermia; see Chapter 23). Temperature should be monitored throughout the transfer.

Equipment and monitoring

It is vital that hospitals identify suitable transfer equipment as part of their advanced planning for critical care transfers. It should be readily available, checked regularly and fully charged (see Chapter 3). All equipment should be durable, lightweight and able to operate on battery as well as mains power. Spare batteries should be available.

During transfer, children should be monitored according to the recommendations of the Association of Anaesthetists of Great Britain and Ireland (AAGBI). This should include the items listed in Table 24.2.

Table 24.2. Basic monitoring.

- ECG
- Pulse oximetry
- Capnography
- Temperature
- Non-invasive and invasive blood pressure
- Clear illuminated display screen
- Audible and visible alarms on all values

Other equipment needed includes:

- Self-inflating bag and mask connected to a dedicated oxygen cylinder
- Portable suction
- Battery-powered infusion pumps.
- Fluid boluses pre-drawn in separate syringes

All equipment should be secured below the level of the patient.

The child must be accompanied by a minimum of two suitably trained people, one of whom will usually be a senior anaesthetist or intensivist capable of securing the airway and managing likely complications during transfer.

Most transfer vehicles will be provided by the local ambulance service and will take place in type B (or equivalent) vehicles. These ambulances have 12 V electric sockets and an oxygen supply. The transfer team should expect to provide all other equipment. Ensure there is plenty of oxygen and battery life.

Safety

The majority of critically ill children are retrieved without the use of 'blue lights and sirens'. However, this may be necessary for time-critical transfers. The aim should always be to complete the transfer swiftly but safely.

Excessive acceleration or deceleration can cause physiological instability and further rises in ICP. The journey should be as smooth as possible. All personnel should be seated and wearing seatbelts. Unforeseen medical interventions should be carried out with the vehicle stopped in a safe place. However, undue delays are likely to be to the detriment of the patient and should be minimized.

What do I need to have organized before departure?

This is best addressed with a checklist, an example of which is given in Table 24.3. A time-out with the team before departure, to go through the checklist, will not add much time to the transfer, and may avoid any undue delays.

Table 24.3. Pre-departure checklist.

1. Patient accepted by neurosurgical centre and destination confirmed (This may be straight to the operating theatre)
2. Referral made to regional paediatric intensive care unit
3. Ambulance service notified of time-critical transfer and confirmed immediate response
4. Appropriate transfer team personnel identified
5. Airway secured, ET tube position confirmed on CXR and C-spine immobilized
6. Adequate IV access: two peripheral cannulae or triple-lumen central line and a dedicated extension line for drug and fluid boluses
7. Adequate monitoring: ECG, SpO_2, $ETCO_2$, temperature, NIBP, IBP (Do not delay departure if unable to insert arterial line)
8. Physiological targets achieved: • $SpO_2 > 95\%$ • Age-appropriate CPP • $PaCO_2$ 4.5–5.0 (or $ETCO_2$ 4.0–4.5)
9. Well sedated and muscle-relaxed
10. Drug and fluid infusions and boluses pre-prepared
11. Essential equipment available: • Self-inflating bag and mask with dedicated portable oxygen cylinder • Adequate oxygen • Portable suction unit and suction catheters • Age-appropriate airway bag • Mobile telephone
12. Case notes, X-rays, CT scan, blood results (including clotting studies)
13. Cross-matched blood if available (in a suitable transport container with appropriate paperwork)
14. Parents fully informed and arrangements made for transport to the neurosurgical centre. Contact details documented
15. Telephone neurosurgical and PICU teams immediately prior to departure

Constant communication with both the neurosurgical and intensive care team is essential, and may best be achieved through mobile telephones with the relevant numbers loaded into their memory.

Summary

A swift and safe transfer of a critically ill child takes planning. It should not be carried out in a rush; instead it should be carried out by senior clinicians in a measured manner. The aim is to bring a child to definitive care in the safest possible way, with minimal delay. Advice should always be available from the local PICU retrieval team even if they are not carrying out the transfer.

Golden rules

- Policies, procedures and equipment must be in place before the event
- Do not delay transfer of the child by undertaking unnecessary procedures
- Suitably skilled personnel must accompany the child
- Good communication is essential
- If in doubt, secure the airway

Further reading

Association of Anaesthetists of Great Britain and Ireland. *Recommendations for the Safe Transfer of Patients with Brain Injury*. London: Association of Anaesthetists of Great Britain and Ireland, 2006.

Association of Anaesthetists of Great Britain and Ireland. *Interhospital Transfer*. London: Association of Anaesthetists of Great Britain and Ireland, 2009.

Nichols DG (ed.). *Rogers' Textbook of Paediatric Intensive Care*, 4th edn., Philadelphia: Lippincott, Williams & Wilkins, 2008.

Anaesthetizing for a surgical emergency

Andy Tatman and Richard Pierson

Introduction

The majority of sick children requiring surgery are transferred to a tertiary centre. However, there may be times when this is not possible; the child may be too sick to move, the surgery may be time-critical or the retrieval team unavailable.

In these situations, high-quality care in the local, non-specialist centre is crucial. Delays in transfer to a tertiary centre and insufficient confidence of the local team to operate have been highlighted in the 2011 National Confidential Enquiry into Patient Outcome and Death (NCEPOD) as contributing factors in paediatric surgical mortality.

The aim of this chapter is to give practical guidance to the non-paediatric anaesthetist on how to manage a sick child requiring emergency surgery.

How do surgical emergencies differ in children and adults?

Preoperative phase

Presentation

Small children often present late in the disease process. Consequently, by the time a child presents to the ED, they may be very sick, with hypovolaemia, acidosis and respiratory distress. They may, for example, have swallowed a great deal of blood from their bleeding tonsillar bed or have been vomiting for several days, from an appendicitis or intussusception.

Children have the ability to compensate for shock to the point of cardiovascular collapse. This compensation is achieved through increased heart rate and vasoconstriction. Hypotension and lethargy are signs of decompensating shock, whereas bradycardia is a sign of impending cardiorespiratory arrest.

Optimization

The key to optimization is to recognize the sick child (see Table 25.1), give high-flow oxygen, control the airway and the breathing and then give rapid fluid resuscitation, followed by prompt surgical correction of the underlying problem.

Children tend not to suffer from degenerative conditions such as atherosclerosis; therefore, adequate resuscitation with oxygen and intravenous fluids usually results in a rapid improvement, without the need for inotropic support or invasive monitoring. If there is any doubt about the adequacy of resuscitation, give a further fluid bolus and reassess the child. Failure to respond to these interventions is a grave sign and should set alarm bells ringing.

Managing the Critically Ill Child, ed. Richard Skone *et al.* Published by Cambridge University Press.

Table 25.1. Recognizing a sick child preoperatively.

System	Preoperative findings	Anaesthetic significance of these problems
Respiratory	Tachypnoea Low saturations Grunting Recession	The child may have these signs as a result of primary lung pathology, secondary to abdominal pathology, or as a compensatory response to a metabolic acidosis Problems may include: • Rapid desaturation on intubation • Difficulty in ventilating • High PEEP requirement • Severe metabolic acidosis
Cardiovascular	Tachycardia Cool peripheries Mottling of skin Poor central capillary refill Hypotension (late) Bradycardia (terminal)	Intense vasoconstriction and tachycardia can compensate for marked hypovolaemia in children Problems in these children include: • Difficult IV access • Decompensation on administration of anaesthetic agents • Multi-organ failure • Hypothermia
Renal	Oliguria (dry nappies)	Oliguria signals an acute kidney injury Problems may include: • Acidosis • Electrolyte disturbance • Difficulty in managing fluid balance • Altered drug handling
Neurological	Drowsiness Lethargy Lack of response to painful stimulus, e.g. cannulation	These signs point to poor brain perfusion, a 'tiring' child, or a marked metabolic disturbance Significance of these signs: • Anaesthetic requirement may be reduced • The child may tire and decompensate before theatre
Other problems	Hypoglycaemia Hypothermia Coagulopathy Thrombocytopenia	These problems will need addressing immediately before or during surgery

Psychology

Younger children who are ill are usually frightened and their fear can be exacerbated by parental and staff anxieties. This is best managed by:

- staying calm
- minimizing the number of people in the room
- explaining what you are doing to the child, parents and staff
- minimizing the number of interventions (cannulae, blood tests, NG tube) to those that are absolutely necessary
- having experienced staff perform interventions.

Reassurance, distraction techniques and the use of local anaesthetic cream should all be considered. However, life-saving interventions should not be delayed by fear of causing transient pain or distress.

Consent

When taking consent for an operation on a very ill child, it is important that the consent process includes a clear, and documented, discussion of the risks, including the risks from complication of central venous access, blood transfusion, admission to intensive care and the risk of death.

Intraoperative phase

Intravenous/intraosseous access

IV access should include a smaller cannula, for drugs and maintenance fluid, and a larger cannula for volume replacement. The size of cannula should be determined by the size of the child and the underlying condition. In an infant, a 24G cannula is useful for drugs and can be used to start resuscitation fluids, but an additional cannula, preferably 22G, should be inserted prior to starting surgery. See Figure 25.1 for suggested sites for insertion.

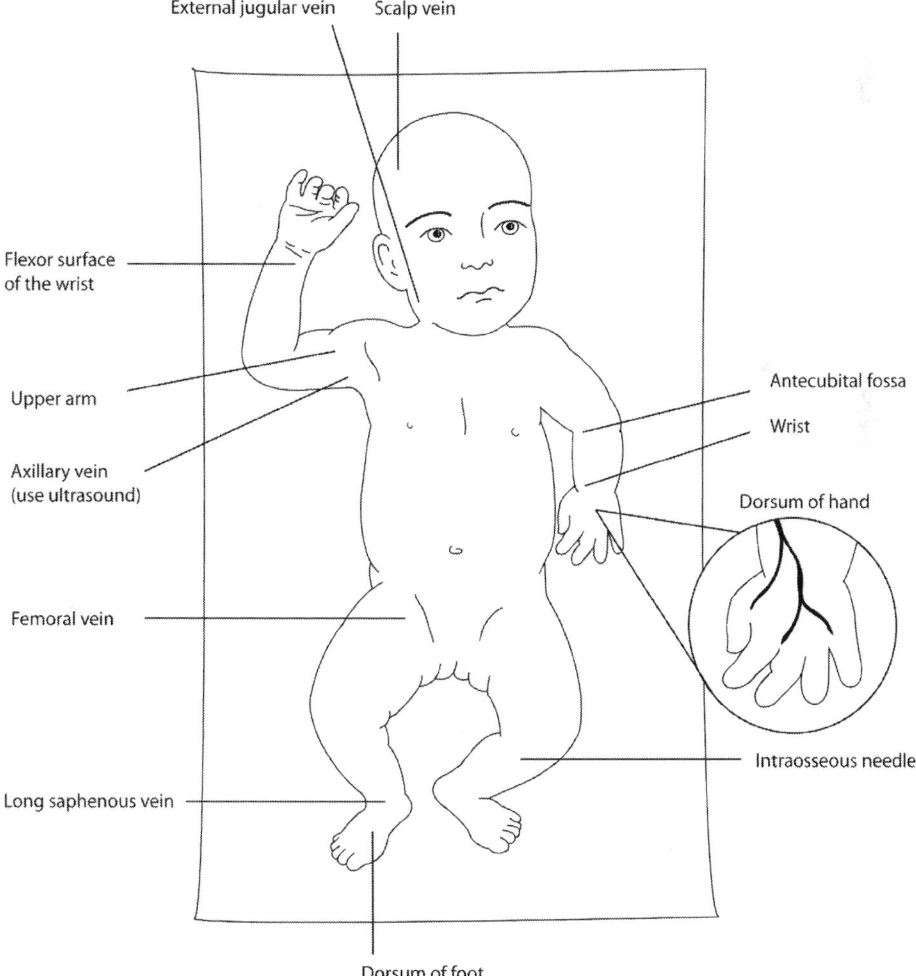

Figure 25.1. Suggested sites for cannula insertion.

If IV access is unsuccessful, intraosseous (IO) access should be considered early, even in a conscious child. It enables early resuscitation and fewer damaged veins, making subsequent IV cannulation easier.

Central venous access is unnecessary in most paediatric surgical emergencies. It should not be the first line of IV access. It should only be performed on an intubated, sedated and paralysed child, unless they are old enough to understand and cooperate with the intervention. A large-bore, single-lumen catheter is more effective than a multiple-lumen catheter for resuscitation.

Intubation and ventilation

The attending physician should have a low threshold for intubation and ventilation in any critically ill or injured child. The indications are well-recognized and may include:

- airway compromise
- cardiovascular instability
- respiratory failure
- reduced consciousness level
- need for investigations or interventions
- surgery
- transfer.

It should be remembered that the presence of a leak around the ET tube is not necessary, and there is no evidence of an increased incidence of post-extubation stridor when there is no leak, provided the tracheal tube passed easily. It is also unnecessary to cut the tracheal tube, as the effect on dead space is minimal.

An example of initial ventilation settings for smaller children is given below:

- pressure-control ventilation (PCV) for small children (uncuffed ET tube)
- rate of 20 breaths per minute
- I:E ratio of 1:2
- pressures of 20/5 cmH_2O
- titrate to a tidal volume of 5–7 ml/kg (up to 10 ml/kg if adequate chest movement is not seen in small children).

PCV will compensate for small leaks around the tracheal tube and will ventilate with appropriately small tidal volumes. Some volume control ventilators may be unable to do this.

Be careful when interpreting the measured tidal volume and $ETCO_2$. If there is a leak around the tube, it is likely that the tidal volume measured on the ventilator will read less than what is being delivered. The $ETCO_2$ will also under-read in this situation. Checking a blood gas will confirm this.

A small infant may require a tidal volume of more than 10 ml/kg to achieve normocapnia ($ETCO_2$ 5.0 to 6.0 kPa), as the tidal volume will include the volume change of the tubing and any dead space in the system. The most important guides to the adequacy of ventilation are chest wall movement and arterial carbon dioxide tension.

Positioning

Gaining access to a child during an operation can be difficult. Figure 25.2 shows how a child might be positioned for abdominal surgery for optimum access and warmth. The hand that has a cannula sited on it should be rested by the child's head, as if saluting. This can provide easy access for assessing capillary refill time and cannula patency.

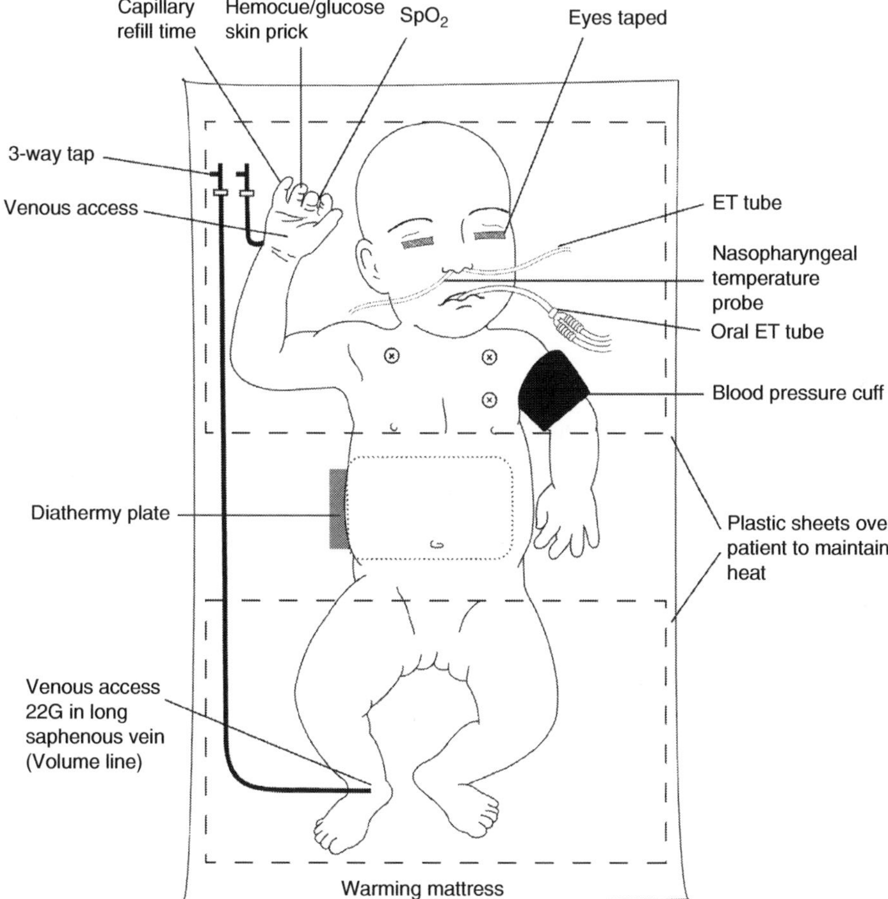

Figure 25.2. Positioning a child for abdominal surgery for optimum access and warmth.

Blood from a finger prick to measure blood sugar and haemoglobin can also be taken easily. A proximal, visible, cannula also reduces the volume of dead space in the IV line when giving drugs

Intravenous fluids

IV fluid therapy can be divided into:

- correction of hypovolaemia, i.e. circulating volume
- correction of fluid deficit, i.e. total body fluid
- maintenance fluids.

When anaesthetizing a sick child for a surgical emergency, it is often difficult to calculate the deficit. In the perioperative period, it is simpler to correct hypovolaemia and replace ongoing losses while ignoring the deficit.

Correction of hypovolaemia

Hypovolaemia should be corrected with 10–20 ml/kg boluses of warmed fluids (0.9% saline, Hartmann's solution or colloid) with attention paid to the response in heart rate, capillary refill time, peripheral temperature and blood pressure. If there is doubt about the adequacy of resuscitation, a further bolus of 10 ml/kg should be given, as the vast majority of problems associated with the adequacy of resuscitation are due to too little volume, rather than too much.

Blood transfusion

An [Hb] greater than 70 g/l, in an otherwise well child who is not actively bleeding, usually does not require transfusion. However, intraoperative [Hb] measurement should be performed at regular intervals.

If a transfusion is necessary, 10 ml/kg of packed cells will raise the child's [Hb] by about 20–25 g/l. Once the child has been exposed to a unit of blood, it is desirable to continue to transfuse from that unit, up to an [Hb] of 120–140 g/l, thereby minimizing the likelihood of requiring a further transfusion, from another donor, later in their hospital stay.

Care must be taken to avoid an excessive transfusion through an open three-way tap. One way to avoid this is to keep a three-way tap in the giving set (closed as the default) and administer the blood aliquots by drawing the correct volume into a syringe before giving it.

Correction of deficit

Do not try to correct the deficit in the operating theatre. The deficit should be corrected over 24 to 48 hours, with the volume and choice of fluid being guided by clinical signs and electrolytes respectively.

Maintenance fluids

Intraoperatively, all IV fluids should be isotonic, with Hartmann's preferred due to its lower chloride content. For small infants, where hypoglycaemia may be an issue, Hartmann's with 2.5% dextrose is an alternative. This can be made up by adding 25 ml of 50% dextrose to 500 ml of Hartmann's solution. See Chapter 32 for calculating fluid maintenance requirements.

Postoperatively, 0.45% saline with 5% dextrose, prescribed at two-thirds maintenance requirements, is a suitable fluid. Fluid losses in excess of calculated maintenance volumes (such as NG and large urinary losses) should be replaced with isotonic crystalloid to minimize the risk of hyponatraemia.

Temperature control

Having a large surface area with small core mass, small children can get cold very quickly. Keep them covered whenever possible, but not at the expense of assessing vital parameters, such as chest movement. Clear plastic sheeting, covering the upper body and legs, is useful in this respect.

Other factors which should be addressed to ensure normothermia are:

- the theatre must be warm before bringing the child in
- blood products and fluids should be administered through a blood warmer
- use external warming devices
- core temperature measurement is essential.

Forced warm-air devices will provide adequate warming for most cases. However, these devices are very powerful, and can result in rapid heating of a small child, with the potential for serious hyperthermia. Electrically heated mattresses will provide adequate heating for children, over 1 year of age, lying supine. The mattresses have a lag time to warm the child, and often the child continues to warm after the mattress has been turned off, so it may be necessary to turn it off before the child reaches the desired temperature. Remember, if there is a leak around the ET tube, the nasopharyngeal temperature probe will under-read, due to cooling, so it is often better to pass it into the upper oesophagus.

Glucose monitoring

Blood glucose should be checked at least once perioperatively in all sick children. Some anaesthetists routinely use Hartmann's solution with 2.5% glucose in infants. If hypoglycaemia is present, this should be corrected with 2 ml/kg of 10% dextrose, and the maintenance fluid changed to a non-hypotonic glucose-containing fluid, such as 5% glucose in 0.9% saline.

Inotropes

Inotropes should be considered if hypotension persists, despite apparently adequate resuscitation. The indications for the choice of inotropes are the same as in adults. Adrenaline should be given via a central line, but if this route is not available it may be given peripherally *in extremis*, as a quarter-strength solution and ideally with the maintenance fluid, to minimize the risk of peripheral ischaemia. It should be changed to a central route as soon as that route becomes available.

Postoperative care

Following emergency surgery, children should be managed in an appropriate environment. This is particularly so at night, when a child may be better cared for on an HDU ward or transferred to a PICU postoperatively.

Examples of surgical emergencies and their management

Postoperative tonsillar bleeding

Postoperative tonsillar bleeding occurs in 1–2% of elective tonsillectomies. It occurs either as primary haemorrhage (within 24 hours) or secondary (usually 5–12 days post surgery).

Common problems with anaesthetizing a child with bleeding tonsils are:

- difficulty in quantifying the degree of blood loss
- potential for significant hypovolaemia

- blood in the stomach, which is emetogenic and results in an increased risk of aspiration
- intubation may be difficult due to an obscured view or laryngeal oedema
- the child and parents may be very anxious
- a general anaesthetic earlier in the day may mean that a child is excessively restless or drowsy.

Table 25.2. Stages in anaesthetizing a patient with a bleeding tonsillar bed.

Phase of management	Actions
Preoperative phase	Resuscitate the child before going to theatre, unless significant haemorrhage • Give 10 ml/kg fluid boluses and monitor response • Repeat fluid boluses as necessary Send a full blood count Cross-match urgently Consider blood transfusion Get help from senior anaesthetist
Intraoperative phase	Prepare anaesthetic room with: • Two suction devices • Two ET tubes (same as previous size and a smaller one) Rapid-sequence induction[a]
Postoperative phase	Pass large-bore NG tube and empty the stomach before extubation Adequate analgesia (taking into account previous anaesthetic) Extubate in left lateral position Consider high dependency care

[a] Effective preoxygenation may be difficult in an anxious child, so gentle positive-pressure ventilation may be necessary, prior to intubation.

Traditionally, bleeding tonsils received an inhalational induction. If the child is hypovolaemic, there is rapid equilibration between the inspired concentration of sevoflurane and the blood, which may result in excessive anaesthetic depth with the potential for severe decompensation and cardiac arrest. The child should be adequately resuscitated before induction of anaesthesia. Most anaesthetists would now advocate performing a rapid-sequence induction (rather than a gas induction) unless there is a specific indication, i.e. previous difficult intubation.

Perforated appendix

Only 5% of cases of appendicitis occur in children under 5 years. However, the risk of perforation is double for this age group, so small children may be very ill when they arrive for surgery.

Table 25.3. Stages in anaesthetizing a child with perforated appendix.

Phase of management	Actions
Preoperative phase	Resuscitate the child before going to theatre If capillary refill prolonged give fluid boluses Ensure antibiotics have been started
Intraoperative phase	Rapid-sequence induction[a] Titrate fluids to heart rate and clinical signs Start maintenance fluid Give gentamicin if faecal contamination of abdomen (7 mg/kg) Manage sepsis and hypotension as in previous chapters
Postoperative phase	Adequate analgesia (usually 100 μg/kg of morphine followed by NCA/PCA) Consider ITU if: • Persistent tachycardia • Tachypnoea • Cool peripheries • Hypotension (despite 30–40 ml/kg fluid) • Temperature > 39°C • Intra-abdominal sepsis

[a] If hypovolaemia is suspected, the dose of induction agent should be reduced accordingly.

The child should stay in recovery until fully recovered, with stable cardiorespiratory parameters. Persistent tachycardia, tachypnoea and cool peripheries are indications that the child needs further resuscitation. Significant systemic sepsis following a perforated appendix is uncommon. Remember that a perforated appendix is a surgical emergency, and delay in getting to the operating theatre can result in a fatal outcome, as was highlighted in the 2011 NCEPOD report.

Intussusception

This presents most commonly in infants. The majority of intussusceptions can be reduced by air enema, thereby avoiding the need for surgery. Those that cannot be reduced will require a laparotomy. Some children, particularly those presenting with a longer history, may have significant fluid loss and be developing sepsis secondary to the presence of necrotic bowel. The management is similar to that for children with perforated appendicitis, with some children requiring 30–40 ml/kg of colloid for resuscitation. Blood transfusion may be necessary, particularly where there is necrotic bowel. These children rarely require invasive monitoring. Usually, by the end of surgery, the child looks remarkably well.

Tertiary hospital advice and transfer

Anaesthetic advice and support is always available from the tertiary paediatric hospital, whether it is just to confirm that the anaesthetic plan is reasonable, or for a more detailed discussion of what to do.

If the child is to be transferred, ensure the patient's notes are up to date and all drugs have been documented, including fluid boluses, inotropes and antibiotics. Document all investigations and results, including radiology and laboratory investigations, and include any imaging, either as a hard copy or on a disk.

Ensure that the tracheal tube is correctly placed and well secured, with the position being confirmed by a CXR. If the child is to be retrieved by the tertiary centre, and is stable, do not feel pressured to put in additional venous access (peripheral or central) prior to the arrival of the retrieval team, as, if unsuccessful, you may make the retrieval team's job more difficult.

Summary

Anaesthetizing a child for emergency surgery in a DGH is rare. If it is needed, the same principles as for an adult anaesthetic apply. The biggest problem is access to a draped child. Take a moment before allowing the surgeons to start to ensure that you have adequate access to the child.

Golden rules

- Ensure adequate access to the child throughout the operation
- Make sure that you can access the cannulae and pay particular attention to temperature and blood glucose
- Make sure that the airway is satisfactory before allowing the drapes to be placed, i.e. not endobronchial intubation
- Pay attention to blood loss, it is easy to underestimate

Further reading

Fleming S, Thompson M, Stevens R, *et al.* Normal ranges of heart rate and respiratory rate in children from birth to 18 years: a systematic review of observational studies. *Lancet* 2011;**377**:1011–1018.

Nafiu O, Voepel-Lewis T, Morris M, *et al.* How do pediatric anesthesiologists define intraoperative hypotension? *Pediatr Anesth* 2009;**19**:1048–1053.

NCEPOD. *Are We There Yet? A Review of Organisational and Clinical Aspects of Children's Surgery*. NCEPOD, 2011

Chapter 26

Managing children on an adult critical care unit

Helga Becker

Introduction

Since the publication of the Department of Health Report titled 'Paediatric Intensive Care: A Framework for the Future' in 1997, a gradual redistribution of surgery for children towards specialized children's hospitals has occurred. In many regions, paediatric referral networks have been developed. These have a lead centre that provides specialist tertiary services and a 24-hour paediatric retrieval service.

Despite the availability of these services, all hospitals that admit children must provide the facilities and expertise to:

- resuscitate children
- deliver high-dependency care
- initiate intensive care
- stabilize prior to transfer to the tertiary centre.

The advent of paediatric retrieval services has reduced the number of paediatric emergency admissions to adult critical care units (ACCU). Often the initial management and stabilization of critically ill children are now performed in the emergency department or on paediatric wards until the arrival of the retrieval team.

Admissions of critically ill children to ACCU do still occur and in selected cases it may be deemed appropriate that such children are cared for on adult units until their need for intensive care support has ceased.

This chapter illustrates the issues surrounding the care for critically ill children in this setting.

Standards for the unit

Any ACCU that agrees to admit critically ill children is well advised to have a basic infrastructure in place to support this. In 2010 the Paediatric Intensive Care Society published standards for the provision of paediatric critical care, including critical care units in district general hospitals (DGH).

In most regions local standards have also been agreed, e.g. 'Standards for The Care of Critically Ill and Critically Injured Children in the West Midlands' (Version 3). A yearly self-assessment to ensure ongoing maintenance of good standards of care and up-to-date facilities should be performed on the critical care unit and within the hospital.

Managing the Critically Ill Child, ed. Richard Skone *et al.* Published by Cambridge University Press.

Multidisciplinary approach

Any ACCU that looks after children should have a consultant with special interest in paediatric critical care. This is often an intensivist who both has a background in anaesthetics and regularly anaesthetizes children electively, or who has had exposure to paediatric critical care during general intensive care training.

Good links with the lead clinician for paediatric anaesthesia, the paediatric lead for high-dependency care and the resuscitation officer will allow the introduction of protocols and equipment specific to paediatric anaesthesia and paediatric critical care. These specialists should be members of a hospital-wide critical care delivery group.

The lead nurse for paediatric critical care needs to work well with the critical care professional development team to ensure adequate training and to provide a link with paediatric ward nursing staff.

Environment

The facilities and environment in an adult critical care unit are adapted to the needs of adults and their relatives rather than children and their care-givers. Facilities are often less than optimally adapted to the care of small children and suitable equipment may not be immediately available or very infrequently used.

Equipment

Any ACCU which accommodates critically ill children will need to maintain a basic stock level of essential equipment such as airway adjuncts and vascular access devices. Simple devices should not be overlooked, such as suitably small NG tubes with the correct compatible adapters for enteral feed, small blood-sampling tubes and blood gas capillary tubes.

Ventilators have to be suitable to ventilate children down to a weight of only a few kilograms. The knowledge of how to set these up and use them for small children is essential if a child is to be cared for safely in an ACCU.

Dosing and infusion regimes for commonly encountered drugs such as sedative agents, muscle relaxants, inotropes, bronchodilators, etc. need to be available. These should be the same as the regimes used at the lead children's hospital so that communication between the two units is simplified.

Despite their design for a different patient group, adult equipment can be surprisingly useful for paediatric care. In the author's unit, we usually nurse children of all ages in an adult critical care bed as opposed to infant beds with high cot sides. This improves the accessibility of the child from all sides. All equipment on the ACCU should be assessed in this way and only be replaced with child-specific equipment if necessary. This reduces a source of error as staff can continue to work with equipment they are familiar with.

Specialist paediatric warming devices should be available, although in most cases it is sufficient to use simple blankets and clothing as long as exposure is reduced to a minimum.

Most other equipment on the general ICU such as syringe drivers, volumetric pumps, invasive monitoring transducers, etc. is suitable for patients of all sizes and therefore will be available.

Discharge

Once the acute critical illness has been treated to a degree that critical care support is no longer needed, adequate step-down arrangements must be in place in the paediatric department, particularly if the critical care outreach service does not routinely extend to paediatric wards.

The decision to manage locally

The decision to treat a critically ill child in an ACCU beyond the initial stabilization period should always be taken in consultation with the local paediatric intensive care unit (PICU) or retrieval service. The treatment plan and progress should be discussed at least once every 24 hours.

Situations when local management in an ACCU may be appropriate or necessary include:

- the age of the child: children between the ages of 14 and 15 years, particularly if physically relatively mature, may be managed on an adult unit for conditions which predictably require only a brief period of ventilation or close observation
- the underlying condition: the classic case would be an infant or child with prolonged febrile convulsions or known epilepsy who required sedation and intubation for (now resolved) SE and who is expected to need ventilation for no more than 24 hours
- the potential for deterioration of the clinical condition, which would require critical care support: a stable patient requiring close observation, e.g. after smoke inhalation or accidental ingestion of sedative medication, etc.
- lack of capacity of paediatric high-dependency beds in the paediatric department
- the lack of availability of PICU beds: despite all efforts to increase PICU capacity nationwide in recent years, this can pose a problem during the winter months and during flu pandemics in particular. During such periods, the tertiary centres have to allocate the available resources carefully, which may lead to a delayed transfer of older children or children with less complex conditions. Some children may have their entire critical care episode within an ACCU. The set-up and available medical expertise in the ACCU in question at the time will also play a role in the decision to deliver care in a DGH.

The challenges to managing a child on an ACCU

Regardless of the reason for the decision to keep the child in the ACCU beyond the stabilization period, the care for these critically ill children in the adult setting poses certain challenges.

Skills

The skills needed are to establish vascular access, sedate, anaesthetize, intubate, ventilate and give inotropic support at appropriate levels. These also need to be weaned when indicated.

Initial stabilization skills have much in common with the generic skills of anaesthesia and are taught on many local and national courses. It is often easier to gain opportunities to intubate children of all ages during elective theatre lists.

The maintenance and weaning of support are skills more specific to paediatric critical care and require a certain amount of experience to be done well. Nursing staff in particular may have little exposure to the maintenance and weaning phases of intensive care provision for a child.

The treatment of some of the conditions for which a child may be cared for in an ACCU also requires relatively specialist paediatric knowledge. It is paramount that good links exist between the paediatric medical and nursing teams in the DGH and critical care.

Exposure

One of the problems a multidisciplinary critical care team in a DGH is faced with when looking after critically ill children on an ACCU is the acquisition and maintenance of sufficient skills and experience. Nursing staff, pharmacists and physiotherapists may encounter children as patients only during a critical illness. This often has a major impact on their confidence in dealing with the particular issues posed by critically ill children of all age groups.

A multidisciplinary approach including paediatric medical input and good working relationships with the paediatric nursing staff is essential to guarantee the best possible standard of care. For neonates and small infants admitted to the hospital from home, input from local neonatal intensive care services will be necessary.

Joint training sessions on specialized equipment used on the neonatal and paediatric high dependency unit such as CPAP and BiPAP machines should be organized.

A professional development plan for nursing and medical staff should be developed locally, in cooperation with the relevant PICU, to ensure that the necessary knowledge is acquired, maintained and practised regularly. This should include:

- participation in regional and national courses, multidisciplinary simulation training
- development of referral pathways taking account of local facilities
- secondment of staff to specialist units.

Often, once a core of medical and nursing staff have undergone this training, the distribution of knowledge and skill on the ACCU takes an exponential course, and the successful management of any critically ill children in this setting enhances the effect greatly.

Parents

Parents are usually allowed access to the bedspace for much longer periods during the day than the relatives of adult critical care patients and are actively encouraged to take part in the personal care for their child.

Ongoing development

Constructive feedback from the local lead PICU is extremely important and a system should be developed with the relevant PICUs or retrieval teams to ensure that this happens on a regular and timely basis. It is important that all members of the local multidisciplinary team including the paediatric, general intensive care and nursing teams are involved. Feedback is essential to reflect on current practice and realize opportunities for improvement.

An ongoing audit of paediatric cases treated on the ACCU is essential to ensure feedback on all cases. This is an important role for the local nursing or medical lead for paediatric critical care.

A good working relationship with the respective PICU and/or retrieval team facilitates communication in the acute situation. It also facilitates establishment of standards and systems development with:

- exchange of knowledge and expertise
- continued medical and nursing education
- advice on equipment acquisition and use
- participation in the development of treatment regimes.

A paediatric critical care network should consist of the local PICUs, the paediatric retrieval team and all the local acute paediatric care providers including the ACCUs providing care for children. Within the network, issues may develop where there is a need for education or the development of guidance or management protocol, which can then be distributed to all participating units. This was recognized during preparation for the flu pandemic.

Within this network, there should also be an atmosphere of collegial cooperation so that no clinician feels any inhibition when asking for advice.

Summary

Paediatric critical care services have been centralized in specialist units over the last few years to focus expertise and achieve best outcomes. This means that ACCU in DGHs with paediatric inpatient departments may be confronted with severely ill children who require resuscitation and critical care support against a background of small case numbers.

To maintain good standards of care for such children, multidisciplinary teamworking and good links between the paediatric, neonatal and critical care specialists are extremely important. Practical, workable and mutually agreed treatment protocols and referral pathways must be in place. The local set-up must include links with the specialist regional centre and retrieval service, a robust governance structure and an effective professional development programme for all staff involved. Under these circumstances, critically ill children can be managed successfully and to a high standard on an ACCU.

Further reading

Edge WE, Kanter RK, Weigle CGM, *et al.* Reduction of morbidity in inter-hospital transport by specialised pediatric staff. *Crit Care Med* 1994;**22**:1186–1191.

http://www.wmsc.nhs.uk/uploaded_media/CIC%20standards%20revision%20D9%2029%207%2009.pdf.

Paediatric Intensive Care Society. *Standards for the Care of the Critically Ill Children*, 4th edn. London: PICS, 2010.

Pollack MM, Alexander SR, Clarke N, *et al.* Improved outcomes from tertiary centre pediatric intensive care. A statewide comparison of tertiary and non tertiary care facilities. *Crit Care Med* 1991;**19**:150–159.

Report from the National Co-ordinating Group to the Chief Executive of the NHS Executive. *Paediatric Intensive Care: A Framework for the Future.* Department of Health, July 1997;**31**.

Chapter 27

Pain management in children

Ursula Dickson

Introduction

In critically ill children pain is often taken care of by the use of morphine as a sedative. However, for any child who is not sedated adequate analgesia is essential in order to:

- gain cooperation
- unmask clinical signs
- minimize the stress response to injury
- treat a child humanely.

Recognizing pain in small children can be very difficult. It should never be assumed that because a child cannot express pain they are comfortable.

As in adults, pain in children has many components which may influence their pain behaviour. These factors can include:

- psychological
- social
- cultural
- previous experiences.

This chapter aims to provide a guide to recognizing and managing pain in children. The medications recommended should be available in all accident and emergency departments and paediatric wards.

Assessing pain in children

When asking children about pain, great efforts should be made to avoid using medical jargon. Take care to explain what you are going to do to help them, and keep to simple terms. It is often useful to ask parents to help you find words that their child or their family uses, e.g. 'hurt' rather than 'sore', and 'Calpol' rather than paracetamol.

Tools used in the assessment of pain need to be quick, reliable and demonstrate low inter-user variability. Pain scores can be used to fulfil these criteria. Depending on the age of the patient, the pain scores used can be observer-based or self-reported.

Observer-based behavioural scores

- FLACC (face, legs, activity, cry, consolability) – for young children
- Neonatal Infant Pain Score – young infants

Managing the Critically Ill Child, ed. Richard Skone *et al.* Published by Cambridge University Press.

The FLACC score

This system has been validated for infants and young children who cannot speak or who find it difficult to quantify pain and emotions. The system scores from 0 to 10, where 0 equates to no pain and 10 to severe pain. A score greater than 7 suggests severe pain.

The FLACC score is also useful in older children who are unable to communicate normally, either because of their illness/trauma or because of pre-existing developmental disorders. The words in italics in Table 27.1 are the terminology developed for children with cognitive impairment.

Table 27.1. The FLACC score.

Categories	Scoring		
	0	1	2
Face	No particular expression or smile	Occasional grimace or frown, withdrawn or disinterested *appears sad or worried*	Frequent to constant quivering chin, clenched jaw *distressed-looking face, expression of fright or panic*
Legs	Normal position or relaxed *usual tone and motion to limbs*	Uneasy, restless, tense *occasional tremors*	Kicking, or legs drawn up *marked increase in spasticity, constant tremors or jerking*
Activity	Lying quietly, normal position, moves easily *regular rhythmic respirations*	Squirming, shifting back and forth, tense *tense or guarded movements, mildly agitated [e.g. head back and forth, aggression], shallow, splinting respirations, intermittent sighs*	Arched, rigid or jerking *severe agitation, head banging, shivering [not rigors], breath holding, gasping or sharp intake of breaths, severe splinting*
Cry	No cry [awake or asleep]	Moans or whimpers: occasional complaint *occasional verbal outburst or grunt*	Crying steadily, screams or sobs, frequent complaints *repeated outbursts, constant grunting*
Consolability	Content, relaxed	Reassured by occasional touching, hugging or being talked to, distractable	Difficult to console or comfort *pushing away care-giver, resisting care or comfort measures*

The NIPS score

The Neonatal Infant Pain Score (NIPS; Table 27.2) is considered a better tool for assessing pain in neonates. The maximum score achievable with this tool is 7. It does have limitations in that a baby who is severely unwell may score falsely low.

Table 27.2. The Neonatal Infant Pain Score (NIPS).

	Score	Finding	Details
Facial expression	0	Relaxed muscle	Restful face, neutral expression
	1	Grimace	Tight facial muscles, furrowed brow, chin, jaw
Cry	0	No cry	Quiet, not crying
	1	Whimper	Mild moaning, intermittent
	2	Vigorous cry	Loud scream, rising, shrill, continuous
Breathing patterns	0	Relaxed	Usual pattern for this baby
	1	Changed	Indrawing, irregular, faster, gagging
Arms	0	Relaxed/restrained	No muscular rigidity, occasional movement
	1	Flexed/extended	Tense, straight arms, rigid, extension/flexion
Legs	0	Relaxed/restrained	No muscular rigidity, occasional movement
	1	Flexed/extended	Tense, straight legs, rigid, extension/flexion
State of arousal	0	Sleeping/awake	Quiet, peaceful, sleeping, or alert and settled
	1	Fussy	Alert, restless, and thrashing

Self-reporting pain scores

Using self-reported pain scores in young children can be prone to errors. For instance, giving a small child a colour-coded system may end up with them picking their favourite colour, rather than one that is representative of their pain score. Children find facial expressions helpful when quantifying their pain. This can be utilized by giving children a modified Wong Baker faces score (Figure 27.1). Scores of 2–6 suggest mild to moderate pain and 8 or more severe pain.

Children may be worried about telling people how much pain they are in because they fear what will happen if they tell the truth.

0
No Hurt
2
Hurts
Little Bit
4
Hurts
Little More
6
Hurts
Even More
8
Hurts
Whole Lot
10
Hurts
Worst

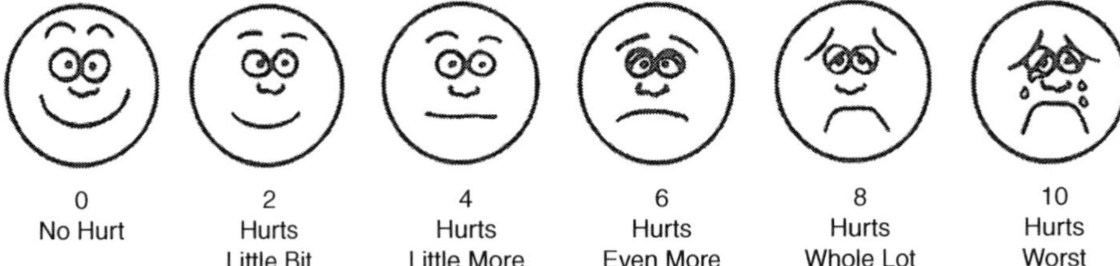

Figure 27.1. The Wong Baker faces chart. From Wong DL, Hockenberry-Eaton M, Wilson D, Winkelstein ML, Schwartz P. *Wong's Essentials of Pediatric Nursing*, 6th edn. St Louis: Mosby, 2001, p. 1301. Copyrighted by Mosby, Inc. Reprinted by permission.

Which analgesics should you give?

The WHO pain ladder is used in children as it is in adults. Mild to moderate pain can often be treated with simple analgesia, whereas severe pain will usually require an opiate. Remember that analgesics that work on different parts of the pain pathway are synergistic. Paracetamol and non-steroidal anti-inflammatories (NSAIDs) should never be stopped purely because an opiate is being given.

Child-friendly preparations should be used where possible, i.e. the drug should ideally be liquid and palatable. Table 27.3 gives dosages based on common practice in children's hospitals and follows the guidelines in the BNFc.

Table 27.3. Dosages based on common practice in children's hospitals and following the guidelines in the BNFc

	PO	PR	IV	Neonates	Frequency	Caution
Paracetamol	20 mg/kg (up to 1 g) max 90 mg/kg/day (up to 4 g)	30–40 mg/kg loading dose then 20 mg/kg max 90 mg/kg/day (up to 4 g)	15 mg/kg over 10 kg (max 60 mg/kg/day)	PO/PR 15 mg/kg (max 60 mg/kg) IV term 10 mg/kg (max 30 mg/kg/day) IV neonates and infants < 10 kg 7.5 mg/kg (max 30 mg/kg/day)	4–6 hourly	Renal impairment Hepatic impairment 10 mg/kg
NSAIDS Diclofenac Ibuprofen	1 mg/kg (max 150 mg/day) 5–10 mg/kg (max 30 mg/kg/day max dose 2.4 g/ 24 h)	1 mg/kg n/a	> 2 years 1 mg/kg bd (max 150 mg/day) n/a	Not < 6 months of age Not < 1 month of age or < 5 kg	8 hourly 6–8 hourly	Asthma – not absolute contraindication Avoid if impaired renal function Bleeding disorders Hepatic impairment
Codeine	1 mg/kg (up to 60 mg)	1 mg/kg (up to 60 mg)	Never	0.5–1 mg/kg	4–6 hourly	Moderate to severe renal impairment reduce dose
Morphine	0.1–0.5 mg/kg	n/a	Bolus dose incrementally > 1 year 100–200 µg/kg Infants 50–100 µg/kg	25–50 µg/kg Oral 80 µg/kg	4 hourly	Moderate to severe renal impairment reduce dose Hepatic impairment – reduced metabolism

Table 27.4. Concentration of the formulations available; drug doses should be sensibly rounded off to match.

	Suspension	Tablets	Dispersible tablets	Suppositories	Melts	IV
Paracetamol	120 mg/5 ml 250 mg/5 ml	500 mg	500 mg	30 mg, 60 mg, 120 mg, 240 mg, 500 mg, 1 g	250 mg	10 mg/ml
Ibuprofen	100 mg/5 ml	200 mg	n/a	n/a	100 mg	n/a
Diclofenac	n/a	25 mg, 50 mg	50 mg	12.5 mg, 25 mg, 50 mg	n/a	75 mg (see BNFc for administration guidance)
Codeine	15 mg/5ml	15 mg, 30 mg, 60 mg	n/a	1 mg, 2 mg, 3 mg (requests) 5 mg, 10 mg	n/a	n/a
Morphine	10 mg/5ml	10 mg, 20 mg	n/a	n/a	n/a	10 mg/ml 50 mg/50 ml

Paracetamol

This is a centrally acting drug that is a cyclooxygenase inhibitor. It also has a mode of action via 5HT receptor agonism and possibly a weak cannabinoid effect.

Paracetamol is used as an antipyretic as well as an analgesic in children. It can be given IV, PO or PR. Absolute contraindications include a history of allergy and liver failure.

Caution should be exercised in the following cases:

- liver disease
  - reduce dosage as there may be reduced glutathione stores to deactivate toxic metabolite
- renal disease
  - reduce maximum daily dosages due to reduced excretion of glucuronide metabolites.

Ibuprofen

This is the NSAID drug that has the best safety profile in children. It is a nonspecific cyclooxygenase inhibitor.

It is recognized that in a few patients NSAIDs can trigger bronchoconstriction. However, in children with well-controlled asthma it can usually be given safely, with no reporting of wheeze or increased inhaler usage. On testing in adults, only 2–5% of asthmatic patients react to skin testing for NSAIDs. It can be given as an oral suspension or as melts.

Ibuprofen should not be given if the patient has any of the following:

- impaired renal function
- hypovolaemia
- acute bleeding

- brittle asthma
- severe sepsis
- liver failure
- history of gastric bleeding
- coagulation abnormality
- history of allergic reaction to any NSAID.

Codeine

This is a weak opiate. It is easy to administer orally or rectally and is well tolerated. Codeine causes less nausea and vomiting than morphine in children.

There is a great deal of genetic variability in people's ability to metabolize codeine to its active morphine form via the CYP2D6 part of the cytochrome P450 system. This may render it of little use in some patients. Also, if a patient is in severe pain it may not be converted to enough morphine to be effective in everyone. If its administration is evaluated as ineffective, oramorph or IV morphine should be given instead.

Morphine

Many people may have concerns about the use of morphine in children. Ultimately, it is very safe as long as you give the right dose, and the patient is adequately monitored. Incremental IV boluses of morphine allow optimal titration in acutely ill patients. A morphine bolus will usually last about 2–4 hours. It can be given PO, IV, PR or intranasally (as diamorphine).

Respiratory depression is a side effect most feared by doctors prescribing morphine. However, this is easily reversible with the opiate antagonist naloxone if it becomes problematic. This does not mean that morphine should be given carelessly. Naloxone should be prescribed (as required) for any child on an opiate infusion who is self-ventilating. If it is given then the patient should be monitored closely as the half-life of naloxone is shorter than that of morphine, so it may wear off sooner.

If a child becomes nauseous or starts vomiting then the serotonin antagonist ondansetron should be given as a first-line anti-emetic: 0.1 mg/kg intravenously up to 8 hourly.

Itching is common in children when using opiates. The histamine antagonist chlorphenamine is a good antidote to this (0.1 mg/kg intravenously), although it may exacerbate drowsiness. Patients experiencing excessive histamine release from morphine may be better on the synthetic opioid fentanyl.

Patient/nurse-controlled analgesia (PCA/NCA)

If a patient is likely to need a strong opiate for many hours after an IV bolus has been given, it is best to start either a patient-controlled analgesia or a nurse-controlled analgesia regime (PCA/NCA) with a background infusion (if your unit has the experience with appropriate protocols and pumps), or a plain morphine infusion.

To avoid dosing errors when administering morphine infusions, the patient's body weight in kilograms should be converted to milligrams and the equivalent dose of morphine should be made up to 50 ml using normal saline, i.e. a 45 kg child should have a 50 ml solution with 45 mg of morphine. Each millilitre of the ensuing solution will then contain

20 μg/kg. For any patient in severe pain who needs a 100 μg/kg loading dose, a 5 ml bolus from this solution can be given to achieve an adequate plasma concentration of morphine.

Neonates and infants are more sensitive to opiates; therefore it may be wise to manage their pain with a 25–50 μg/kg initial bolus, followed by a continuous infusion of 10 μg/kg/h (0.5 ml/h).

Table 27.5. A guide for morphine loading doses and infusion rates according to age.

Patient age group	Bolus – loading dose	Infusion rate if breathing spontaneously	Infusion rate if ventilated
Neonate or ex-premature baby	25–50 μg/kg	0.1–0.5 ml/h	0–2 ml/h
Child 1 month – 1 year	50–100 μg/kg	0.1–1 ml/h	0–3 ml/h
Child older than 1 year	100–200 μg/kg	0.1–2 ml/h	0–5 ml/h

Fentanyl

Fentanyl is 100 times more potent than morphine, so the usual dose is 1 μg/kg.

When administered as a single bolus, its duration of action is only 20–30 minutes. As with all opiates, incremental boluses are the safest way to administer to a spontaneously ventilating patient.

Fentanyl can be given by infusion (after a loading dose) in patients with renal failure, as it has no active metabolites that depend on renal excretion (unlike morphine). However, this should only be done in centres that are experienced in its use.

Intranasal diamorphine

Over the last few years, many accident and emergency departments have written protocols for administration of intranasal diamorphine. It provides an easy, quick way of administering potent analgesia to a child who does not have IV access. Diamorphine should be diluted in a small volume (0.2 ml) of saline and then either sprayed into the nostril via a mucosal atomization device or dripped onto the nasal mucosa. It is usually effective within 5 minutes.

Most EDs have a chart detailing how to make up the diamorphine solution according to the child's weight so that they receive a dose of 0.1 mg/kg.

Topical anaesthesia

A topical anaesthetic agent should be applied (and given time to work), if time permits, prior to cannulation and phlebotomy. Ametop (amethocaine), emla (lignocaine mixed with prilocaine) and LMX4 (4% lignocaine) are the commonest available formulations for application to the skin. If there is not enough time to allow these to work then consider using ethyl chloride spray to numb the desired area.

Entonox

This is a mixture of the gases nitrous oxide and oxygen. It produces analgesia and anxiolysis for procedures such as plaster application. The patient has to be old enough to self-administer it through a one-way mouthpiece. It is considered safe because if a child becomes sedated they will stop breathing the gas. However, Entonox may cause nausea, vomiting and disinhibition.

Entonox should not be used if the child has, or is suspected to have:

- a head injury
- a pneumothorax
- a distended abdomen
- maxillo-facial injuries
- air embolus.

Nerve blocks

In skilled hands a femoral nerve block can provide effective analgesia for a fractured femur and, once working, facilitates the application of traction and a Thomas splint. The femoral nerve lies immediately lateral to the femoral artery. It can be easily visualized with an ultrasound machine. After negative aspiration for blood, a 0.5 ml/kg slow bolus injection of 0.25% of chirocaine around the nerve should provide analgesia within 15–20 minutes and should last for several hours. However, this procedure should only be performed after adequate training.

Summary

The principles of pain relief in children are the same as those in adults. A calm, common-sense approach is essential. The two situations commonly seen in children are giving too little analgesia, or giving too much.

Although the temptation might be to jump straight in to try to alleviate pain in a child immediately, incremental doses of opiates are the safest way of administration. Remember the adage that 'you can always give more, but you can't take away what you've given'.

Golden rules

- Pain needs to be managed proactively in small children
- Morphine can be used safely in children – use incremental doses
- Use simple language when assessing pain
- Explain your management plan clearly and simply to both the child and parents

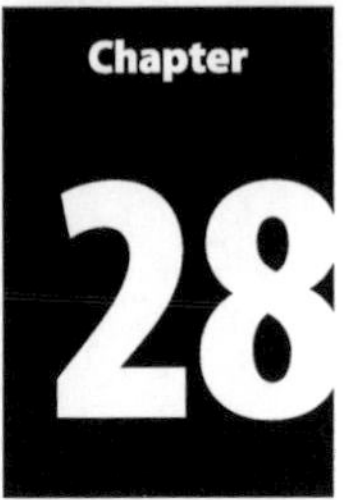

Children with complex needs and disability

Kate Skone and Ian Wacogne

Introduction

Children with complex medical problems pose particular challenges to the clinical team. The family members and carers are often expert in their child's condition, have frequent visits to hospital and may have very specific expectations.

Despite the fact that these children can have very complicated background medical problems they are still most likely to present with one of three problems:

- respiratory infection or respiratory failure
- seizures
- systemic infection.

Children with complex needs will be managed along the same principles as detailed in the other chapters in this book. The aim of this chapter is to highlight two important factors that should be considered in these children; namely, how to access information about the child and to consider which other professionals should be involved in the child's care. It will also discuss how children may deviate from the usual care pathways in some circumstances.

Differences in children

Although the vast majority of the conditions encountered are very rare individually, children with some form of disability are relatively common. The Office for Disability Issues reports that approximately 1 in 20 children have a disability. This equates to approximately 700 000 children across the UK suffering from physical disabilities, learning difficulties or a combination of both.

Children with complex needs differ from adults with multiple co-morbidities in:

- the types of pathology
- the challenges of learning difficulties and communication at different developmental stages
- the network of professionals involved in looking after the child.

Often children with a disability may have conditions that cause chronic health problems as well as disability. In children, long hospital stays and complex medical problems can have significant effects on growth and development.

Managing the Critically Ill Child, ed. Richard Skone *et al.* Published by Cambridge University Press.

The care package

Primary carers

Children with complex medical problems and disability will have the majority of their care carried out by their parents and extended family but may have professional carers involved to provide respite or regular nursing support. The family may be very used to their child being unwell and have had many hospital stays or visits to intensive care.

Care-givers may be responsible for delivering quite complex medical care for their children including:

- home ventilation
- tracheostomy changes
- chest physiotherapy
- nasogastric feeding
- administration of medications, in some cases intravenous.

They will often continue to deliver care while the child is in hospital.

Medical input

Children with disabilities and complex needs will have a lead paediatric consultant who may be community- or hospital-based. The children may well be known to a number of other paediatric teams, either locally or specialists in the nearest children's hospital. They are often well known to medical and nursing staff on paediatric wards, especially if they are regularly admitted with medical problems.

Community input

In the community setting, children are often well known to community and school nursing teams. They are likely to have regular contact with therapists, who may also have information about a child's usual function.

Respite care

Children may have regular respite care and may have carers outside the family who also know them well. Children may be brought to hospital by respite carers who understand the medical issues. However, carers will not have parental responsibility and cannot consent to treatment. In the absence of parents emergency treatment should be administered working under the principle of 'best interests'.

It is important to inform and involve the lead clinician or the paediatric team when the child presents unwell, and to consider other members of the team involved when seeking information. Many local paediatric departments keep information about children who have complex health problems readily available, for example in a file on the ward. This can be a useful source of information, provided the information is up to date.

Communicating with children

It can be difficult to communicate with young children, especially when they are frightened and unwell. It may be more difficult with children who have underlying disability. It is essential to discover the child's normal level of function and understanding.

Children with disabilities will communicate in a wide range of ways, and use certain forms of sign language, e.g. Makaton in the UK. They may have hearing impairment and may wear hearing aids, which should be used even if they are critically unwell. A parent or carer may need to be involved. This aspect of care should not be neglected.

Particular conditions to consider

Respiratory conditions

The practical management of respiratory problems in children with disability is no different from that in other children. However, children with underlying disease may get more unwell more quickly.

Respiratory infections

The management of respiratory infections in children has already been covered in Chapter 7. Several different mechanisms may make some children prone to recurrent, severe, chest infections (see Table 28.1).

Table 28.1. Common precipitants of illness in children with complex illnesses.

Mechanism	Examples
Lung disease with colonization or poor reserve	Bronchopulmonary dysplasia Bronchiectasis
Recurrent aspirations	Tracheostomy (microaspiration) Chronic neurological disease Neurodegenerative conditions, e.g. mitochondrial disease Epilepsy
Neurological disease with poor respiratory effort	Cerebral palsy Hypotonia Scoliosis Muscular dystrophy
Immunocompromise	Malignancy Asplenism

Choice of antibiotics

Children with frequent chest infections may be on prophylactic antibiotics during the winter months or all year round. These children are often colonized with unusual flora. It is important to look at previous microbiology reports, as this will guide antibiotic choice. If there is doubt a discussion with their respiratory clinician or microbiologist may be useful.

Prophylactic measures

In children under 1 year the most significant viral illness is usually respiratory syncitial virus (RSV). The presenting features and management of RSV have been discussed elsewhere (see Chapter 7). Children with complex medical problems may be treated with palivizumab, a monoclonal RSV antibody that may prevent severe pathology from RSV infection. Passive immunization against RSV requires monthly IM injections. Current UK guidelines from the Department of Health recommend giving palivizumab:

- according to gestation at birth and presence of chronic lung disease at times of high RSV prevalence
- to premature infants with haemodynamically significant acyanotic congenital heart disease
- to children younger than 1 year old who are on long-term ventilation
- To children suffering from certain immune deficiency syndromes, e.g. SCID.

Tracheostomy

There are a number of children in the population with long-term tracheostomies. These may have been inserted to manage:

- structural airway problems, such as subglottic stenosis following intubation
- congenital airway abnormalities such as Pierre Robin sequence
- long-term respiratory disease such as bronchopulmonary dysplasia
- children who require home ventilation.

Parents and carers will have been trained in tracheostomy management but they may present with problems to the emergency department. Tracheostomies may become blocked or dislodged. It is likely that paediatricians will be less confident with tracheostomy care than anaesthetists. All children with a tracheostomy are expected to have an appropriate-sized replacement and a suction machine with them at all times.

Home oxygen

The commonest reason for children to require home oxygen is prematurity. This is usually to treat chronic lung disease. Babies are discharged from the neonatal unit with low-flow oxygen, usually delivered by nasal prongs. In general this is in continuous use and it is unusual for this to be above 0.5 l/min.

Lung maturation continues, with new alveoli developing, during the first few years of life. It is unusual for premature babies to need oxygen therapy after the age of 2 years. The need for oxygen therapy is assessed by regular sleep studies, which are monitored by a neonatal physician or respiratory team.

The physiology of these children can be compared to adults with chronic obstructive airways disease in that they often have a compensated respiratory acidosis. It is not uncommon to see a high $PaCO_2$ of up to 10–12 kPa with a compensatory high bicarbonate level.

Children with limited respiratory function

While some children have limited reserve because of poor gas transfer at an alveolar level, others may suffer from an inability to mount a respiratory response to infection or acidosis. These children may have neurological conditions such as cerebral palsy or muscular dystrophy.

The important thing to note in these children is that they may not look as if they are in respiratory distress. Signs such as intercostal recession may not be present if they have poor muscle function. If there is any doubt, a capillary or arterial blood gas analysis should be performed to evaluate the effectiveness of their ventilation.

Neurological problems

Seizures

The standard management of seizures in children has been covered in Chapter 10.

Children with complex epilepsy will often have frequent seizures at home. The manifestation of seizures may be very variable. Some children can present obviously in convulsive status epilepticus with generalized tonic clonic seizures, whereas others may have more subtle seizures causing facial twitching or eye deviation. To complicate matters, children with neurological disorders may have other abnormal movements that do not represent seizures, for example tics or dystonic movements.

In children with severe disabilities it can be difficult to assess how alert the child is and what is abnormal for them. Parents and carers will be able to describe the various seizures that their child has and how the current seizures differ. Sometimes the only way to identify whether repetitive abnormal movements are seizures is to use EEG monitoring.

Clusters of seizures, even partial seizures, may require IV anticonvulsants. Children may also present in non-convulsive or subclinical status; features that suggest this include:

- reduced conscious level
- behavioural or mood changes
- sleep disturbance
- loss of skills or developmental regression.

This is usually confirmed on an EEG. It may require intervention with intravenous anticonvulsants, most commonly benzodiazapines. This will be managed on the advice of a paediatrician or neurologist but may necessitate respiratory support on intensive care.

Many families of children with epilepsy will have been taught to administer buccal midazolam at home. In many cases the parents will have been instructed to present to the ED whenever they use midazolam. In others, buccal midazolam may be used frequently and parents will only bring the child into hospital if it has not been effective.

Individualized management plans

Many children with difficult to manage seizures have individualized management plans written by their lead clinicians. Parents are likely to have a copy of this and it should also be available in the child's notes. It is usually developed after many previous successes and failures and may avoid the need for intubation and ventilation. As well as detailing the drugs that work, the management plan will contain information about which drugs to avoid; for example, some children have profound respiratory depression with benzodiazepines which often results in admission to ICU.

Many children do end up with frequent ICU admissions when their seizure control decompensates; however, it is important to make use of the individualized management plan and if possible discuss the child with the clinicians who know them to try and optimize further management.

Some children with complex needs may have an advanced care plan regarding escalation of treatment, e.g. admission to ICU or palliative care (see Chapter 29).

Ventriculoperitoneal shunt

Ventriculoperitoneal (VP) shunt drains fluid from the ventricles of the brain. They may become blocked, leading to an accumulation of CSF and a rise in ICP. This may or may not be associated with infection. The symptoms and signs of a blocked shunt may be subtle, especially in non-verbal children. They include:

- headaches
- increase in frequency of seizures
- vomiting
- reduced conscious level
- full and tense fontanelle
- irritability.

If there is any suspicion of a blocked shunt a CT scan should be requested and the child discussed with their neurosurgical team. Infections of a VP shunt are more likely within the first 6 months after insertion and may present with meningism.

Infection

Management of sepsis has been covered in Chapter 5. In children with complex medical problems the signs of sepsis may be subtle. In searching for a source of infection it is important to remember about indwelling devices as a source.

Children may have long-term vascular access for numerous reasons:

- chronic respiratory conditions, e.g. those with cystic fibrosis or bronchiectasis may have regular courses of IV antibiotics
- chronic gastro-intestinal diseases, e.g. those with short gut syndromes or malabsorption syndromes may need parenteral nutrition and have a central line for this
- dialysis lines
- malignancy and chemotherapy.

Children on chemotherapy will be immunocompromised and are at risk of being neutropenic. Therefore any child with a malignancy presenting with fever should be treated with IV antibiotics. The central lines should only be accessed using a sterile technique, and only if necessary. Ideally the antibiotics should be given within the first hour of presentation as this has been demonstrated to be associated with reduced morbidity and mortality. If there is any doubt, consideration should be given to removing the CVC. This should be discussed with the team responsible for the child's ongoing care.

Table 28.2. Potential sources of infection.

Device	Examination	Investigations
Ventriculoperitoneal shunt	Shunt can normally be felt running behind the ear and down the back of the neck	Shunt series to look for fractured shunt (plain X-rays of shunt tubing, CT head) Tap of shunt (see Chapter 19)
Central line	Tunnelled line usually palpable on the chest; examine under the dressing for infection and along the path of the line	Blood cultures from each lumen Swab of line insertion site
Implantable long-term venous access device, e.g. Portacath	Palpate port, usually on chest wall, and examine along the course of the palpable line	If access is possible then send cultures from the port
Percutaneous endoscopic gastrostomy	Remove dressings over percutaneous endoscopic gastrostomy and examine surrounding skin	Swab of site
-ostomies	Examine site	Swab Send samples to laboratory
Urinary catheter	Contents of urine bag Abdominal examination	Send urine specimen

Management and sources of information

Often the most complex aspect of management of children with complex needs is communication. It is important to ensure that information is available to the intensive care team who are involved in looking after the child.

The paediatric team should be leading and coordinating the fact-finding. Sources of information about the child will include:

- the family themselves; they may carry recent letters from appointments with their community paediatrician that summarize their care
- the hospital notes, which should be accessed early, particularly if there is a need for transfer elsewhere
- notes or recent letters, which many paediatric departments will keep available on the ward for children who present frequently
- patient-held notes, which some departments are piloting; which means that the family may carry some of the medical notes with them.

The child's regular clinician should be involved with any significant decisions about changes to the long-term treatment plan.

After initial stabilization

The admission of a child to hospital may be an opportunity to review the child's medication. Often children are on many drugs and, on admission, errors in drug doses are discovered. This is often particularly important for anti-epileptic medication, where the child may have outgrown their dose.

The admitting team should not change a child's long-term medications without discussion with the primary team; however, taking a detailed history may give an idea as to the precipitating cause of the problem. This can then help guide the ongoing management.

Discussing with parents

Although they may be used to the process of having their child admitted to hospital, parents of children with complex needs will need a lot of support when their child is critically ill. The admissions do not stop being scary.

The parents may wish to continue carrying out aspects of their care. They may also have had previous experiences when their child has been unwell which affect their expectations.

When informing them of the management plan for their child take time to listen to any worries that they may have. Address each question, and give a clear explanation of what is going to happen next.

Although many are knowledgeable about their child, the majority of parents who have a child with a rare condition will not expect you to know everything about their disease. It is very easy to come unstuck if you are not open with them about the level of your knowledge of their child's condition.

Preparation for transfer

When transferring a child to another hospital there should be as detailed as possible a transfer letter so that the team looking after the child understand the medical problems. The local paediatric team should produce this, especially if they are well known to them. It should include:

- any recent background letters
- any information about advanced care plans, which should be clear and discussed with the family
- all investigations performed on this admission (including radiology)
- information about who is going to inform the primary teams involved in looking after the child.

Summary

Managing a child with complex needs can be daunting. However, the majority of management principles are the same as for any other child. If it is possible to get parents 'on board' early, then the management of the child becomes a lot easier. The main aim of management is to gather as much information as possible while managing the child's presenting problem. In reality, the paediatricians present at an emergency will be collecting the information quickly, while the emergency physicians deal with the acute problems.

Golden rules

- Gather as much information as possible from the parents
- Do not exclude parents from the resuscitation area if they wish to be present
- In the absence of any other information treat the child as you would a less complicated paediatric patient
- Be clear about your management plan
- You do not need to be an expert in the child's condition – most parents will not expect it
- Phone the parent team/retrieval team early for advice

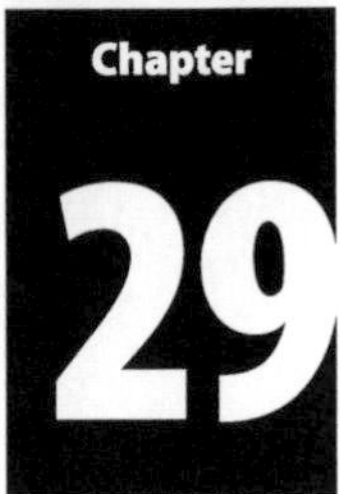

When a child dies

Fiona Reynolds

Introduction

A dying child should be afforded the comfort and dignity which good palliative care provides. ED doctors and anaesthetists are likely to be involved in the care of children at the end of life either during failed resuscitation attempts or when children on a palliative care pathway are brought into hospital because of a sudden deterioration.

Children with 'end of life plans'

Unplanned admission

For children with end of life plans hospice admission may be the most appropriate way to support care-givers and children. Sometimes, however, care-givers may bring their child to a hospital as they become scared and feel they cannot cope at home with a child at the end of life. Good planning and palliative care should prevent children who are receiving palliative care at home from needing to be admitted to hospital.

Setting the environment

Care-givers should be supported and allowed to be present when their child is dying. If they do not want to be present, they should not be pressured to do so. Most care-givers choose to be present and ultimately find comfort in being close to their dying child. Care-givers may need support to be there and may find comfort from the presence of a senior nurse; other care-givers may want privacy to say goodbye with only family members present.

Medical and nursing staff who seldom deal with dying children may find this especially difficult. Staff may experience a mixture of emotions and may find it difficult to perform their duties. Care-givers and families often remember a variety of acts or words from professional staff during this time. While it is acceptable for staff to be sad and to look sad, it is important that professionalism is maintained, as there is a very important job to do when a child is dying.

Withholding or withdrawal of life-sustaining therapy

Decisions about withdrawal of intensive therapy require a sound knowledge of the condition, treatment and the child's prognosis. They also require a working knowledge of

Managing the Critically Ill Child, ed. Richard Skone *et al.* Published by Cambridge University Press.

ethical and legal aspects of withholding and withdrawing life-sustaining therapy. The Royal College of Paediatric and Child Health and the General Medical Council in the UK publish a professional framework for end of life care. It discusses both ethical and legal aspects of practice.

Medicine relating to withdrawing and withholding life-sustaining therapy

Senior medical and nursing staff should be involved in the medical decisions about the diagnosis, possible treatments and prognosis for critically ill children. These individuals should be expert in the appropriate area of medicine and should know the patient's clinical details. Decisions about treatment should involve care-givers: this applies whether it is continued active treatment or the withholding or withdrawal of life-sustaining therapy.

Decisions about withholding or withdrawal of life-sustaining therapy should be made by consensus between the senior professionals involved, the care-givers and child if he or she is able to participate in the decision. Decisions are based on the 'best interests' of the child. If there is no consensus a second opinion should be requested and may be useful as an independent review of the child's treatment and prognosis. If no consensus can be reached ultimately a court may have to decide on whether to continue active treatment or to withhold or withdraw life-sustaining therapy.

Many children with life-limiting disorders who are expected to die have an advance care plan. This plan outlines the actions to be followed in the event of acute deterioration. The treatment plan may range from an attempt at active resuscitation to a plan for comfort care and to allow natural death to occur. It is important that clinicians are aware of the local paperwork which supports advance care or 'Do not attempt cardiopulmonary resuscitation' plans.

Ethics relating to withdrawing and withholding life-sustaining therapy

The duties of a doctor underpin their professional actions. Deontological ethics judges the morality of an action based on adherence to rules or performance of duties. The duties of a doctor are considered to be:

- autonomy: respect for a person to decide about themselves
- beneficence: to do good
- nonmaleficence: to do no harm
- justice: addresses the question of distribution of scarce healthcare resources.

The primary duties of a doctor are to 'do good' in trying to preserve life but the other duties of a doctor may challenge the duty of beneficence. A doctor also has a duty to recognize the dying patient so as not to prolong the process of dying with an unnecessary burden of treatment, which will not improve the outcome but cause suffering whilst not allowing natural death to occur.

Law relating to withdrawing and withholding life-sustaining therapy

Allowing natural death or the process of withdrawing or withholding life-sustaining therapy is both legal and ethical when further treatment is considered futile or not in the best interests of the patient. Withdrawal or withholding intensive therapy requires a consensus between the medical teams treating the patient and the care-givers. If no consensus can be reached a second opinion may help the care-givers with an independent objective view.

If a consensus cannot be reached, ultimately a court may need to decide on the issue of withdrawal of intensive therapy. This is rare; most care-givers' initial resistance is part of a journey of grief, which often starts with denial, but eventual acceptance can allow a consensus to be built and an agreement to switch to comfort care.

Deaths in the emergency department

Most children who die in ED are admitted with cardiopulmonary resuscitation in progress. Occasionally a child who is known to have a terminal illness is admitted *in extremis* and subsequently dies. Most ED have a system to support care-givers while resuscitation is in progress.

All sudden or unexpected deaths in children have to be reported to the coroner, who will establish the cause of death. Most sudden unexpected deaths in childhood are due to natural causes or the result of accidents. A minority of deaths are the result of non-accidental injury.

When the cause of death is not clear, there are often local arrangements for the ED to take blood and small biopsy samples with the coroner's permission to look for infection or inherited diseases which may be the cause of death. These samples are often best taken as soon as possible after death.

If the coroner is to hold a post mortem or an inquest, he or she will be responsible for issuing the death certificate rather than the hospital.

Witnessed resuscitation

In the UK it is now common practice to allow care-givers to be present during attempts at resuscitation if they wish. This may be in the ED, on the children's ward or in the PICU. A senior member of staff should support the care-givers if they wish to be present during resuscitation. The member of staff should explain what is going on and answer any questions that the care-givers have.

Although it may be distressing at the time, there is evidence that parental presence during resuscitation attempts reassures care-givers in the long term that everything possible was done for their child.

Talking to care-givers after the death of a child

This can be particularly stressful for a doctor who is not used to dealing with this situation. Care-givers often do not remember much of what is said but will remember kindnesses and people who take the time to talk to them and show empathy after the death of a child. Being honest particularly about the things that are not understood, e.g. the cause of death or why an accident happened, is particularly important.

Siblings

There are no rules about what to say to siblings, or whether they should visit or see a dying sibling. Many children will have created an impression of what is happening to a loved sibling. Visiting their sick brother or sister and seeing the reality of what is happening may bring comfort as the child's imagination may have created a more distressing image.

Bereavement counselling and follow-up

Bereavement counselling can be accessed through either hospital or community services. Care-givers may find this useful immediately after the death of a child or in the months or years afterwards. Counselling can be accessed through voluntary organizations or the family doctor.

Care-givers frequently have unanswered questions after the death of a child. An individual who can act as a point of contact at the hospital to signpost care-givers to an individual who can answer questions is important. Most hospitals offer care-givers an opportunity to return after a few weeks so that the results of any tests or post mortem examination can be shared with them and to discuss any questions they may have. Unanswered questions can make grieving more difficult and where answers are available they should be given to care-givers so that they understand as much as possible about what happened to their child.

Organ donation

Children may donate organs after death. This usually occurs when patients die in PICU following brainstem death after neurological injury. Organ donation is done with the consent of the care-givers.

Organ donation is also possible after cardiac death when the patient has a non-survivable condition or injury and withdrawal of intensive care results in cardiac arrest. Kidney, liver, lung, corneas, heart valves and small bowel may be donated. However, in these circumstances heart transplantation is not possible.

In the UK organ donation does not usually occur in children under 6 months of age. In the USA there is no lower age limit.

Further reading

Beauchamp TL, Childress JF. *Principles of Biomedical Ethics*. Oxford University Press, 2008.

General Medical Council. *Treatment and care towards the end of life. Good practice in decision making*. July 2010.

Royal College of Paediatrics and Child Health. *Withholding or Withdrawing Life Sustaining Therapy. A Framework for Practice*, 2nd edn. 2004.

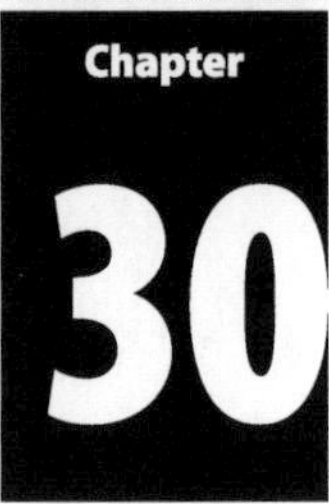

Child protection

Kate Skone and Geoff Debelle

Introduction

It is estimated that around 1% of injuries seen in EDs are not accidental. Children of any age are at risk of assault and non-accidental injury (NAI). However, NAI is commonest under 1 year of age. A Welsh study in 2002 estimated that approximately 1 in 880 babies are abused in the first year of life. The mode of injury, particularly NAI, should be considered in all critically unwell children.

The majority of sudden unexpected deaths in infancy (SUDIs) are due to natural causes; only a small minority are homicides. The sudden unexpected death of a child or infant will automatically initiate an investigation into the cause of death. This will include looking for evidence of NAI by the investigating team. The priorities in the management of child protection issues include:

- involving the sudden unexpected death in infancy (SUDI) team as soon as concerns are raised
- ensuring documentation is detailed
- taking appropriate samples and using the correct procedures when handling samples.

The management issues in a child where NAI is suspected and the protocols associated with the death of a child will be described in this chapter.

Documentation standards

The medical notes for a child who has died may well form evidence in court. However, documentation standards for child protection purposes are no different from standards for all clinical notes (see Table 30.1).

Table 30.1. Minimum standards for documentation.

Name, designation, GMC number on every page
Name, hospital number of patient, date of birth of patient on every page
Date and time of writing notes (24-hour clock)
Full names of others present – clinical staff and family members
Detailed description of clinical events
Any clinical or family history obtained
Any direct quotes from family that are relevant in full

Managing the Critically Ill Child, ed. Richard Skone *et al.* Published by Cambridge University Press.

The paediatric team will complete a detailed assessment, usually on a pre-printed proforma, that includes a detailed history, past medical history, social history and family history. In addition they will carry out a full and detailed examination that is recorded on a body map diagram. If it is possible, consent for this assessment should be taken from a person with parental responsibility.

There will be many other team members involved in the care of a critically ill child. In cases of NAI, the responsible consultant paediatrician will usually write the medical reports that are sent to the police. However, they may not be present when the child arrives in hospital. The police, therefore, often request reports from all of the clinicians involved in the care of the child. All reports should be reviewed by the consultant paediatrician or, in the case of a death, the consultant leading the SUDI team, before submission.

A key responsibility of every team member is therefore accurate and contemporaneous documentation of their observations and the resuscitation.

It is possible that, following investigation, a case may go to court and the court may contact all clinical staff involved in the case. However, the responsibility for attending court and providing medical information usually falls to the lead consultant paediatrician.

Management of laboratory samples – the 'chain of evidence'

All samples should be taken to the laboratories using a 'chain of evidence'. A chain of evidence is a legal concept that requires the names of all persons handling a sample, and the places and conditions of storage, to be documented. The form accompanying each sample will include:

- the person handling the sample's signature
- the time and date
- place of storage or transfer.

This is to ensure that samples are not tampered with. If a chain of evidence is not started when a sample is taken, it is invalid. Chain of evidence proformas should be available in all EDs and PICU.

Critically ill children where NAI is suspected

It is important to consider NAI when looking after a seriously ill or injured child. The clinical scenario will dictate how high on the list of differential diagnoses this may be considered. An inconsistent history or worrying patterns of injury should alert staff to the possibility of harm being inflicted on a child.

History

After the initial stabilization of a sick child an experienced clinician, probably a paediatrician, will need to take a history of events. There may be information from other healthcare professionals, such as paramedics, which may indicate that NAI should be considered.

When the history is taken the following factors may increase suspicion of NAI:

- history that does not seem to fit with the pattern of injuries
- inconsistent history between family members
- injuries that are attributed to a child or sibling and are not commensurate with their developmental stage
- delay in presentation to healthcare.

Examination

If a child presents with any of the injuries in Table 30.2 it is important to consider whether they are inflicted injuries and take a careful history (see above).

Table 30.2. Injuries that should prompt consideration of NAI as a cause.

Complex skull fractures (bilateral, stellate, crossing suture lines)
Abdominal trauma without any history of abdominal injury
Multiple clusters of bruises
Bruises away from bony prominences such as ears, face, chin, buttocks, trunk and posterior thigh
Bruises in the shape of objects
Drowning (in infants)
Human bite marks
Poisoning, such as methadone ingestion, that may present as non-traumatic coma
Burns – forced-immersion scalds, contact burns, burns in unusual areas and burns from house fires
Fractures • Long bone fractures in infants < 18 months • Multiple fractures • Fractures in unusual sites (scapula, sternum) • Occult fractures such as rib or metaphyseal
Torn labial or lingual frenulum

Abusive head injury is the commonest inflicted life-threatening injury. Features that would raise concerns of NAI in a head injury include:

- subdural haemorrhages in children under 1 year old, particularly multiple subdurals
- associated hypoxic ischaemic injury and cerebral oedema
- no evidence of impact injury
- co-existing acute encephalopathy (with apnoea, seizures and collapse)
- other injuries to the head and neck or long bone fractures
- multiple retinal haemorrhages through all layers of the retina, may be unilateral.

Management

Non-clinical

The principal differences in the care of a child when NAIs are suspected are the additional medical investigations and social enquiries that are carried out. It is important to inform the parents of each step in this process. This process will include referral to children's social services. Parents should also be informed about this, unless this action will put the child at increased risk.

Any members of the team who have concerns about child protection must make sure that these are communicated to the team leader and the child safeguarding teams so that they can be investigated appropriately. The child must not be discharged home without a clear decision being made and documented.

Clinical

When managing a child with suspected NAI it is important to remember that the child may have additional unseen injuries. They should therefore be managed as a trauma patient. The important sites to consider are:

- abdominal injury: there may be no signs of external injury but visceral trauma may result in the patient becoming cardiovascularly unstable
- intracranial injury: children with abusive head injury may have multiple subdurals, parenchymal contusions and generalized cerebral hypoxic ischaemia with brain swelling
- limb injuries: children who have been assaulted may also have new or old fractures that will be revealed on a skeletal survey.

Additional investigations

Alongside the important clinical management, additional investigations will be necessary to assess for further injuries or look for medical causes that explain the illness or injury (see below).

Ongoing child protection issues

Once the child has been stabilized ensure that the child is in a place of safety and that they are kept free from further harm. A critically ill child is likely to go to intensive care. Police and social services have powers at their disposal to keep children in a place of safety and limit or supervise visitors.

Once a referral has been made to social services and the police are involved in ongoing investigations a range of court orders can be used to ensure the child is kept safe. These can be initiated immediately, and are then continued by the family courts. It is the responsibility of social services to set these up but the team looking after the child need to know if the child is under a court order, who is allowed to visit, and if the visits need supervising.

Police and social services need to be involved early as there may be other children who need to be in a place of safety.

Sudden unexpected death in children and infants (SUDI)

The investigation of deaths in children is always a difficult and sensitive issue. Over 300 babies a year die suddenly and unexpectedly in the UK. Following several recent high-profile cases it is an area that is under a great deal of scrutiny. Government guidance has led to the structure and organization of child protection services being tightly legislated.

Children may have a sudden and unexpected death either in hospital or as an out-of-hospital cardiac arrest. Every ED and paediatric department will have a local protocol for the assessment and management of the sudden, unexpected deaths. The SUDI team and the on-call paediatric consultant should be involved in all of these cases. This team is also involved in investigating traffic accidents, suicides and children who have a pre-existing life-limiting condition who are deemed to have died unexpectedly.

When a child is found dead resuscitation is usually attempted and is often ongoing on arrival at hospital. The police are informed by the ambulance crew and are often present when the child is brought into hospital. The police are responsible for leading the investigation, along with children's services.

The role of the health professionals is to provide appropriate medical care. If the child dies they must carry out the relevant investigations into the cause of death and produce a medical report. This medical report will be written by the paediatric consultant involved in the case or by the named doctor for child protection. As part of the investigation the SUDI team will carry out a 'rapid response' investigation that may include a home visit by a senior clinician. These home visits can provide a wealth of information for the subsequent investigations. This is always carried out when a child dies and may also be appropriate following an 'out-of-hospital arrest'.

Medical investigations to consider in a critically ill child or following a SUDI

The investigations carried out in each case of critical illness or death will be dictated by the clinical situation. The results may form part of a criminal investigation, and should therefore be managed with a 'chain of evidence' (see above).

If a critical illness or death is unexpected the purpose of investigations is to look for a medical cause, including rare causes, or to provide evidence of inflicted injury. This usually includes detailed imaging and extensive investigations for infection, toxicology, metabolic disease and inherited conditions. The majority of these additional investigations can be carried out after the child has been stabilized.

A medical investigation into the cause of an unexpected death will involve a post mortem. Any samples taken during resuscitation may also be important in determining the cause of death. There are also investigations that need to be sent off immediately after death.

The RCPCH Child Protection Companion is a valuable source of suggested investigations in children who present with particular patterns of injuries; an example of investigations for abusive head trauma can be seen in Table 30.3.

Table 30.3. Investigations in abusive head trauma.

Formal indirect opthalmoscopy through dilated pupils for retinal haemorrhages using RETCAM
Neuroimaging: • CT scan of head as soon as stable on presentation • If CT head abnormal then MRI head and spinal cord on day 3–5 • Following MRI if abnormalities at 3–6 months after injury
Skeletal survey when stable and repeat survey or chest film in 14 days
Coagulation studies – full blood count and film, PT, APTT (not INR), thrombin time, serum fibrinogen, factor VIIIc, VWF antigen and activity, platelet glycoproteins Ib, IIb/IIIa or PFA closure time with epinephrine and ADP, factor XIII screen (if under 3 months)
Blood for carnitine and acyl carnitine profile
Blood cultures to exclude sepsis
Urine for toxicology and metabolic screen

Some children who present seriously unwell to the ED may go on to die on PICU. Samples taken at the time of presentation can be vital in investigating the cause of death; for example, it is important that coagulation studies are done before administering blood products where possible, or toxicology is taken immediately at the time of presentation. Every region will have a list of recommended investigations that will be carried out following a SUDI; an example of these is detailed below from the West Midlands SUDI protocol (Table 30.4).

Table 30.4. Example of investigations undertaken following a SUDI (from West Midlands SUDI protocol).

Blood should be taken ideally within 30 minutes of death and not more than 4 hours after death. All the sites of sampling should be documented and a cardiac stab may be necessary. The investigations include tests for infection, toxicology, metabolic causes and genetic causes of death
Blood cultures
Full blood count (consider carboxyhaemoglobin)
Electrolytes, renal and liver function
Serum for toxicology
Blood for a Guthrie card (if available) for inherited metabolic diseases
Cytogenetics
CSF for culture and microscopy
Nasopharyngeal aspirate for microbiology and virology and immunofluorescence
Swabs from any identifiable lesions for microbiology
Urine for culture, toxicology and inherited diseases
Throat swab for culture and microscopy
Skin biopsy for fibroblast culture
Skeletal survey; it is important that parents do not have unsupervised access to the body prior to this happening

Organ donation

The process of investigation does not exclude the possibility of organ donation. However, coroners may differ in their response. Some may allow donation of organs if the paediatric and forensic pathologist is present in the operating theatre to ensure that no evidence is lost in the process. If organ donation is a possibility then the regional donor transplant coordinator should be involved as soon as possible.

What do I need to have organized before departure to PICU?

In suspected NAI, the clinical management of a critically ill child takes priority. In order to ensure that any necessary investigations are carried out as smoothly as possible the most important thing to do is to ensure that the contact information for the local paediatrician who is going to lead on the child protection investigation is available. The local paediatric team will be involved in any child protection investigations and they will liaise with social services, the police and the ICU as child protection investigations continue.

It is important to keep parents and carers informed of all steps in the child protection process and investigation.

Summary

Child protection is the responsibility of the local paediatric team but careful documentation and management of samples is crucial. This chapter has detailed the child protection management that will occur alongside the stabilization of a sick child.

Golden rules

- Documentation must be scrupulous
- Samples must be transported with a chain of evidence
- Samples should be taken for coagulation studies before any blood products are given
- Treat a child who has been assaulted as a trauma patient and remember to look for additional injuries
- Families must be handled sensitively

Further reading

Craft A. *Child Protection Companion*. RCPCH, 2006. (Revised edition to be published 13 March 2013.)

http://www.core-info.cardiff.ac.uk.

RCoA child protection guidelines. http://www.rcoa.ac.uk/document-store/child-protection-and-the-anaesthetist-safeguarding-children-the-operating-theatre.

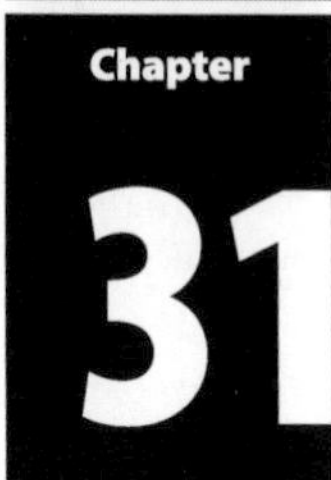

Ventilation

J. Nick Pratap

Introduction

Critically ill children often require ventilatory support as part of their intensive care management. Indications include:

- prevention of airway soiling
- reversal of failing gas exchange
- overcoming airway obstruction or protecting airway structures
- reduction in the work of breathing, e.g. advanced circulatory failure
- access for suction of secretions
- initiation of therapies, such as bronchial lavage in burns, or surfactant administration in prematurity.

Considerations when ventilating children

Physiology

A respiratory membrane capable of gas exchange develops by 22–23 weeks' gestation, but true alveoli only develop after 30 weeks. Very premature birth, especially before 26 weeks, disrupts lung development. This can be compounded by factors such as pneumonia, oxygen toxicity and the mechanical effects of artificial ventilation, leading to chronic lung disease (CLD) of prematurity.

Smaller children

There are a number of physiological differences between infants and older children/adults, including:

- at term there are only a third to half the adult number of alveoli
- they have a high oxygen requirement per unit body weight and low relative functional residual capacity (leading to rapid desaturation)
- respiratory muscles of young children have a low proportion of high-endurance muscle fibres, so they tire more readily than adults
- apnoeas are often accompanied by bradycardia and desaturation.

Managing the Critically Ill Child, ed. Richard Skone *et al.* Published by Cambridge University Press.

For premature babies, the difference is even greater:

- surfactant is not secreted in adequate quantity until approximately 30 weeks (may be stimulated earlier by exogenous corticosteroids if given to the mother prenatally)
- control of breathing is not fully matured in preterm infants – central apnoeas occur in response to a wide range of insults.

The work of breathing is higher in spontaneously breathing young children, consequently establishing mechanical ventilation can substantially reduce these demands.

Ventilators and associated equipment in PICUs

Ventilators

Children requiring ventilation on PICU can vary from below 500 g to more than 100 kg in weight. No single ventilator is ideal for the whole range. NICU ventilators often work well for infants up to 5–10 kg. Above this adult ventilators are often suitable, although paediatric software upgrades may be needed.

Humidification

For PICU ventilators active humidification is standard, often composed of a hot water bath with heating wires in the inspiratory limb to reduce condensation. For transport purposes heat and moisture exchange (HME) filters are suitable.

End-tidal capnography

This may reduce the need for blood gas analysis, but is less accurate with small tidal volumes and fast respiratory rates. Main-stream analysers are less affected than side-stream, so may be better in small children. Care needs to be taken to ensure the weight of the sensor does not kink the endotracheal tube (ET tube).

Suction

ET tube blockage is a problem, especially with the smaller sizes necessary in newborns; urgent re-intubation may be necessary. An inability to pass an endotracheal suction catheter (in French gauge, twice the internal diameter of the ET tube) may be the first sign, but the problem should also be considered in the face of increasing ventilator pressure requirements or an obstructive $ETCO_2$ trace.

When suctioning the trachea in children, many prefer to limit passage of the catheter to the end of the ET tube, to avoid damaging the fragile mucosa.

Ventilator therapies

Non-invasive ventilatory support (NIVS)

In this instance NIVS is used to cover both CPAP and non-invasive ventilation (NIV). Ventilation support that avoids intubating the trachea may reduce both the risk of respiratory infection and the need for sedation. Problems when using NIVS in children include:

- lack of cooperation – careful use of sedation can help
- skin trauma – may develop rapidly, but can be ameliorated by application of colloid dressings

- gastric distension and diaphragmatic splinting – inserting a gastric tube (via the oral route if using nasal NIVS) helps overcome this
- difficulty clearing lower respiratory tract secretions – can be overcome with effective physiotherapy
- it may not be possible in cases of orofacial trauma or congenital anomaly, such as choanal atresia.

In neonatal practice NIVS is commonly chosen as a first-line support, mainly in the form of nasal CPAP, as it is useful for apnoeas related to both prematurity and respiratory infection. Infants with very immature lungs are often extubated early to CPAP after intratracheal administration of surfactant, to protect the lungs from iatrogenic damage.

Some of the indications for NIVS in children are given in Table 31.1. However, it tends to fail in patients who meet ARDS criteria or have multi-organ dysfunction, due to severity of underlying disease.

Table 31.1. Indications for NIVS in children.

Condition	Comments
Neuromuscular disease	Useful with intercurrent pneumonia – avoids risks and complications of intubation, including ventilator dependence
Obstructive sleep apnoea	Usually nocturnal support only
Immunocompromise	Intubation associated with poor outcome
Sickle-cell acute chest syndrome	Use in combination with good analgesia
Cardiomyopathy/ myocarditis	Supports myocardium through cardiopulmonary interactions and avoids cardiovascular system decompensation at intubation
Laryngomalacia	Helps overcome upper airway obstruction
Post-extubation	May avoid need for reintubation if ongoing CVS or RS compromise, such as impaired cardiac function or post-surgical diaphragmatic paresis

Continuous positive airway pressure (CPAP)

A face mask, covering both nose and mouth, is often used to deliver CPAP, but nose-only masks and helmets have a role too. For infants the nasal route is preferred, with short, binasal prongs shown to be more effective than a single nasopharyngeal prong.

Bi-level ventilation

Non-invasive bi-level ventilation can be used instead of CPAP, particularly if CO_2 clearance is a problem. Generally a flow trigger is used, as this is most sensitive to small respiratory efforts. A backup rate may also be provided. Typical set pressures are 10–20 cmH_2O and 5–10 cmH_2O for inspiratory and expiratory phases, respectively.

Invasive positive-pressure ventilation

For the majority of children with normal lungs, such as postoperative surgical cases, conventional pressure-controlled ventilation is ideal. This is because it compensates better than volume-control for a leak around an uncuffed ET tube. Typical ventilator parameters are set as follows:

- peak inspiratory pressure (PIP) of 14–18 cmH_2O
- positive end expiratory pressure (PEEP) 5 cmH_2O
- I:E ratio around 1:1.5–2
- respiratory rate in the low normal range for spontaneous breathing in that age group (see Chapter 35).

When adjusting the ventilator to ideal settings, change the PIP to achieve a tidal volume of 5–7 ml/kg. If the child should start breathing, it may be more comfortable for the child to set a SIMV or bi-level version of the mode.

Displayed tidal volumes may be inaccurate in small children as ventilator tubing distends with increased pressure, giving a falsely high reading. A visual check for adequate chest movement along with assessment of end-tidal and arterial CO_2 should always be performed. In order to achieve adequate chest movement, tidal volumes up to 10 ml/kg may be used.

In synchronized (spontaneous) modes flow rather than pressure triggers are preferred, as less respiratory effort is required. Although there may be concern about the work of breathing through a narrow ET tube, studies have shown this to be negligible, even for small infants.

A pressure-generated volume guarantee mode (such as pressure-regulated volume control, PRVC) is also suitable, especially where it is desirable to maintain a stable $PaCO_2$ or where compliance and resistance may change rapidly.

As with adults, permissive hypercapnia may be an appropriate strategy, if not contra-indicated. Following the influential ARDSnet study of lung-protective ventilation, respiratory acidosis is tolerated as long as the pH remains above 7.15.

High-frequency oscillatory ventilation (HFOV)

HFOV is frequently used in PICU, with the aim of avoiding ventilator-induced lung injury and improving oxygenation. The ventilator generates compressions and rarefactions in the inspired gases, similar to sound waves but below the threshold of human hearing. As the 'tidal volumes' generated are smaller than the anatomical dead space, gas transport to the respiratory membrane depends on non-physiological mechanisms.

The main adjustable parameters used are:

- mean airway pressure (MAP)
- frequency (f) of oscillation
- amplitude or power (ΔP) of oscillation

To improve oxygenation MAP (and FiO_2) can be altered whereas ΔP and f govern CO_2 clearance.

HFOV is most frequently used following failure of adequate oxygenation or CO_2 clearance on conventional ventilation. It may also be used if high inspiratory pressures and FiO_2 are required to maintain oxygenation with conventional ventilation, or the patient has developed an air leak.

Disadvantages of HFOV include:

- elevation of intrathoracic pressure – avoid in intracranial hypertension
- drop in BP when HFOV initiated, by reducing venous return – fluid bolus often needed
- ET tube suction leads to lung derecruitment
- no clinical information from auscultation and $ETCO_2$ measurement.

Initiating HFOV should be learned in a practical session and follow local guidelines. The following is provided as a guide.

- Ensure a relatively straight path from the ventilator to the patient. Avoid even minor kinks of the ET tube and ventilator tube. Do not use an angle connector.
- Frequency should be set at 10–12 Hz for a preterm neonate, 8–10 Hz for an infant, and 5 Hz for a larger child.
- MAP should be set 2–4 cmH_2O higher than the MAP on conventional ventilation.
- Set the ΔP at 10, then increase whilst directly observing the chest of the patient until adequate 'bounce' is seen.
- Perform an arterial blood gas within 20 minutes as a precipitous drop in $PaCO_2$ is common.
- Perform a CXR within the first few hours. Over-distension of the lung may occur. This is associated with suboptimal gas exchange and barotrauma. The diaphragm should be at the level of the eighth rib posteriorly.
- MAP should remain unchanged until the FiO_2 has been weaned to 0.5 or less.
- CO_2 levels can be adjusted through the ΔP and the frequency (reducing f increases CO_2 clearance).

Increasing the MAP to improve oxygenation only works until the lung is over-distended. If increasing the MAP worsens oxygenation then reduce the pressure and reassess. Over time the lung compliance will change on the oscillator; this means that the original MAP may become an 'over-distending' pressure over time. Repeated CXRs and clinical monitoring of the patient should avoid this.

HFOV works better in diffuse lung disease and less well in unilateral disease, due to the risks of over-distending normal lung.

Aids to ventilation

Inhaled nitric oxide (iNO)

iNO dilates the blood vessels associated with ventilated alveoli. This may be useful in both pulmonary hypertension and parenchymal lung disease where there is substantial ventilation/perfusion mismatch. There is minimal systemic vasodilatation as nitric oxide (NO) is readily inactivated by binding to haemoglobin in the pulmonary circulation.

iNO concentrations greater than 10–20 parts per million (ppm) have no additional benefit. Intensivists tend to start at 20 ppm and reduce according to response. Because habituation occurs within a few hours, NO must be weaned slowly, even if there is no clinical benefit. There is a risk of methaemoglobinaemia with prolonged use, so arterial blood co-oximetry should be performed at least daily to identify this. Nitrogen dioxide is inevitably delivered with iNO due to reaction with oxygen. The concentration should be monitored and not allowed to rise above 2 ppm due to the potential for pulmonary toxicity.

Specific ventilatory strategies for different conditions

Preterm neonates

Extremely preterm infant lungs are deficient in surfactant. This increases the work done with each breath to re-open collapsed, poorly compliant alveoli. When combined with minimal airway resistance, this means the time constant (τ) of the respiratory system (compliance × resistance) is low. Neonatology practice reflects this, with a preference for a short inspiratory time (0.4–0.5 s). Meta-analyses confirm that this is associated with lower incidence of air leak syndromes and even a decrease in mortality.

Pressure-controlled ventilation is traditionally used, but volume-targeted modes can result in earlier extubation, and a reduction in both pneumothorax and severe intraventricular haemorrhage rates. Synchronized ventilatory modes show benefit in terms of air leak and duration of ventilation. From large meta-analyses it is clear that choosing conventional ventilation or HFOV does not affect long-term respiratory or neurological outcome.

In severe necrotizing enterocolitis (NEC) patients suffer overwhelming Gram-negative sepsis and develop respiratory failure similar to ARDS. They may also have a tense abdomen, causing considerable mechanical compromise of ventilation. In these patients a longer inspiratory time is often necessary to maintain oxygenation.

The target for oxygenation in premature neonates is lower than in older children in order to reduce the risks of oxygen toxicity, including CLD and retinopathy of prematurity (ROP). However, there are dangers of insufficient oxygenation in this group too, notably patent ductus arteriosus, developmental delay and even increased mortality. The precise at-risk group is not yet defined, but it seems prudent to exercise caution with infants born below 32 weeks or birthweight less than 1.5 kg. An oxygen saturation target of 92–94% is appropriate below 32 weeks of age, thereafter a higher target of 94–99%.

Current practice supports extubation of premature infants from a low ventilator rate without a trial of CPAP. However, electively putting infants on nasal CPAP reduces extubation failure risk.

There has been considerable research into pharmacological strategies to reduce length of ventilatory support and to decrease the incidence of CLD. Diuretics do not appear helpful in this regard. Postnatal steroids have benefits in terms of CLD reduction, but may be associated with worse neurobehavioural outcomes. Antenatal steroid administration to the mother and early postnatal surfactant do improve outcomes.

Chronic lung disease of prematurity

Premature infants requiring 'aggressive' ventilation, or with a genetic predisposition, may suffer scarring and overinflation of the lungs, particularly involving the bronchioles and alveolar septi. This bronchopulmonary dysplasia may be so severe that the infant remains ventilator-dependent for months or even years.

Some children receive long-term ventilatory support in hospital, whilst others are discharged home, often with a tracheostomy. Exacerbations of lung disease may be triggered by common respiratory viruses and can be life-threatening, so PICU admission is common. Aspiration pneumonia is frequent in this population, as long periods of intubation tend to disrupt the usual protective laryngeal mechanisms.

Asthma

Ventilation of children with asthma follows similar principles to that in adults. Slow rates are preferred to allow adequate time for expiration. PEEP should be matched to the patient's intrinsic PEEP, which may vary considerably over time (see Chapter 8 for more details).

Barotrauma and air leaks are very real risks, so pressure-control modes are advisable. A higher than normal maximum peak inspiratory pressure can be tolerated (up to

35 cmH_2O), as this is not transmitted to the alveoli, due to increased airway resistance. Hypercapnia is usually well tolerated.

Bronchiolitis

The pathophysiology of viral bronchiolitis is narrowing of the small airways. It is commoner in young children than asthma, but the principles of mechanical ventilation are broadly similar as it is an acute obstructive lung disease.

Many of the worst affected infants have pre-existing cardiac or lung disease, particularly chronic lung disease of prematurity. HFOV is sometimes used, if conventional ventilation fails.

Tracheobronchomalacia (TBM)

Floppiness of tracheal and/or bronchial wall cartilage results in a tendency for the airway to collapse during active expiration. The key role of the intensivist in TBM is to consider this diagnosis in the infant who is failing a respiratory wean, particularly if they suffer cyanotic spells when agitated.

The diagnosis is best made by bronchography or flexible bronchoscopy. The condition may result from a developmental abnormality of the airway cartilage, from prolonged ventilation (particularly in premature infants) or secondary to external compression by a cardiovascular malformation. High CPAP levels following extubation act as a pneumatic splint for the airways. Surgical treatment or stenting is sometimes required.

Congenital diaphragmatic hernia (CDH)

In this condition the fetus develops with abdominal viscera within the thoracic cavity. Repair of CDH has become a relatively straightforward surgical procedure. However, the increasing success of surgical intervention has highlighted the major cause of morbidity and mortality in these children as pulmonary hypoplasia and pulmonary hypertension. In fact, the pulmonary hypoplasia may be a primary event during the formation of a CDH and not just a consequence. Management following delivery includes:

- avoiding positive-pressure ventilation by face mask
- immediate intubation and ventilation with paralysis to prevent air swallowing and bowel distension
- decompression of the stomach with an NG tube (may be seen to loop back up into the chest on CXR)
- high $PaCO_2$, which is often tolerated and may be necessary to avoid ventilator-induced lung injury (even in the presence of pulmonary hypertension).

Decisions regarding therapy, particularly consideration for extracorporeal membrane oxygenation (ECMO), are complicated by prognostic uncertainty, as the quantity of healthy lung tissue may be inadequate for a good long-term outcome.

Surgical repair of the CDH is usually delayed until pulmonary hypertension is under control and the long-term outlook is clearer.

Congenital heart disease

While standard principles of ventilation apply to most children with congenital heart disease, there are important considerations in certain pathologies.

When there is unrestricted flow between the pulmonary and systemic circulations the proportion of blood flow that passes to each depends on the balance of the pulmonary vascular resistance (PVR) and the systemic vascular resistance (SVR). Connections that can allow unrestricted flow include:

- VSD
- ductus arteriosus
- Blalock–Taussig shunt/aortopulmonary window.

In these patients the oxygenation of arterial blood is dependent on the following factors:

- gas exchange in the lung
- the ratio of pulmonary to systemic blood flow
- degree of mixing of arterial and venous blood.

There are two corollaries of vital importance.

- The usual target of oxygen saturations in the high 90s may be dangerous, as it would require such high pulmonary blood flow that systemic perfusion would be compromised.
- Should the child's oxygen saturations change, it is necessary to consider both the lungs and cardiovascular system as possible causative factors.

'Balancing' circulations

In patients with univentricular physiology, maintaining good lung function is vital. It is desirable to prevent atelectasis. Low levels of CPAP or PEEP should be used routinely. Excessive intrathoracic pressure impedes pulmonary blood flow, so high PEEP is best avoided. To prevent a precipitous drop in PVR and therefore systemic perfusion, FiO_2 is kept low, targeting oxygen saturations of 75–85%. Indeed it is common to ventilate in air. For the same reason, $PaCO_2$ is often kept towards the upper end of the normal range (see Chapter 6).

Children with surgical shunts

As children with surgically 'shunted' physiology grow, their shunts do not. The ratio of pulmonary to systemic blood flow progressively reduces. When pulmonary blood flow is insufficient, further intervention is required.

Failing right heart

Restrictive right heart failure

Acute right heart failure is sometimes seen postoperatively. A classic example occurs after surgical correction of tetralogy of Fallot. This 'restrictive' physiology is exquisitely sensitive to loading conditions, including intrathoracic pressure.

Univentricular systems

For most children with univentricular hearts the Fontan circulation (total cavopulmonary connection) represents their final physiology. To achieve this, following a cavopulmonary shunt, the inferior vena cava is anastomosed to the pulmonary arteries. In these children, all systemic venous blood bypasses the heart and passes directly to the lungs. The absence of a right ventricle can be thought of as an extreme form of right heart failure.

Both the above groups of patients are kept on low PEEP (usually 5 cmH_2O) when intubated. Spontaneous modes and early extubation are preferred where possible, since the negative intrathoracic pressure generated by spontaneous ventilation promotes better pulmonary blood flow. Patients are very dependent on adequate circulating blood volume. Hypovolaemia must be considered should either blood pressure or systemic oxygen saturations drop.

The child who is difficult to ventilate

When difficulties are encountered in achieving adequate gas exchange the following initial steps should be undertaken:

- muscle relaxation (with adequate sedation) – metabolic oxygen requirements are minimized and unhelpful respiratory efforts abolished
- review the CXR for correct ET tube position, lung expansion, areas of collapse and evidence of fluid overload
- optimize cardiac output with fluids and inotropes
- consider changing ET tube, especially in infants, as partial ET tube blockage is hard to detect
- correct anaemia (or increase Hb if cyanotic CHD)
- review the target for oxygenation and $PaCO_2$ depending on underlying conditions (e.g. CLD and CHD) and evidence of tissue oxygenation (e.g. lactate and mixed venous oxygen saturation)
- prone positioning may be beneficial and is usually easy in young children, though care must be taken with lines and tubes.

If the child remains difficult to ventilate, a therapeutic trial of HFOV may be performed. iNO can be tried if severe hypoxaemia remains. Exogenous surfactant administration has been shown to reduce mortality in ventilated children with acute respiratory failure.

Bronchoscopy may elucidate uncertain diagnoses in ventilated children. It also facilitates instillation of the mucolytic agent deoxyribonuclease (DNase), with reports of success in conditions such as lobar collapse, asthma and acute sickle-cell chest crisis.

Refractory respiratory failure

Extracorporeal life support (ECLS) is the subject of renewed interest following trial evidence of good outcome in adults in whom ventilatory strategies fail to achieve adequate gas exchange. Extracorporeal membrane oxygenation (ECMO) is the most common modality. The principle is similar to cardiopulmonary bypass, but the circuit is optimized for longevity. Percutaneous cannulae are used and generally inserted by surgeons. Two types of treatment are available:

- veno-venous ECMO – blood is both drained and returned to the right atrium
- veno-arterial ECMO – blood is drained from the right atrium and returned to the aorta.

The latter does not depend on native myocardial function, so is ideal for cases of cardiogenic shock or where high inotrope doses are needed.

Weaning and extubation

No single mode of ventilation or weaning protocol has been shown to facilitate ventilatory weaning in paediatric critical care. Many PICU patients can be extubated successfully without protracted weaning, although no clinical test adequately predicts readiness for extubation.

Upper airway obstruction accounts for around one-third of PICU extubation failures. Unfortunately, there is no reliable way of predicting this. Dexamethasone, started at least 6 hours before planned extubation, reduces the need for re-intubation, but is usually reserved for those most likely to benefit, such as prolonged intubations, difficult airways or patients with trisomy 21.

Weaning difficulty

Achieving successful extubation can be a challenge in paediatric practice, for a number of reasons:

- neuromuscular weakness may occur in very ill children with a prolonged PICU stay
- undiagnosed congenital conditions may be present in newborns
- residual shunts, valvular lesions or myocardial failure occur following cardiac surgery
- airway compression by abnormal vascular structures may cause airway obstruction and tracheobronchomalacia
- phrenic or laryngeal nerve lesions may occur after thoracic surgery.

Flexible bronchoscopy may reveal unanticipated airways problems. As in adults a tracheostomy may facilitate weaning, but this is less frequently employed, as it needs to be performed surgically. A good way to consider the causes of failure to wean is to think of the six 'Fs':

- failure of organ systems
- fluid balance
- feeding
- fever
- fear, pain and anxiety
- farmacology (*sic*).

Summary

The need for ventilation is common in critically ill children. By fully understanding their different physiological and pathological considerations, it is possible to undertake this safely and effectively.

Golden rules

- Always ventilate children when indicated – don't delay as they can decompensate very rapidly
- The majority of children can be managed with similar ventilatory strategies to adults
- Avoid interventions that may cause harm to the patient or their lungs

Further reading

Essouri S, Chevret L, Durand P, *et al.* Noninvasive positive pressure ventilation: five years of experience in a pediatric intensive care unit. *Pediatr Crit Care Med* 2006;7:329–334.

Newth CJL, Venkataraman S, Willson DF, *et al.* Weaning and extubation readiness in pediatric patients. *Pediatr Crit Care Med* 2009;**10**:1–11.

Saugstad OD, Aune D. In search of the optimal oxygen saturation for extremely low birth weight infants: a systematic review and meta-analysis. *Neonatology* 2010;**100**:1–8.

Stocks J. The respiratory system. In Bingham R, Lloyd-Thomas A, Sury M (eds.), *Hatch & Sumner's Textbook of Paediatric Anaesthesia.* London: Hodder Arnold, 2008.

Chapter 32

Fluid therapy

Adrian Plunkett

Introduction

Acutely ill children often present with derangements in water and electrolyte homeostasis. Although these presentations frequently fall into recognized patterns, an individualized approach to fluid therapy is required to correct deficits safely and establish appropriate maintenance therapy.

A clinician who does not encounter paediatric patients in his or her daily practice may feel daunted when faced with a requirement to prescribe fluid therapy for a sick child. However, an understanding of basic physiological principles and knowledge of some important potential pitfalls are sufficient to inform safe fluid therapy prescribing.

The main aim of this chapter is to describe a structured and simple approach to paediatric fluid therapy, using physiological principles. Prior knowledge of the concepts of osmolarity and tonicity and an understanding of the composition of common IV fluid preparations are assumed (see Tables 32.1 and 32.2 for a summary). There is also a small section on feeding, which is less relevant to the acutely ill child, but important to consider if the child subsequently requires intensive care.

Table 32.1. Osmolarity and tonicity.

Concept	Definition
Osmolarity	The number of osmoles (particles exerting an osmolar effect) per litre of solution
Tonicity	The sum of the concentrations of the solutes which exert an osmotic effect across a cell membrane, i.e. the 'effective osmolarity'. The in vivo tonicity of 5% dextrose is zero, because the dextrose is rapidly metabolized after infusion

Managing the Critically Ill Child, ed. Richard Skone *et al.* Published by Cambridge University Press.

Table 32.2. Osmolarity and tonicity of common intravenous fluid preparations.

Fluid	Sodium ion (mmol/l)	Osmolarity (mOsm/l)	Tonicity, in vivo (mOsm/l)
5% dextrose	0	278	0
0.18% sodium chloride and 4% dextrose	30	300	60
0.45% sodium chloride	75	154	154
0.45% sodium chloride and 5% dextrose	75	432	154
0.9% sodium chloride	154	308	308
0.9% sodium chloride and 5% dextrose	154	586	308

How does fluid therapy differ in children?

The principles of fluid therapy are consistent across all ages. However, it is important to recognize certain physiological differences between adults and children when prescribing fluid therapy. These differences are more pronounced in younger age groups, so particular caution is required when prescribing fluid therapy for infants and newborns. Some important physiological differences between children and adults are listed below.

Energy expenditure (metabolic rate)

The relationship between metabolic rate and body mass is not linear; at smaller mass the metabolic rate is considerably higher. Maintenance water and electrolyte requirements are directly related to energy expenditure as maintenance requirements are replacement for the physiological losses of metabolism. For this reason children require higher rates of maintenance fluid therapy relative to their body size, compared with adults. Quantitative estimates of water and electrolyte maintenance therapy are based on estimates of metabolic rate (see Table 32.4).

Urinary concentrating ability

Newborns typically pass isotonic urine but are only able to concentrate the urine to levels of approximately 500–700 mOsm/l (approximately 50% of maximal adult urine concentration). Along with the greater metabolic demands, this renders newborns and small infants susceptible to dehydration. The urinary concentrating ability typically reaches adult levels by 1 year of age.

Distribution of body water

The proportion of body mass made of water decreases with age until adulthood. Newborn body mass is approximately 75–80% water, compared with adult values of approximately 60%. The extracellular fluid compartment is particularly large in newborns, and undergoes significant contraction in the first few days of life, resulting in physiological weight loss of up to 10% of birth weight. Thus, fluid therapy in the first few days of life should be restricted to avoid fluid overload.

Energy stores

Small children and infants have minimal energy reserves. Maintenance fluid therapy should therefore include adequate glucose to prevent the onset of hypoglycaemia and catabolism.

Non-osmotic release of antidiuretic hormone (ADH)

This is common in sick children. Under normal conditions, ADH is secreted in response to increased serum osmolality, hypotension and hypovolaemia. However, it is also secreted in response to a variety of non-osmotic stimuli, including illnesses such as pneumonia and meningitis. ADH reduces the ability of the kidneys to excrete electrolyte-free water. In the presence of non-osmotic ADH secretion, administration of hypotonic maintenance fluid and failure to restrict water intake will result in hyponatraemia.

Surface area to volume ratio

Because of their high surface area to volume ratio, infants and small children are more susceptible to dehydration secondary to increased evaporative losses of water.

Estimations of fluid and electrolyte therapy – how much to give, and how fast to give it

Acutely ill children often have deficits of water and electrolytes due to their presenting illness. Fluid therapy is composed of three main elements:

- restoring deficits – treatment of shock, or correction of dehydration
- maintenance therapy – providing adequate water, electrolytes and energy to replace the normal losses resulting from metabolism
- replacement of ongoing, non-physiological losses – replacement of excess loss from a pathological process such as diarrhoea.

A fourth category would be replacement of circulatory volume, as in active haemorrhage.

Ideally, each of these three components of fluid therapy should be calculated separately and combined to make a fluid prescription. It is important to remember that these calculations will necessarily be based on gross estimates. Regular assessment of clinical signs, with appropriate alterations to the fluid therapy, is therefore necessary to optimize therapy.

Restoring deficits

Expansion of circulating volume in shock

Some patients present in shock and require rapid resuscitation. The goal of this stage of therapy is to rapidly expand the circulating volume. Initial therapy should consist of isotonic crystalloid or colloid, given in aliquots of 20 ml/kg as a rapid bolus. Repeat this until haemodynamic stability is achieved.

If shock is still present after 60 ml/kg, further haemodynamic support is required, and the patient is likely to require mechanical ventilation, central line insertion and inotropic support.

Choice of fluid for volume expansion

Use an isotonic fluid. Current evidence does not support a preference regarding crystalloid or colloid. Most clinicians favour using crystalloid over colloid as the initial therapy, although colloid may be preferred in septic shock. Resuscitation fluid should not contain potassium or glucose.

Correction of dehydration

The goal of this stage of therapy is to replace water and electrolyte deficits more slowly, over 24–48 hours. Fluid deficit is normally presented as a percentage of body weight, as any short-term reduction in weight is due to fluid loss alone. Estimate of severity of dehydration and calculation of replacement therapy can be done in two ways:

- clinical signs can be used to estimate the severity of dehydration as a proportion of body weight (see Table 32.3)
- a recent, reliable body weight (e.g. from an outpatient appointment) makes a more accurate estimation of dehydration possible.

The rate of fluid deficit replacements and the type of fluid used depend on the plasma sodium level but, in general, the fluid deficit should be replaced slowly (usually 24–48 hours), avoiding rapid changes in plasma sodium levels. Regular electrolyte monitoring is therefore essential.

Remember to include maintenance fluid and replacement of ongoing non-physiological losses in addition to this fluid regimen.

Table 32.3. Clinical signs and symptoms of dehydration.

Degree of dehydration	Mild	Moderate	Severe
Clinical signs and symptoms	Restless, thirsty; no clinical signs of dehydration	Lethargic or irritable; postural hypotension; tachycardia; sunken eyes and fontanelle; dry mucous membranes; decreased urine output	Lethargic or comatose; shocked; hypotensive; grossly sunken eyes and fontanelle; anuria
Deficit as % of body weight	3–5%	6–9%	10% +
Deficit in ml/kg	30–50	60–90	100 +

Fluid choice to correct dehydration according to sodium level

Isonatraemic dehydration (plasma sodium between 130 and 150 mmol/l)

This is the commonest type of dehydration, usually due to gastroenteritis. There has been net loss of isotonic fluid, so replacement therapy should comprise isotonic, or near isotonic, electrolyte solution (e.g. 0.9% saline or Hartmann's solution).

Hypernatraemic dehydration (plasma sodium >150 mmol/l)

In this situation water loss has exceeded sodium loss, so it would seem logical to replace fluid losses with hypotonic fluid. However, there is a danger of reducing the plasma sodium too rapidly, resulting in rapid influx of water to the intracellular compartment, potentially causing fatal cerebral oedema. Infants and small children are particularly susceptible to this event, due to the relatively high ratio of cerebral intracellular volume to skull-vault volume.

A safer approach is to commence replacement fluid therapy with isotonic fluid, and consider reducing the tonicity (e.g. 0.45% saline + 5% dextrose) if the plasma sodium level is not falling after 6 hours.

The rate of decline in plasma sodium should be carefully monitored (1–2 hourly sampling initially) aiming for a fall of no greater than 1 mmol/l every 2 hours.

Worked example of fluid deficit calculation in dehydration:
a case of a 10 kg child with 10% dehydration; plasma sodium is in the normal range; isonatraemic dehydration diagnosed.

- In this situation, there has been net loss of isotonic fluid
- Isotonic fluid should be used for deficit replacement
- Aim to replace the deficit over 24 hours, with 50% in the first 8 hours
- The deficit is 1000 ml (10% of 10 kg, or 1 kg fluid). Replace 500 ml over the first 8 hours, and the remaining 500 ml over the next 16 hours
- Maintenance fluid and replacement of ongoing non-physiological losses should be added to this prescription

Hyponatraemic dehydration (plasma sodium < 130 mmol/l)

Here, sodium loss has exceeded water loss. Neurological symptoms due to cerebral intracellular water influx may occur if the hyponatraemia is severe (< 120 mmol/l) or the fall in sodium is rapid.

If this is the case, urgent correction of hyponatraemia is required with hypertonic fluid (e.g. 1–3 ml/kg 3% saline over 30 minutes). This is an emergency and the patient should be managed in PICU. Consider intubation and ventilation if neurological symptoms are present.

Chronic hyponatraemia may be tolerated better and can be corrected more slowly.

In less severe hyponatraemic dehydration the deficit may be adequately replaced with isotonic fluid.

The ongoing, non-physiological losses of sodium (e.g. diarrhoea) will also require replacement as part of the overall fluid prescription – see 'Replacement of ongoing non-physiological losses' below.

Maintenance fluid therapy

This is the replacement of physiological losses of fluid and electrolytes incurred as a result of metabolism. It includes both sensible losses (e.g. urine) and insensible losses (e.g. sweat). Electrolytes are always lost with fluid, so both must be replaced.

Fluid replacement

Metabolic rate is influenced by multiple factors, including underlying disease processes. Therefore, estimation of the patient's metabolic rate, and hence the maintenance fluid requirement, is imprecise. The most widely used method for estimation of metabolic rate in hospitalized children is the Holliday and Segar method (Table 32.4):

- it is a simplified formula using body weight, based on the calorie requirements of the average hospital patient
- the method separates patients into convenient groups according to body weight, and assumes 1 ml of water is required for every 1 kcal expended
- it is applicable to all age ranges, including adults
- whilst the method is convenient and simple, it provides only a gross estimate of energy expenditure and thus fluid requirements
- this method gives rise to the 4–2–1 rule of hourly fluid requirement (as long as one assumes a 25-hour day).

It is essential to adjust the maintenance fluid according to individual factors that are likely to influence energy expenditure or water and electrolyte requirements. For example, non-osmotic ADH may significantly reduce the ability to excrete water. The requirement for water per kcal expended will then be less than 1 ml, so restriction of water intake is required. Other factors influencing energy expenditure and water requirement are shown in Table 32.5.

Table 32.4. Holliday and Segar simplified method for calculating maintenance fluid requirements, based on estimated energy expenditure.

Body weight (kg)	Maintenance fluid requirement
Up to 10 kg	100 ml/kg/day
10–20 kg	1000 ml plus 50 ml/kg/day for each kg above 10 kg
Over 20 kg	1500 ml plus 20 ml/kg/day for each kg above 20 kg

Table 32.5. Approximate adjustments to resting energy expenditure (and thus fluid requirement) required for certain factors.

Factor	Resting energy expenditure adjustment (approximate)
Fever	+12% per °C above 37°C
Hypothermia	−12% per °C below 37°C
Pharmacological paralysis	−30%
Humidified ventilation gases	−25%
Non-osmotic ADH	−30–50%
Prematurity	+20%
Normal activity	+50%

Electrolyte replacement

Electrolyte maintenance replacement for a child under normal conditions is 3 mmol of sodium and 2 mmol of potassium per kcal of energy expended. Thus, a solution of 0.18% saline with 20 mmol/l of potassium chloride should provide adequate maintenance of electrolytes.

Until recently, this was the moot common IV fluid therapy in hospitalized children. However, if the energy expenditure and water requirement are overestimated, there is a risk of iatrogenic hyponatraemia, as the solution is hypotonic. Consequently, it is now rarely used for this purpose. Current recommendations for paediatric maintenance IV fluid therapy are to use either 0.45% saline or 0.9% saline (or other near-isotonic fluid, such as Hartmann's solution).

Use of these higher-tonicity fluids reduces the risk of hyponatraemia, at the expense of exposing the patient to a larger sodium load. In most situations, the renal function is capable of excreting the excess sodium, so the risk of hypernatraemia is low.

Dextrose replacement

Glucose requirement is related to body weight. For small children and infants a solution containing 5% dextrose will usually provide adequate carbohydrate to avoid hypoglycaemia and catabolism.

For neonates, a higher dextrose solution is usually required (e.g. 10% dextrose). Although IV dextrose will provide some caloric input, catabolism will ultimately ensue if enteral feeding is not established. Therefore, if a patient requires IV fluid therapy for more than 48 hours and enteral feeding is not possible, consideration should be given to commencing parenteral nutrition.

Replacement of ongoing non-physiological losses

Acutely ill children may have ongoing non-physiological fluid losses, necessitating further adjustment to their individualized fluid regimen. A thorough clinical assessment will allow anticipation of these losses. Knowledge of the composition of various body fluid compartments will aid in the prescription of replacement fluid; aim to replace like for like. See Table 32.6 for electrolyte composition of various body fluids. Examples of clinical scenarios with ongoing fluid losses are:

- diarrhoea
- osmotic diuresis (e.g. glucose)
- gastric losses (e.g. pyloric stenosis)
- sweat and increased evaporative losses in fever
- burns.

Table 32.6. Examples of body-fluid electrolyte composition.

Body fluid	Sodium (mmol/l)	Potassium (mmol/l)	Chloride (mmol/l)
Gastric	20–80	5–20	100–150
Ileosotomy	45–135	3–15	20–115
Diarrhoea	10–90	10–80	10–110
Sweat	10–30	3–10	10–35
Burn	140	5	110

Monitoring, warning signs and pitfalls

Estimation of fluid and electrolyte requirements is a blunt tool, so the clinician should carefully monitor the response to therapy. Regular assessments of clinical and biochemical endpoints will inform ongoing therapy.

Clinical monitoring in shock

During urgent treatment of shock with volume expansion, improving clinical signs such as capillary refill time, heart rate, blood pressure and urine output are the goals against which to judge initial therapy. Failure to respond to volume expansion signifies the need to escalate therapy or change the treatment strategy (e.g. provide inotropic or vasopressor support).

Continuous clinical assessment by an experienced clinician is mandatory in these patients.

Biochemical markers

Biochemical markers form useful goals against which to judge maintenance and replacement fluid therapy, outside the setting of urgent treatment of shock.

A normal plasma sodium level should be targeted, and maintained. Care should be given to avoiding rapid changes in plasma sodium concentration, particularly in the case of hypernatraemic dehydration. Compartment shifts of water should be anticipated when giving fluid therapy for a hyperosmolar state. Regular monitoring of plasma sodium and plasma osmolality will help identify rapid changes, but the clinician should also be vigilant for clinical signs of cerebral oedema (e.g. irritability, drowsiness and seizures).

See Tables 32.7 and 32.8 for a list of causes of hypernatraemia and hyponatraemia and important implications for fluid therapy.

Table 32.7. Hypernatraemia: causes and clinical implications for fluid therapy.

Cause	Implications for fluid therapy
Relative water deficit:	
Diarrhoea	Treat dehydration, but recognize ongoing non-physiological loss of water and electrolytes in the stool
Burns	In addition to the burn losses, patients often lose insensible water due to hyperthermia
Osmotic diuresis (e.g. DKA)	Monitor and replace ongoing losses
Diabetes insipidus	May respond to ADH analogue therapy (e.g. desmopressin), depending on the type of diabetes insipidus. Seek expert advice from endocrinologist
Inadequate feed intake (e.g. newborn infant with inadequate breast-feeding)	History may provide clues to this diagnosis
Excess sodium administration:	
Salt poisoning	Rare. Usually affects infants on formula feeds. Patients are unwell but not dehydrated. High urinary fractional excretion of sodium and water. Seek expert opinion (paediatric nephrology or endocrinology)
Iatrogenic administration (e.g. hypertonic saline or hypertonic sodium bicarbonate infusions)	Consider reducing sodium administration in maintenance fluid

Table 32.8. Hyponatraemia: causes and implications for fluid therapy.

Cause	Implications for fluid therapy
Iatrogenic (e.g. administration of hypotonic fluid in excess of water requirement)	Avoid very hypotonic fluids (0.18% saline), and regularly reassess effect of fluid regimen on sodium concentration. Can be managed by fluid restriction alone
Non-osmotic ADH	Restrict fluid therapy to 50–75% of calculated maintenance and avoid very hypotonic fluid, if risk factors for non-osmotic ADH (e.g. pneumonia, meningitis, bronchiolitis, sepsis)
Gastrointestinal losses (e.g. hyponatraemic dehydration due to diarrhoea)	Adjust replacement of losses to provide more sodium
Adrenal failure (rare) – e.g. congenital adrenal hyperplasia, Addison disease	Other signs of adrenal failure may be present (e.g. hyperkalaemia, shock, hypoglycaemia). Will require steroid therapy and referral to paediatric endocrinology

Other hyperosmolar states

Be aware that hyperosmolar states can exist without a raised plasma sodium level, e.g. diabetic ketoacidosis (DKA – see Chapter 11), where the hyperglycaemia exerts a significant effect on osmolality. Other examples are uraemia and hyperlipidaemia.

Slow correction of the hyperosmolar state should follow the same principles as treatment of hypernatraemic dehydration. It can be useful to calculate the corrected sodium level to monitor these cases, although sodium normally self-corrects once the underlying cause has been treated.

Specialist advice should be sought for management of these cases (e.g. paediatric intensivist).

Hypoglycaemia

Hypoglycaemia (blood glucose < 2.6 mmol/l) is common in small infants after only short periods of starvation. Hypoglycaemia in newborns may manifest as drowsiness, lethargy, apnoeas or seizures, therefore delays in administering IV fluid therapy should be avoided in sick neonates and regular monitoring of plasma glucose is required.

If the plasma glucose levels are below 3 mmol/l then the dextrose delivery should be increased. Symptomatic (or ventilated) babies should receive a bolus of 2 ml/kg of 10% dextrose in addition to the increase in background rate of dextrose. The background rate of dextrose can be increased by increasing the rate of maintenance administration or by increasing the concentration of dextrose in the fluid.

Some newborns exhibit hyperinsulinism, e.g. secondary to maternal diabetes mellitus. These children require significantly greater amounts of glucose to avoid hypoglycaemia, sometimes necessitating infusions of fluid containing very high dextrose concentration (e.g. 15–20%) via a central venous catheter.

Feeding on the PICU

Patients requiring intensive care often become catabolic due to increased metabolic demands and inadequate calorie delivery. Every effort should be made to satisfy the patient's nutritional requirements at the earliest opportunity. The options available are enteral feeding, parenteral feeding or a combination of both.

Enteral feeding

This is the preferred option in most patients. It is technically easier, has fewer side effects and is cheaper than parenteral nutrition. Contraindications may include:

- necrotizing enterocolitis
- short-gut syndrome
- low cardiac output states (especially with cyanotic congenital heart disease)
- chylothorax unresponsive to medium chain triglycerides (MCT) feed
- feed intolerance (vomiting and diarrhoea)
- high-output enteral fistula.

Different standard feed formulae are available. The choice depends on the availability of breast milk as an alternative, the age and calorie requirements of the patient. Dietetic advice should be sought to identify the best feed for the patient.

Most feeds are delivered continuously, as this is better tolerated by patients with respiratory compromise. It also allows assessment of feed absorption, without risking large gastric aspirates and potential regurgitation or vomiting. Feed intolerance is common and related to a number of factors including:

- gastric stasis
- drug effects, e.g. opioids or anticholinergics
- bowel obstruction
- paralytic ileus.

This can be overcome by reducing feed volumes, adding in drugs to increase gastric emptying (e.g. domperidone), administering other prokinetics (e.g. erythromycin) or passing a nasojejunal tube.

In certain situations special feeds are required. These include thickened feeds (for gastric reflux), modular feeds (e.g. MCT feeds in chylothorax), lactose-free feeds, pre-digested feeds or calorie-loaded feeds when volumes are limited or growth poor.

Tolerance of feeds should be ascertained on a regular basis by aspiration of the NG tube. It is common to aspirate some feed, but this can be replaced if the volume is not too great (< 5 ml/kg). Indications that feed is not being tolerated include:

- persistent, large NG aspirates
- nausea and vomiting
- abdominal distension
- abdominal pain
- diarrhoea.

Once respiratory function has improved, problems such as hunger and hypoglycaemia can be addressed by introducing bolus feeds. At first these are 2 hourly, but the interval can be increased to 3–4 hourly, as long as the patient is absorbing the feed and can tolerate the increased volumes.

Parenteral feeding

Patients who do not tolerate enteral feeding or in whom it is contraindicated need to receive total parenteral nutrition (TPN). Ideally, this involves feeding through a central venous line (central or peripheral long line). It is possible to administer TPN through a peripheral cannula. However, this rarely provides sufficient calories, as the glucose concentration is limited to 12.5%. It should, therefore, only be used for short-term nutritional support.

The main components of TPN are:

- glucose
- amino acids (as Vamin)
- fat (as Intralipid)
- electrolytes, trace elements and vitamins.

Most TPN is bespoke and manufactured for the patient on a daily basis. However, 'standard' bags are available for times when it is not possible to manufacture TPN. The complicated process of prescribing TPN is increasingly being devolved to specialist nutritional support teams or pharmacy departments. The general principles are:

- calorie requirements differ with age – growing children require more, e.g. 90–120 kcal/kg/day in neonates compared with 30–60 kcal/kg/day in a sedentary adolescent
- most daily calories are provided by glucose (60–70%)
- fat is also a valuable source of calories and requirements range from 3–4 g/kg/day (infants) to 0.5–1 g/kg/day (adolescents)
- protein requirements are for growth and healing, not calories – again requirements vary with age from 3–3.5 g/kg/day in infancy to 1–1.5 g/kg/day in older children.

In patients with hypercapnoea, it may be possible to reduce CO_2 production by reducing the glucose concentration in the TPN and replacing it with fat or Vamin.

The lipid component of TPN is administered separately and interruption of the infusion for 4 hours per day is commonly done to reduce some of the pathophysiological effects on the liver. Regular monitoring of the patient on TPN is vital and should include:

- blood sugar
- electrolytes
- urea and creatinine
- liver function tests
- phosphate
- triglycerides
- trace elements.

TPN should be replaced with enteral nutrition at the earliest opportunity, but increasingly we are seeing patients on the PICU who are TPN-dependent, so a good understanding of the principles and problems involved with administering it are essential to those working there.

Summary

Fluid therapy should be an individualized prescription based on an assessment of the patients' deficits, maintenance requirements and ongoing non-physiological losses. Fluid prescriptions are based on gross estimates, and therefore regular monitoring of clinical and biochemical end-points should take place to inform alterations in fluid therapy. The goal is to restore and maintain homeostasis.

No single IV fluid solution is perfect for every paediatric patient, across all phases of illness. However, avoidance of very hypotonic fluids will reduce the risk of hyponatraemia.

Golden rules

- Fluid therapy does not conform to a 'one size fits all' protocol
- Ongoing assessment is essential
- Normal blood glucose levels should be maintained at all times
- Electrolytes should be checked on a regular basis

Further reading

Behrman RE, Kliegman RM, Jenson HB. *Nelson's Textbook of Pediatrics*, 16th edn. WB Saunders, 2000.

Coulthard MG. Will changing maintenance intravenous fluid from 0.18% to 0.45% saline do more harm than good? *Arch Dis Child* 2008;**93**:335–340.

Holliday MA, Segar WE. The maintenance need for water in parenteral fluid therapy. *Pediatrics* 1957;**19**:823–832.

NPSA. *Patient safety alert 22: reducing the risk of hyponatraemia when administering infusions to children*. National Patient Safety Agency, 2007.

Taylor D, Durward A. Pouring salt on troubled waters. *Arch Dis Child* 2004;**89**:414–418.

Chapter 33

Pharmacology in children

Rhian Isaac

Introduction

Drug therapies in children require individualization, because of their size and immature metabolic pathways. This is usually done by calculating doses in direct relation to body size (weight or body surface area) or by using a surrogate for normal size (e.g. age). The critically ill child will also show variation in pharmacokinetics and pharmacodynamics as a result of their disease process.

Although the dosing of drugs can seem daunting, especially in time-critical circumstances, it is helped by some general rules; for example, it is rare to require a dose above the adult maximum dosage recommendations. This is particularly important to avoid overdosing the adolescent age group or the obese child. In these populations a dose for age banding is usually more appropriate.

This chapter aims to provide a brief synopsis of how drugs commonly used in paediatric intensive care affect critically ill children. It also serves as a brief reminder of how paediatric pharmacology differs from that of adults.

Pharmacokinetic and pharmacodynamic differences throughout childhood

Pharmacokinetics relates to how the body alters the absorption, distribution, metabolism and elimination of a drug. The differences in the pharmacokinetics seen in small children are summarized in Table 33.1.

Absorption

Oral route

Oral absorption of drugs is mainly affected by pH-dependent passive diffusion and/or gastric emptying. Usually a drug needs to be in the un-ionized (lipophyllic) form to cross membranes. Gastric pH is relatively elevated in the neonatal period, reaching adult values by 2 years of age. This increased gastric pH (i.e. more alkaline environment) will increase the absorption of weak bases and decrease that of acidic drugs (see Figure 33.1). Also, the slower gastric emptying time seen in neonates will increase the time a drug takes to reach its peak levels. Gastric emptying times will shorten by 6–8 months of age.

Managing the Critically Ill Child, ed. Richard Skone *et al.* Published by Cambridge University Press.

Intestinal transit time is prolonged in neonates due to decreased motility and peristalsis, whereas motility in the infant may exceed adult values. In neonates the dosing of drugs that have a high intestinal absorption needs to take account of:

- slower gut motility increasing absorption for some drugs that are actively absorbed via specific transporters
- increased permeability of immature intestinal mucosa
- decreased intestinal enzyme activity.

Enterohepatic recirculation (or reabsorption) is a process whereby a drug or its conjugate metabolites are excreted via the biliary tree and then reabsorbed in the lower intestine. Critical illness may reduce drug recirculation in children because of decreased bile salt production or reduced bacterial colonization of the gastrointestinal tract (GIT) (required to cleave the conjugate for reabsorption). These bacteria are absent during the first few days of life and following administration of broad-spectrum antibiotics.

Many medicines, such as newer anticonvulsants, are only available in oral form. Where there is dubious absorption from the gut due to decreased blood flow or oedematous gut, regular oral medication will require changing to the parenteral form.

Table 33.1. The physiological parameter changes during childhood that affect pharmacokinetic and pharmacodynamic processes compared with the adult.

Physiological parameter	Neonate	Child	Post-pubertal adolescent	PK/PD affected
Gastric pH	↑	↔	↔	A
Gastric emptying	↑	↔	↔	A
Skin absorption	↑	↔	↔	A
Total body water	↑	↑	↔	D
Intracellular fluid	↓	↓	↔	D
Extracellular fluid	↑	↑	↔	D
Adipose tissue	↓	↑↓↔	↑↓	D
Albumin concentration	↓	↔	↓↑↔	D E
Albumin binding/affinity	↓	↔	↔	D E
Enzyme capacity	↓↑	↓↑	↔↓	M E
Renal function	↓	↔	↔	E
Glomerular filtration rate (GFR)	↓	↔	↔	E
Tubular secretion	↓	↔	↔	E
Receptor sensitivity	↓↑	↑↓	↔	PD
Blood–brain barrier (BBB) permeability	↑	↑↔	↔	PD

PK, pharmacokinetic; PD, pharmacodynamic; A, absorption; D, distribution; M, metabolism; E, elimination.

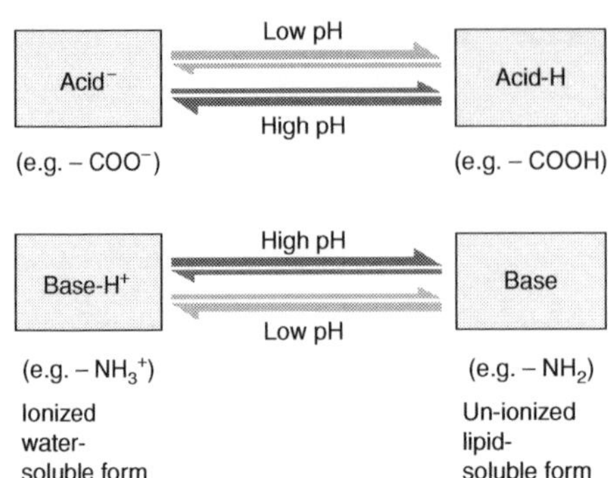

Figure 33.1. Effect of pH on ionization status of drugs.

Rectal route

Rectal absorption is variable in neonates due to reduced GI motility. For all ages, the depth of insertion of rectal drugs will alter bioavailability. Drugs placed in the upper rectum will undergo first-pass metabolism, whereas those placed in the middle and lower sections may bypass the liver, as the inferior rectal veins drain into the vena cava, rather than the portal vein.

The drugs most commonly administered rectally in critically ill children are paracetamol, chloral hydrate and diazepam. Lack of availability of suitable-sized suppositories may make the rectal route less practical. Cutting suppositories is not advisable, as the drug may not be evenly distributed throughout the excipient.

Distribution

For a drug to have an effect, it must reach its target by being distributed to the appropriate compartment. Distribution is dependent on both drug and patient factors (see Table 33.2). Smaller molecules and lipophilic drugs tend to distribute widely, i.e. they have a higher volume of distribution.

Table 33.2. Factors affecting distribution of a drug.

Drug factors	Patient factors
Protein bound (%)	Total body water (%)
Lipophilicity	Ratio of extracellular to intracellular water
Molecular size	Adipose tissue Plasma protein levels Affinity of plasma proteins to bind with drug Uraemia/bilirubinaemia Acid–base status

Distribution can be affected by:

- blood loss
- fluid accumulation
- changes in plasma protein levels.

The increase in extracellular water seen in critically ill children can lead to a higher proportion of hydrophilic compounds being limited to the extracellular compartment. This results in lower concentrations of a drug in the interstitial tissues with standard doses (e.g. β-lactams and aminoglycosides). This can be overcome by an adequate loading dose followed by standard maintenance dosing. It should be remembered that steady state will not be achieved for 4 to 5 half-lives of the drug unless an adequate loading dose is given.

Protein binding

Only the unbound drug is free to act at the receptor site. Albumin is the plasma protein that binds mainly acidic drugs, while α-1-acid glycoprotein tends to bind basic drugs.

Critically ill and very young children may have a lower than usual concentration of albumin in their blood. As a result, the albumin binding sites can become saturated with a given drug. Other plasma proteins have a lower affinity for binding drugs and endogenous circulating agents such as bilirubin may displace them from their binding sites. This is compounded in burns, stress, trauma, and liver and renal impairment, where there is a further decrease in plasma proteins.

If protein binding decreases, the free fraction of a drug available to act at receptor sites increases. This increases the free fraction of a drug and amplifies the pharmacological response to a given dose. It also increases the risk of adverse drug reactions. Conversely, in sepsis, there is an increase in α-1-acid glycoprotein which can lead to a decrease in the free fraction of basic drugs.

Clearance

If a drug is cleared at a high rate then there is less time for the drug to distribute to the target compartment. Many interventions for the critically ill can increase the clearance of a drug, such as renal replacement therapy and forced diuresis.

Blood–brain barrier

The volume of the CNS is relatively large in children, reaching adult values by 4–6 years. It also receives a higher amount of the cardiac output. The blood–brain barrier (BBB) is thought to be more permeable in the younger infant and may allow passage of non-lipid-soluble drugs. Whilst this can be beneficial, it can also increase the risk of CNS side effects (e.g. cerebral irritation), such as when giving higher doses of the penicillins for CNS infections. Sepsis, hypoxia and acidosis also increase the BBB permeability. Acidosis in the critically ill child will also increase the permeability of the BBB to acidic drugs due to an increase in the un-ionized fraction.

Metabolism

Metabolism is the process by which the body breaks down or converts drugs into alternative, sometimes active, products. Each individual isoform of the enzymes involved in phase I and II metabolism has its own developmental profile; reaching and in some cases exceeding adult values throughout childhood.

Depending on the profile of the enzymes involved, drug metabolism may be limited by either the capacity of the enzymes (saturation-limited) or delivery of the drug to the relevant organ (perfusion-limited). There is a decrease in cytochrome-oxidase-mediated drug metabolism in sepsis and during an inflammatory response which may cause a drug's metabolism to be saturation-limited. Perfusion-limited metabolism may occur if the liver blood flow is decreased, such as in:

- hypotension
- hypothermia
- shunting of blood, e.g. through a patent ductus arteriosus in neonates can impair blood flow to both the liver and kidneys.

An increase in metabolic activity occurs with age and can lead to an improved clearance of a drug. For example, morphine clearance increases six-fold from birth to 6 months due to increased biotransformation to its glucuronide metabolites.

Elimination

Drugs are usually eliminated via the kidneys or the biliary system. Critically ill children, as with adults, commonly suffer from impairment of these organs. Drug elimination may, therefore, be affected. Hypoxic episodes in neonates will decrease GFR and tubular function; therefore doses should be modified accordingly or levels ascertained before repeat dosing.

Drugs that are haemodynamically active, such as inotropes, may improve renal blood flow and as a result can increase the clearance of certain drugs. This is only usually significant in drugs that have a high unchanged moiety when cleared by the kidneys.

Considerations with parenteral routes of administration in children

Intravenous administration

Most medicines are not licensed for use in children and therefore the technical information provided with the medicine does not offer paediatric parameters, increasing the risk of unsafe administration. The age and weight of a child must be taken into account when determining the volume for dilution, diluents and rate of administration. For example:

- to maintain the higher glucose intake for a neonate, continuous infusions may require dilution in 10% glucose
- the volume and sodium load of the drugs and flushes can add up to a considerable amount in the smaller child
- in adults the maximum rate of phenytoin administration is 50 mg/min, which would have serious consequences if applied to a small child, where the maximum rate for treatment of SE is 1 mg/kg/min
- in neonates, many antibiotics have a longer infusion time depending on the dose, such as high-dose benzylpenicillin, which should be given as an infusion to minimize cerebral irritation.

Intraosseous (IO) route

When IV access is difficult to obtain the IO route may be used in the resuscitation situation. The same dose as the IV route should be used. Bolus administration or small-volume doses can result in a depot-type effect, due to the drug remaining in the medullary cavity, leading to lower serum peak concentrations and a longer time for drug distribution. This can be overcome by giving a flush of 5–10 ml after the dose.

Common drugs used in critically ill children that differ from adults in pharmacokinetics

Paracetamol

Paracetamol is metabolized principally via the glucuronidation pathway in children and adults; approximately a third undergoes sulphonation. Small amounts are oxidized by the CYP450 enzymes to a toxic metabolite, which causes necrosis to liver cells unless neutralized or scavenged by glutathione. With higher doses of paracetamol, more drug is oxidized and the glutathione stores become depleted, leading to hepatocyte damage. In infants less than 3 months old the sulphonation pathway is dominant and the oxidation pathway less developed. As a result production of the toxic metabolite is less likely. In addition, neonates synthesize more glutathione than adults; hence hepatic damage from overdose is less likely. Paracetamol has dosing differences for each age group, indication and route, thus the prescriber should refer to a reputable formulary, such as the BNFc.

Morphine

Morphine is metabolized via the glucuronidation pathway to active metabolites morphine-3-glucuronide (an antanalgesic) and morphine-6-glucuronide (10–20 times more potent than morphine). In the first 2 months of life glucuronidation by the UGT2B7 enzyme is immature. There is also a decrease in hepatic and renal clearance. This accounts for the higher respiratory depression seen in the younger infant. Clearance reaches approximately 80% of adult values by 6 months of age and 100% by 1 year.

Whilst morphine is not considered lipid-soluble, the increased permeability of the BBB in the younger infant allows greater CNS penetration and thus increased sensitivity. When giving morphine to children, lower doses and closer monitoring and observations should be applied to those under 1 year of age. This should not, however, discourage the use of morphine as an analgesic or sedative when appropriate in these children (see Chapter 27).

Midazolam

Midazolam is water-soluble as a commercial formulation, but becomes lipid-soluble at physiological pH. In the latter state it is able to cross the blood–brain barrier. It is extensively metabolized by CYP3A4/5 liver enzymes to an active and equipotent metabolite (1-hydroxymethylmidazolam). This metabolite is then conjugated to a minimally active glucuronide for renal clearance. The dose of midazolam should be reduced if renal function is impaired.

The half-life of midazolam in children is approximately four times longer than in adults, and is extended further in critically ill children, due to their decreased ability to metabolize the drug. Common drugs used in the critically ill child that will increase midazolam levels include fluconazole and omeprazole.

Hypotension as a result of midazolam administration is commonly seen in neonates and infants; the risk is increased further with rapid IV bolus administration. Because of this, and the variable metabolism and clearance seen in this age group, midazolam is rarely used as a sedative in the young infant population (< 3 months).

Drugs used commonly in the critically ill child that you may not be familiar with

Prostaglandin E1 and E2

These are potent vasodilators used to maintain the patency of the ductus arteriosus in the neonate awaiting surgery for correction of a duct-dependent cardiac abnormality. In the fetal circulation the duct is kept open by the effects of low PO_2 and the high concentration of prostaglandins (particularly prostaglandin E2). After birth, the smooth muscle constricts as arterial oxygenation increases and placental concentrations of prostaglandin decrease. This can be counteracted by giving continuous infusions of prostaglandin.

Alprostadil (E1) and dinoprostone (E2) are interchangeable (alprostadil is the licensed version). Initial higher doses may be required (50–100 ng/kg/min) to open the duct, but the lowest dose should be used where possible, due to the risk of apnoeas and hypotension. A dose of 5–10 ng/kg/min is usually sufficient for most patients. Prostaglandin E1 and E2 have half-lives of minutes and therefore interrupting the continuous infusion should be avoided.

Milrinone

Milrinone is a phosphodiesterase III inhibitor which produces a positive inotropic effect and vasodilatation. Inhibition of phosphodiesterase III leads to an accumulation of cyclic adenosine monophosphate cAMP in the cardiac cell and in the vascular muscle. The effects are dose-dependent (continuous infusion of 0.25–0.75 μg/kg/min). The main advantage of milrinone in children, when compared to other inotropic agents, includes increasing cardiac output without effects such as:

- excessive increases in heart rate (more of a problem in adults)
- increased myocardial oxygen consumption
- down-regulation of β-adrenoreceptors
- increased systemic vascular resistance.

In infants and children milrinone has a higher volume of distribution and increased renal clearance. However, the half-life appears to be longer in infants compared with children and adults. As with the catecholamines, it does carry a risk of arrhythmias and may exacerbate hypotension if given too fast.

Whilst many texts suggest a loading dose, this should be avoided or reduced in patients at risk of hypotension. Milrinone is cleared by the renal route, so the dose should be decreased in renal impairment.

Chloral hydrate

This is a non-barbiturate hypnotic metabolized by the liver to active trichloroethanol. It is used as an oral or rectal sedative in PICU. It has minimal effects on the respiratory system and in lower doses (30 mg/kg) is haemodynamically stable. There is an increased risk of myocardial depression, apnoeas and arrhythmias in children younger than 3 months old.

Drugs that should be avoided in children

Propofol

Prolonged use of propofol for sedation in children under 16 years old is contraindicated due to the increased risk of the potentially fatal 'propofol infusion syndrome'. This is characterized by:

- arrhythmias
- severe metabolic acidosis
- rhabdomyolysis
- hepatomegaly
- lipaemia
- myocardial failure
- hyperkalaemia.

Multiple drug therapy used in the critically ill child can alter propofol metabolism. During stress children are more dependent on fatty acid metabolism for energy; propofol is associated with mitochondrial respiration failure and defects in fatty acid oxidation.

It can be used for short procedures such as dressing changes, but due to its lack of analgesic properties an opioid is usually required.

Drug dosing in renal impairment

Use of the GFR or creatinine clearance has limitations in critically ill children and therefore makes dosing of renally cleared drugs challenging; where possible drug levels should be used to guide therapy. Baseline creatinine, and subsequent increases, along with decreased urine output, should be used to highlight when drug therapy and dosing require scrutiny.

Drug dosing in renal replacement therapy

Literature regarding drug dosing in paediatrics is scarce. Renal dosing books do not often differentiate between high and low ultrafiltration rates which can lead to under- or overdosing of medicines. As a result, the prescriber may be required to estimate the dose reduction or whether supplemental doses are required. Table 33.3 highlights some of the factors affecting dosing.

Table 33.3. Factors affecting drug removal in CVVH.

Drug factors favouring removal by CVVH	High % renal eliminated Low protein binding Low volume of distribution Molecular weight of 1000–5000 Anions
CVVH factors favouring drug removal	Synthetic membranes Large membrane surface area High ultrafiltration rate Post-dilution ultrafiltration
Patient factors that may affect drug removal	Liver impairment Low albumin, increased free drug Fluid overload, potentially larger volume distribution Deranged acid–base status

If the indication for continuous veno-venous haemofiltration (CVVH) is acute renal impairment, further dose adjustments may be required when stopping CVVH depending on the degree of renal impairment. Consideration should be given if there is a lack of clinical response, especially with antimicrobials, to whether the patient is being under-dosed. In these circumstances the adverse effects in accumulation versus the benefits of therapy should be discussed. The pharmacists should be consulted to assist with drug dosing in continuous renal replacement therapy (CRRT).

Summary

Prescribing drugs to children can be a complex and difficult task. Consideration needs to be given to contraindications, the patient's underlying illness, co-morbidity, physiology, and patient maturity and size. The dose of many drugs needs to be modified in children, particularly in the infant age group. There are a number of very helpful reference formularies that can be used to aid the process but, as always, if in doubt, seek expert advice from an intensivist or pharmacist.

Golden rules

- Never exceed the adult dose of a drug, unless there is a specific indication
- Always consider co-morbidity when prescribing in critically ill children
- Always double-check doses in children, particularly if it is a drug you are not used to prescribing
- Give a loading dose if a desired drug level needs to be achieved quickly

Further reading

Kearns G, Alander S, Leeder J. Developmental pharmacology – drug disposition, action, and therapy in infants and children. *N Engl J Med* 2003;**349**:1157–1167.

Krishnan V, Murray P. Pharmacological issues in the critically ill. *Clin Chest Med* 2003;**24**:671–688.

Pea F, Viale P, Furlanut M. Antimicrobial therapy in critically ill patients. *Clin Pharmacokinet* 2005;**44**(10):1009–1034.

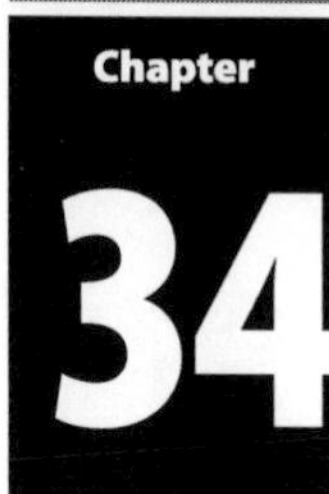

Neonates

Richard Skone

Introduction

A neonate is a term that describes any child from birth up to 28 days old. Paediatric intensive care unit interactions with neonates tend to be limited to those with surgical problems, e.g. congenital diaphragmatic hernias, or congenital heart disease. However, units will also look after babies who have been discharged from neonatal units and subsequently need re-admission.

This chapter will address the common principles in managing neonates on PICUs although cardiac problems have been mentioned in an earlier chapter. Greater attention will be paid to conditions seen on PICU, rather than on neonatal intensive care units (NICU). The first part will focus on the day-to-day practicalities of intensive care management. The latter part will describe common conditions seen on PICU.

Managing a neonate on PICU

When compared to looking after adults on intensive care units the approach to neonates is one of having a 'light touch'. For much of the time in PICU a great deal of effort is made in not disturbing the child. However, vigilance is needed as the signs of significant pathology can be very subtle. Sepsis, for instance, may only be heralded by brief episodes of desaturation and bradycardias.

Calculating the age of a neonate

As babies may be born significantly preterm, their corrected gestational age (CGA) is important. It is unfair to compare two children at 1 month old if one was born at 24 weeks while the other was born at term.

Until a prematurely born child reaches the date on which they were predicted to be born their age is usually referred to as their gestational age, i.e. 32 weeks post menstrual age. After the child crosses their 'due date', the age is often 'corrected', counting their 'due date' as day 1; e.g. a child aged 3 months but born at 32 weeks would be referred to as being 'an ex-32 week neonate currently 4 weeks corrected gestational age'.

The more premature a child, the greater the significance of the correction as a baby born at 24 weeks when 4 months old chronologically will only (to a certain extent) be the size and maturity of a normal newborn.

Managing the Critically Ill Child, ed. Richard Skone *et al.* Published by Cambridge University Press.

Intubation

Size of ET tube

There are no reliable equations for calculating the size of ET tube needed for children this small. It is therefore useful to remember that a full-term (3 kg) neonate will usually be intubated with a size 3.5 mm ET tube. The size of the tube should be adjusted according to the size of the baby. It is important in babies to have a variety of ET tube sizes available at the time of intubation as some of the neonates will have been ventilated on NICU previously and may suffer from sub-glottic stenosis.

Although conventional teaching has been against cuffed ET tube in neonates due to the risk of subglottic stenosis, the development of high-volume, low-pressure cuffs has meant that they are now used for specific conditions. The indications are rare in neonatal practice and include burns or trauma.

Length of ET tube

The distance from vocal cords to the carina in a term neonate may be as little as 5 cm (shorter in premature babies). Endobronchial intubation is, therefore, a common problem. The most useful guide to the appropriate length of an ET tube is the intubation depth mark present on many ET tubes. ET tubes are often secured by elastoplast or tape 'strapping' in an attempt to minimize movement of the ET tube once the appropriate distance is decided upon.

Because of the short length of ET tube distal to the vocal cords unplanned extubation can occur in neonates if great care is not exercised. It is possible to have a child who is saturating adequately but difficult to bag who has managed to expel the ET tube into the pharynx.

Nasal ET tube

Children are often intubated nasally on PICU (after an initial oral intubation) as nasal ET tubes are better tolerated than oral ones. The sinuses are not fully developed in young children; hence sinusitis does not occur as it does in adults.

ET tube blockage

One of the problems associated with the use of small ET tubes is the risk of blockage. This may manifest as:

- increased airway pressures
- a changing or unstable $ETCO_2$ dioxide level
- a baby who is 'fighting the ventilator'
- desaturation.

This situation should be treated urgently as desaturation can be rapid and precipitous. Most problems can be treated by changing to a T-piece to ventilate the patient manually, and passing a suction catheter down the ET tube. If this does not work, and chest expansion or breath sounds do not appear convincing, then a decision about whether to change the ET tube should be made promptly. As with adults, if you are doubtful about the ET tube (and the child has been intubated in a straightforward manner previously) then remove the ET tube and resort to mask ventilation.

Ventilation

Setting the ventilator

Inspiratory (I) time

Children on neonatal units are often ventilated with an inspiratory time (I-time) of 0.3 seconds. This is based on the neonates having an alveolar time constant of 0.1 seconds. There is also some evidence that long I-times in neonates can adversely affect outcome. However, a significant number of young babies are admitted to PICU with conditions such as bronchiolitis or RDS from sepsis. It is therefore reasonable to assume that the time constant for their alveoli is prolonged (although not necessarily homogeneously in some conditions). The I-time on PICU is therefore more often set to 0.5 seconds, or longer in larger babies. This should be altered for the very low birthweight neonates.

Pressure

As with adults, barotrauma can cause long-term problems in children. Although a healthy neonate has a more compliant chest than an adult, this may be altered by disease states. Ultimately ventilator pressures should be set similar to those seen in adults.

Positive end-expiratory pressure is also used to the same effect, although it may cause more cardiovascular instability if excessive. If lung disease is mild or moderate without oxygenation difficulties a PEEP of 4–6 is generally used. In more severe lung disease the lower point of inflection of the compliance curve should be estimated and the PEEP level set above it.

Volume

Volutrauma also causes long-term problems in neonates. Tidal volumes should aim to deliver between 5 and 7 ml/kg. This can be difficult to measure in small babies. The values displayed on many ventilators reflect the volume change of the ventilator circuit, not the actual volume delivered to a child. Some ventilators will compensate to an extent for the volume of compression within the ventilator circuit when ventilating small infants. The baby needs to be assessed clinically for adequate chest movement. Volume-controlled ventilation with pressure limitation is often used to ventilate neonates on PICU. If this is ineffective or problematic then pressure-controlled ventilation can be used.

Dead space

This is often a major preoccupation for many anaesthetists. In practice the length of an ET tube does not often compromise ventilation. It is important, however, that appropriately sized HME filters and $ETCO_2$ monitors are used. The most important factor in managing ventilation in neonates is to be aware of the potential for re-breathing. If the arterial $PaCO_2$ continues to rise in spite of what appears to be adequate ventilation, then attempts should be made to minimize the dead space within a circuit.

End-tidal carbon dioxide monitoring

This can prove very difficult to monitor in neonates due to the small tidal volumes generated; however, $ETCO_2$ monitoring is still the least invasive and best way of helping to confirm correct ET tube placement.

In the absence of an arterial line, capillary gases can be used as an indicator of arterial CO_2 tension.

Circulation

Blood pressure

As a rule of thumb, for premature babies (up to 40 weeks) it is often useful to *aim for a mean arterial blood pressure (in mmHg) which is equal to the baby's gestational age in weeks.* This gives a rough idea of an adequate blood pressure. As with adults, adequate pressure does not always equate to adequate flow so it should only be used in conjunction with other clinical observations.

Fluid boluses

Received wisdom is that blood pressure in neonates is largely heart-rate dependent. This is not always reflected in clinical situations. Hypotension is still best treated with fluid boluses, which are usually administered as 5–10 ml/kg fluid boluses, with clinical response monitored. Similarly sepsis and vasodilatation will also require adequate fluid resuscitation and vasoconstrictors, much as in adults. The choice of fluid is still controversial, and the colloid vs. crystalloid debate continues with the same vigour in paediatrics as in adults.

Remember that a 5 ml flush through a neonatal cannula will constitute a 'fluid bolus'!

Inotropes

The choice of inotrope is one area which can confuse adult physicians. There are arguments for and against the use of dopamine in neonates. What is certain is dopamine may be an adequate initial inotrope which can be administered peripherally. Most PICUs will be happy to use more familiar inotropes and vasoconstrictors on very sick babies. Adrenaline and noradrenaline are used for the same indications as in adults. Correcting ionized calcium in neonates is very important. This is because of the lower stores of intracellular calcium within the sarcoplasmic reticulum of the myocardium.

Renal function

The kidneys, like other neonatal organs, are immature. They have decreased urine-concentrating ability which renders neonates susceptible to fluid overload or dehydration if not managed carefully. Fluid overload in neonates can compromise ventilation in severe cases as the oedema can compromise chest wall compliance.

Because of the poor urine-concentrating ability of neonates, it is usual to aim for an hourly urine output of 1 ml/kg/h. Neonates have a high calcium output in their urine which is exacerbated by the use of calciuric drugs such as furosemide. This can lead to nephrocalcinosis if care is not taken. Fully developed function of the kidneys does not occur until approximately 1 year old.

When taken in combination with immature liver function, great care must be taken in prescribing drugs to neonates. A neonatal pharmacist should be consulted when prescribing for premature babies.

Access

Cannulae

Cannulae of 24 gauge are often used as a means of gaining access in neonates. The size and fragility of veins does, however, mean that care is required in order to avoid extravasation injuries even in well-sited cannulae.

Long lines

Longer-term central access is often acquired using 'long lines'. These are narrow, peripheral lines that are sited under aseptic technique and are fed through until the tip sits in the great veins. The diameter of these lines can be as little as 28 gauge (1 French). They can be used for TPN or inotropes, or for giving high-concentration infusions. Traditional, triple-lumen central venous catheters are also used, but the large diameter of the catheters means that they are often associated with complications such as venous obstruction and clot formation.

Arterial lines

For arterial lines, as with adults, peripheral lines are preferred at sites where good collateral flow ensures adequate perfusion. Typically 24G cannulae are used in the radial or posterior tibial arteries. Brachial artery cannulae are associated with a high level of morbidity in premature babies and are therefore avoided where possible. Palpating and fixing an artery in a neonate can be difficult. One technique used in neonates is to transillumintae the arm or foot with a 'cold light'. These lights minimize the risk of thermal injury while showing the arteries or veins as black threads which can be targeted.

Capillary gases

In the absence of an arterial line, capillary gas samples are used as a way of monitoring the status of a child. There are important caveats to interpreting capillary gas samples. When they have been difficult to sample, it is possible to get spuriously raised:

- potassium
- lactate
- hydrogen ion levels (lower pH).

The PaO_2 on a capillary gas does not necessarily reflect the arterial PaO_2. Unusual results, which do not correlate with the state of the patient, should be interpreted with care.

Umbilical lines

Some babies may arrive on PICU from neonatal units with umbilical artery (UAC) or venous (UVC) catheters *in situ*. These can act as a method of invasive arterial monitoring or central venous access respectively. Care should be taken in their management in terms of positioning and infection-control measures.

Sedation

Morphine is used as a sole agent for sedation in neonates. It is usually diluted in 5% or 10% dextrose and started at a dose of 40 μg/kg/h (titrated to effect). Morphine metabolism is underdeveloped in neonates and differs slightly from that of adults (see Chapter 33).

Midazolam is rarely used in children younger than 3 months old (CGA) as its cardiovascular depressant activities are significant. There are also concerns that it may worsen neurological outcomes on NICU.

As with adults, environment plays a large part in successful sedation of neonates. Incubators have been shown to amplify sounds of any tapping or knocking on their surface. This noise can agitate neonates, causing them to experience apnoeas or bradycardias or to desaturate. Opening and closing incubator doors can also cause a significant level of distress.

Feeds/maintenance fluids

Enteral feeding

An approximation to the usual feeding regime aims to give neonates a daily calorie intake of 100 kcal/kg. Formula and breast milk contain approximately two-thirds of a kcal per ml. Therefore babies are usually allowed 150 ml/kg/day if enteral feeds are used.

Breast milk provides the gold standard form of nutrition for neonates due to the additional benefits of maternal enzyme and antibody transfer (passive immunity). Many neonates will be too ill to manage breast-feeding directly, so most PICU and NICU will have facilities for breast milk expression by mothers. This can then be administered via an NG tube.

High-risk feeding groups

Certain groups of children are kept nil by mouth for fear of precipitating necrotizing enterocolitis (NEC) (see below). These include children with cardiac defects where bowel perfusion may be compromised, e.g. coarctation of the aorta. A combination of highly concentrated (hyperosmolar) feeds and bowel ischaemia can precipitate NEC.

Fluid maintenance

A neonate who is nil by mouth, receiving IV crystalloid maintenance fluid, needs to be monitored very closely. A child receiving 100 ml/kg/day of IV fluid may get overloaded over a period of days, and iatrogenic electrolyte imbalances are easy to manufacture. When giving the fluid it should be remembered that the requirements are:

- sodium 1–3 mmol/kg/day
- potassium 1–2 mmol/kg/day
- glucose 4–6 mmol/kg/min.

One of the reasons that many drugs are made in high-concentration dextrose fluids is that, using the above fluid regime, a 2 kg neonate will be allowed 8.3 ml/h of maintenance fluid. This can be easily exceeded if a child is on sedation, multiple inotropes, and drugs which need to be diluted in large volumes, e.g. antibiotics. In paediatric practice drug infusions are included in the total hourly fluid allowance. In order to meet the child's glucose requirement and restrict fluid appropriately it may be necessary to:

- increase the concentration of drugs in infusions
- increase the concentration of glucose in the infusions
- keep to essential drugs.

Hypoglycaemia

The lack of carbohydrate reserve and the catabolic nature of critically ill neonates make them prone to hypoglycaemia. Regular checking of blood sugars is therefore essential with blood sugars of less than 2.6 mmol/l (or higher if symptomatic), prompting intervention; i.e. give 2 ml/kg of 10% dextrose and increase basal glucose delivery. As can be seen, lower blood glucose is tolerated in stable neonates compared with the other children mentioned in this book.

Glucose requirements in neonates may rise as high as 12 mg/kg/min in some neonates. If the requirement is greater than this then a 'hypoglycaemia screen' should be performed while the child is hypoglycaemic (if there is no need for urgent intervention). The purpose of this screen is to look for conditions such as inborn errors of metabolism or hyperinsulinism, e.g. Beckwith–Wiedeman syndrome (see Chapter 9 for a list of tests). Do not forget to include the drug infusion fluids when calculating the amount of dextrose that a neonate is receiving.

TPN

For neonates where enteral feeding is not possible or advisable most PICUs have a low threshold for starting parenteral nutrition in order to sustain growth and development. They will be aiming for a growth rate of 10 g/kg per day.

Temperature

Thermoregulation is a significant problem for premature neonates compared to term babies. This is due to:

- large surface area to volume ratio
- fewer subcutaneous fat deposits
- less brown fat
- immature development of neurological response to cold.

Great effort has to be made therefore to maintain an appropriate temperature at all times. This can be accomplished by:

- not taking the baby out of the incubator unless essential
- placing the neonate on a warming device if they have to be taken out of the incubator
- keeping the baby well wrapped
- avoiding long procedures
- temperature monitoring.

Surgical pathologies

There are a large number of surgical conditions that can affect neonates. The most common ones are detailed below.

Necrotizing enterocolitis (NEC)

NEC is the most common surgical problem affecting neonates. Risk factors for NEC include:

- prematurity
- very low birthweight
- congenital heart disease/patent ductus arteriosus
- poor umbilical blood flow *in utero*
- perinatal asphyxia.

Its exact cause is uncertain and it is likely to be multifactorial. The idiopathic nature of the condition has led to speculation that it is a perfusion/reperfusion problem; it may also be due to dysregulation of the pro-inflammatory cascade, while some epidemiological patterns point to a possible infective cause.

As the name suggests NEC affects the GI tract. It typically presents with feed intolerance, abdominal distension and bilious aspirates from the NG tube, although signs can be much more subtle. The disease can range in its severity from feed intolerance through to multi-organ failure. The condition can be managed conservatively in the majority of cases. This involves keeping the child nil by mouth for 7–10 days ('gut rest') and giving appropriate antibiotics. However, surgical review should be sought, especially if there are signs of perforation or systemic sepsis.

Findings on the abdominal X-ray can include:

- fixed dilated loops
- bowel wall thickening
- intramural gas
- perforation.

Blood results may show:

- metabolic acidosis
- thrombocytopenia
- white cell count may be raised or worryingly low
- raised lactate.

Supportive therapy may be necessary for multi-organ failure and bacterial translocation. TPN will also be necessary to try to maintain an anabolic state in these very small babies, in an attempt to encourage growth.

Surgical intervention often involves a defunctioning colostomy/ileostomy and/or resection of diseased bowel. This can be extensive. Postoperatively it is important to take note of the extent of gut resection ($<$ 40 cm of remaining small intestine is associated with an increased chance of short gut syndrome, although shorter can be tolerated if the ileo-caecal valve remains in place). Premature neonates deemed too sick for surgery may have intra-abdominal drains sited on the unit instead of surgery. The mortality from NEC can be up to 30% depending on weight and gestation.

Patent ductus arteriosus (PDA)

Persistence of the ductus arteriosus (DA) after day 10 of life is termed a PDA. The duct closes in two stages. Usually the duct undergoes functional closure at about 15 hours, by smooth muscle contraction, followed by true anatomical closure, which can take a couple of weeks. Persistence of the duct is suggested by:

- a characteristic continuous 'machine like' murmur
- a low diastolic blood pressure
- pulmonary overcirculation.

The impact of a PDA depends on the size of the lesion. The signs can be subtle, and so a high degree of suspicion is essential to avoid complications such as:

- heart failure
- pulmonary hypertension
- NEC.

Management can be conservative. Indomethacin is given in an attempt to block production of prostaglandins which maintain patency of the duct. This is, however, associated with an increased risk of GI bleeds, perforation and NEC. If conservative management fails then children may be referred for a surgical ligation of the duct. This is performed without the need for cardiac bypass, through a left-sided thoracotomy incision.

Congenital diaphragmatic hernia (CDH)

As the name suggests, this condition involves development of a fetus with abdominal viscera within the thoracic cavity. Eighty-five per cent of CDH are left-sided; the remainder are either right-sided or bilateral. Over time the repair of CDH has become a relatively straightforward surgical procedure. However, increasing success of surgical intervention has highlighted that the major cause of morbidity and mortality in these children is pulmonary hypoplasia and pulmonary hypertension. In fact the pulmonary hypoplasia is thought to be a primary event during the formation of a CDH (not just a consequence). Up to half of children with CDH will have it as part of another syndrome; therefore a thorough plan of investigation is needed before surgery.

As with other neonatal surgical conditions the timing of surgery is important. Children may initially need HFOV, inhaled nitric oxide and even ECMO. Where possible these will need to be weaned prior to surgery. Predicting outcome in CDH preoperatively can be attempted using the oxygenation index as a means of assessing pulmonary function (being mindful of the site of ABG sampling due to the likely presence of a DA).

Intracranial haemorrhage (ICH)

ICHs are relevant to PICU because children will either develop them during the course of their illness or present for surgery to decompress obstructed CSF drainage by creating a shunt.

Premature neonates are at increased risk of developing intracranial bleeds. This is due to the immature nature of the germinal matrix. The germinal matrix is a highly vascular region of the brain, from which cells migrate outwards during development. Extravasation of blood from the matrix leads to periventricular or intraventricular haemorrhage (PVH/IVH). Other types of intracranial haemorrhages can occur in neonates, e.g. subdural haematomas, but are now less common as obstetric practice improves.

The majority of neonates with ICH are managed conservatively, with correction of coagulopathy and supportive treatment for any consequence of the bleed. Outcome in these children largely depends on the severity of the bleed but is difficult to predict in individuals. IVH and parenchymal bleeding can be diagnosed on ultrasound due to the window provided by the anterior fontanelle.

An intracranial bleed should be suspected in any neonate who:

- shows signs of cerebral irritation
- appears floppy or lethargic
- has a change in neurology associated with a significant drop in haemoglobin
- shows any signs of focal neurological changes.

Although the above gives a list of when to suspect a PVH/IVH, essentially it is prudent to suspect it in any premature neonate who is seriously unwell. It is also wise to remember that any 'ex-prem' child who presents with neurological problems, e.g. meningitis, should be examined carefully for a VP shunt, as this may be driving a CNS infection. Hence a detailed birth history can be of use even in older children.

Prenantal diagnosis of surgical conditions

Prenatal diagnosis of conditions such as gastroschisis, exomphalos and oesophageal atresia has advanced the management of many neonatal surgical conditions. It enables neonatologists to plan the care of neonates, prior to delivery, in a way that minimizes harm and facilitates prompt management. It also allows time to search for associated pathologies; for instance children with conditions such as exomphalos are likely to suffer from other congenital abnormalities (such as trisomies 13, 18 and 21), while oesophageal atresia can be seen in the VACTERL association.

Conditions associated with prematurity

Respiratory distress of the newborn (RDS)

RDS increases in incidence the more premature the neonate. Diagnosis is based on clinical observation, blood gases and a CXR that shows diffuse 'ground glass' type changes. RDS has similarities to adult RDS in terms of being exacerbated by overenthusiastic ventilation and benefiting from early recruitment of collapsed airways. There are, however, major differences. RDS in neonates is a disease of lung immaturity and surfactant deficiency. As such, two interventions that help to decrease the incidence of RDS in newborns are antenatal steroid administration and the early administration of surfactant to 'at risk' neonates. Complications of RDS include:

- pulmonary and intracranial haemorrhage
- PDA
- progression to chronic lung disease.

Once it has developed, management is as mentioned above coupled with supportive care and protective lung ventilation strategies.

Chronic lung disease (CLD)

CLD in neonates is defined as supplemental oxygen dependence at 36-week post menstrual age or 28-day postnatal age in conjunction with persistent clinical respiratory symptoms and compatible abnormalities on CXRs. Although management of this condition is improving, the increased survival of younger preterm babies means that this condition still forms a large burden. Many children with chronic lung disease will have clinically undetectable long-term consequences from CLD, although others will demonstrate a rise in pulmonary vascular resistance, arterial carbon dioxide tension and respiratory rate as well as a lower arterial oxygen tension.

The definition of CLD is also changing as many more babies survive being born at 23 and 24 weeks gestation. This is because these babies will often be oxygen-dependent 28 days after delivery, when their corrected gestational age is still only 27 or 28 weeks. However, they may not require oxygen by the time they are discharged.

Other terminology used in describing lung pathology includes:

- bronchopulmonary dysplasia (BPD) – a term which has had various definitions in the past. It refers to children with chronic lung disease who have been ventilated with IPPV
- pulmonary interstitial emphysema (PIE) – a condition in which air tracks out into the peribronchial space causing obstruction to airflow, pneumothoraces and pneumomediastinum.

Retinopathy of prematurity (ROP)

ROP is a condition that affects premature neonates. Abnormal blood vessels grow in the retina, causing scarring and blindness. Normal retinal vascular growth in the fetus is complete by 36 weeks; however, prematurity, periods of hypoxia and the use of supplemental oxygen before completion of development of the vessels can lead to abnormal growth. Laser therapy can improve outcome and reduces the risk of visual impairment in ROP. It can be performed on very small and sick neonates on PICU.

ROP is one of the reasons that neonatologists previously targeted oxygen saturations of 88–92% on their units as a routine. However, recent evidence points to higher saturations (91–95%) improving outcomes in premature neonates.

Seizures

The causes of seizures in neonates are legion. Searching for a cause requires significant neonatal experience. However, basic correctable causes and life-threatening treatable causes need to be diagnosed quickly. As with adults the basic management of a seizure is straightforward (see Chapter 10). Many of the metabolic causes of seizure activity in a neonate can be detected on a blood gas analysis. They include blood sugar, ionized calcium or plasma sodium concentrations. The first two can be corrected quickly, while the latter needs acute management of the seizure followed by a gradual correction of the sodium (see Chapter 32). Intracranial causes of seizures in neonates include infection and haemorrhage.

A ventilated child may demonstrate seizure activity through autonomic changes. A sharp jump in heart rate and blood pressure coupled with dilated pupils may be the main presentation. Conversely sudden bradycardias in the absence of hypoxia or vagal stimulation may also herald a seizure.

Infection

Although sepsis is often managed on NICU there are occasions when a neonate with sepsis may be admitted to a PICU. Primarily these are when:

- the child has been discharged home prior to acquiring the infection
- when the infection leads to a need for surgical intervention, e.g. congenital HSV causing fulminant liver failure
- the sepsis is associated with a surgical pathology, e.g. volvulus or NEC.

Neonates are more susceptible to infections than older children due to the relative immaturity of their immune system. Premature neonates are at an even higher risk. The commonest organisms affecting neonates can be thought of according to timing of presentation. Early-onset (within 6–72 hours of birth) infections tend to be caused by organisms acquired intrapartum. These include:

- group B *Streptococci*
- Gram-negative enteric bacilli
- *Haemophilus influenzae.*

The pathogens causing later-onset sepsis in a neonate are more likely to have been acquired from the environment. The management of sepsis in neonates follows the same principles as for other children (see Chapter 5). Remember that care should be taken with neonates to pay particular attention to blood sugar and temperature.

Summary

It is impossible to cover the whole of neonatology in one chapter. While there are some similarities in the approach to ITU in neonates to that in adults, the differences become most marked as the child becomes younger. There are fewer 'hard' signs than in older children and treatment often feels as if it is blind. Probably the hardest thing to remember in neonates is that being aggressive in your day-to-day management is not always for the best. A quiet, warm incubator with as few lines as possible, while ensuring adequate caloric intake, is often the best approach. The caveat to this is for time-critical conditions such as sepsis or bleeding.

Golden rules

- Signs of a deteriorating neonate can be very subtle
- ET tubes can block easily due to their narrow lumen
- Flushing cannulae can be the equivalent of a fluid bolus if care is not taken
- Do not take a neonate out of an incubator for practical procedures without some way of keeping them warm
- Despite all of the above, minimal interference and a delicate touch are needed in order to avoid apnoeas and bradycardias in premature neonates

Further reading

Lissauer T, Fanaroff AA. *Neonatology at a Glance*, 2nd edn. Wiley-Blackwell, 2011.

Golden Rules

Quick reference for emergencies

Kasyap Jamalapuram

Normal physiological paramaters

Age	Respiratory rate range (breaths per minute)	Heart rate range (beats per minute)	Systolic blood pressure range (mmHg)
< 1 year	30–60	110–150	70–90
1–5 years	20–40	90–120	80–100
5–12 years	15–30	80–120	90–110
> 12 years	15–25	60–100	100–130

Common equations in emergencies

Weight

- (Age + 4) × 2 = weight in kg

Adrenaline dose in an arrested patient

- 0.1 ml/kg of 1:10 000 concentration

Defibrillator

- 4 × weight = joules (ventricular fibrillation)

Endotracheal tube

- Age/4 + 4 = mm (internal diameter)

Managing the Critically Ill Child, ed. Richard Skone *et al.* Published by Cambridge University Press.

Paediatric Glasgow Coma Scale (child/infant)

Eye opening (E)	
4	Spontaneous
3	To verbal stimuli
2	To painful stimuli
1	No response
C	Eyes closed due to swelling/bandage

Verbal		Grimace	
5	Alert, babbles, coos, words or to normal ability	5	Spontaneous normalfacial/oro-motor activity
4	Less than usual ability or spontaneous/irritable cry	4	Less than usual spontaneous ability or only response to touch stimulus
3	Cries inappropriately	3	Vigorous grimace to pain
2	Occasionally whimpers and/or moans	2	Mild grimace to pain
1	No response	1	No response
T	Intubated		

Motor	
6	Normal spontaneous movements
5	Withdraws to touch
4	Withdraws to painful stimuli
3	Abnormal flexion to pain
2	Abnormal extension to pain
1	No response to pain

Section 5 Golden Rules

Chapter 36

Drug infusions

Kasyap Jamalapuram

Table 36.1. Commonly used drugs for critically ill children.

Drug	Dose to draw up	Dilute to 50 ml total volume with:	Rate/dose equivalents	Dose range
Adrenaline (central)	0.3 mg/kg	5% Dex/10% Dex/NS	1ml/h = 0.1 μg/kg/min	0.01–1.0 μg/kg/min
Adrenaline (peripheral – discuss with PICU)	¼ of above strength (0.07 5 mg/kg)	5% Dex/10% Dex/NS	1ml/h = 0.025 μg/kg/min	0.01–1.0 μg/kg/min
Noradrenaline (central)	0.3 mg/kg	5% Dex/10% Dex/NS	1ml/h = 0.1 μg/kg/min	0.01–1.0 μg/kg/min
Dobutamine (central)	15 mg/kg	5% Dex/10% Dex/NS	1ml/h = 5 μg/kg/min	1.0–20 μg/kg/min
Morphine	1 mg/kg	5% Dex/10% Dex/NS	1ml/h = 20 μg/kg/h	10–40 μg/kg/h
Midazolam (> 33 kg)	100 mg	5% Dex/10% Dex/NS	(wt × 0.03) ml/h = 1 μg/kg/min	0.5–3.0 μg/kg/min
Midazolam (< 33 kg)	3 mg/kg	5% Dex/10% Dex/NS	1 ml/h = 1 μg/kg/min	0.5–3.0 μg/kg/min
Prostaglandin E1/E2	50 μg	5% Dex/10% Dex/NS	(wt × 0.3) ml/h = 5 ng/kg/min	5.0–20 ng/kg/min
Salbutamol (peripheral)	10 mg	5% Dex/NS	(wt × 0.3) ml/h = 1 μg/kg/min	1.0–2.0 μg/kg/min
Aminophyline (> 50 kg)	1250 mg	5% Dex/10% Dex/NS	(wt/50) ml/h = 0.5 mg/kg/h	0.5–1.0 μg/kg/h
Aminophyline (< 50 kg)	25 mg/kg	5% Dex/10% Dex/NS	1 ml/h = 0.5 mg/kg/h	0.5–1.0 μg/kg/h
Insulin for DKA (> 20 kg)	50 units	5% Dex/10% Dex/NS	(wt/10) ml/h = 0.1 units/kg/h	005–0.1 units/kg/h
Insulin for DKA (< 20 kg)	2.5 units/kg	5% Dex/10% Dex/NS	2 ml/h = 0.1 units/kg/h	005–0.1 units/kg/h

Peripheral-strength adrenaline needs to be used with great caution. Only in emergency, via a good IV cannula (to avoid extravasation). Consider IO administration instead.

Managing the Critically Ill Child, ed. Richard Skone *et al.* Published by Cambridge University Press.

Table 36.2. Drugs used to lower plasma ammonia in IMD.

Drug	Mode of action	Conditions	Dose	Notes
Sodium benzoate	Scavenges ammonia by converting to hippuric acid, which is excreted in urine	Urea cycle disorders Organic acidurias with hyperammonaemia, e.g. PA, MMA, IVA – when carglumic acid 250 mg/kg PO/NG is not available	250 mg/kg loading dose over 90 min then 250 mg/kg/day	Maximum peripheral concentration 50 mg/ml
Sodium phenylbutyrate	Scavenges ammonia by converting to phenylacetic acid, which is excreted in urine	Urea cycle disorders	250 mg/kg loading dose over 90 min then 250 mg/kg/day	Maximum peripheral concentration 50 mg/ml
L-Arginine	Replenishes urea cycle for continued function despite enzyme block	Urea cycle disorders	150 mg/kg loading dose over 90 min then 150 mg/kg/day	Double dose can be used in citrullinaemia and argininosuccinic aciduria

References

KIDS. West Midlands regional retrieval service website: http://kids.bch.nhs.uk/wp-content/uploads/2011/10/KIDS-Infusion-guideV1.pdf.

KIDS drug calculator: http://kids.bch.nhs.uk/wp-content/uploads/2011/10/Drug_Calculator_V1.pdf.

Chapter 37

Top tips for practical procedures

Steven Cray

Airway management

- If the airway is compromised for non-infective reasons, always consider a nasopharyngeal airway or placing the child in the prone position
- Paediatric colleagues and the local retrieval service are a resource of useful information, e.g. whether the child is syndromic and a potentially difficult intubation
- Difficult laryngoscopy is rare in children and usually predictable – if in doubt keep them breathing
- Don't overextend the head when managing the airway and intubating infants or children
- Placing a NG tube before induction in a neonate and infant facilitates stomach decompression
- Preoxygenation may be ineffective in children – don't be afraid to gently ventilate following induction, even if an RSI
- A roll under the shoulders of an infant may aid laryngoscopy
- Laryngeal pressure is a useful means of improving laryngoscopic view in young children
- Incorrectly applied cricoid pressure may make laryngoscopy more difficult – don't be afraid to remove it
- The paediatric larynx is funnel-shaped; a circular motion of the tip of an ET tube will help its passage
- The tongue is your biggest enemy when intubating children – make sure you get it out of the way during laryngoscopy
- The epiglottis is long and floppy in younger children – consider placing the laryngoscope blade posterior to the epiglottis when attempting intubation
- Always have a bougie handy to intubate a child with suspected C-spine injury
- Children can desaturate very quickly during laryngoscopy attempts – do not persist too hard or too long to intubate
- The commonest error in ET tube placement is a tube which is too small and too long
- Failed endotracheal intubation is not a disaster – the laryngeal mask airway is a perfectly reasonable, temporary, alternative
- A neutral head position is required for a CXR in order to evaluate ET tube position

Managing the Critically Ill Child, ed. Richard Skone *et al.* Published by Cambridge University Press.

Vascular access and circulation

- Long sapheonous and scalp veins are often easier to access than veins in small arms and hands
- IO needles should be used if IV access cannot be obtained within 90 seconds in a critically ill child
- IO access is the first choice access in a paediatric arrest situation (if no cannula *in situ*)
- Paediatric veins can be transfixed and successfully cannulated – always remove needle and slowly withdraw cannula following an attempt, even if there was no flashback initially
- Always use isotonic fluids for resuscitation in children
- Don't be afraid to administer volume resuscitation quickly in sick children – they tolerate it extremely well
- An increase in blood pressure with gentle pressure on the liver may be an indication of hypovolaemia

Central line

- Ultrasound should be used to identify the vein and during line placement
- Children who have complex past medical histories may have central veins that have been occluded following previous lines. It is important to establish vein patency before attempting insertion
- The internal jugular and femoral veins are most commonly used for central venous access in children. There is no difference in the incidence of infection between the two sites in children
- The internal jugular vein is generally very easily identified with ultrasound. The femoral vein is a smaller vessel and may be more difficult to distinguish from other structures
- For infants a 4.5 or 5FG triple-lumen line is appropriate for internal jugular placement. For femoral access in babies a 4.5FG line is more suitable because of the smaller size of the vein
- A femoral line may be transduced for a central venous pressure measurement; this is generally a good reflection of right atrial pressure
- For femoral venous insertion aim to have the catheter tip at L3 level (below the level of the renal veins). The optimal insertion length (cm) $= 0.45 \times$ body weight (kg) $+ 8.13$. This gives an insertion length of 10 cm in a 4 kg baby, for example
- Reverse Trendelenburg position, hepatic pressure and Valsalva manoeuvre can all increase the diameter of the femoral vein
- Give at least one fluid bolus before attempting central line insertion

Arterial line

- The patient should be positioned carefully. For example for radial artery access the wrist can be extended over a roll of gauze and immobilized with tape. A pad under the bottom will help with femoral access in infants
- A transfixition technique is generally necessary when cannulating an artery in a small child
- Use arteries where you can feel a pulse – don't waste time trying peripherally if the arteries are impalpable. Use the femoral artery (or axillary artery if necessary)
- A Babywire (0.012″) should always be available when attempting arterial cannulation in small children
- The brachial artery should not be cannulated in premature neonates
- 22G is suitable for most infants and children, although 24G is used in premature neonates and small babies
- Seldinger-type cannulae are well suited to the femoral artery as standard cannulae may be too short
- An aseptic technique should be used – especially for femoral arterial lines
- The use of ultrasound should be considered for femoral and axillary sites

Urethral catheters

Age	Weight (kg)	French gauge
0–6 months	3.5–7	6
1 year	10	6–8
2 years	12	8
3 years	14	8–10
5 years	18	10
6 years	21	12
8 years	27	12
12 years	varies	12–14

NG tubes

Age	Weight (kg)	NG tube (French gauge)
0–6 months	3.5–7	8–10
1 year	10	10
2 years	12	10
3 years	14	10–12
5 years	18	12
6 years	21	12
8 years	27	14
12 years	varies	14–16

Chest drains

Age	Chest drain size (French gauge)
Newborn	8–12Fr
Infant	12–16Fr
Child	16–24Fr
Adolescent	20–32Fr

Section 5 Golden Rules

Chapter 38

UK vaccination schedule

Richard Skone

Age	Vaccinations given	Indication
Birth	BCG	Regional variations – usually given if family members from areas where TB is endemic
	Hepatitis B (with/without immunoglobulin within 12 hours of birth)	If mother is a carrier . Boosters at 1 month, 2 months and 12 months
2 months	DTaP/IPV/Hib: diphtheria, tetanus, pertussis, polio, *Haemophilus influenzae* type b Pneumococcus	Routine vaccinations
3 months	DTaP/IPV/Hib Meningitis C	Routine vaccinations
4 months	DTaP/IPV/Hib: Pneumococcus Meningitis C	Routine vaccinations
12 months	Hib/MenC: *Haemophilus influenzae* type b, Meningitis C MMR: measles, mumps, rubella Pneumococcus	Routine vaccinations
Pre-school boosters (3.5–5yrs)	DTaP/IPV: diphtheria, tetanus, pertussis, polio MMR	Routine vaccinations
Girls 12–13yrs	Human papillomavirus vaccine (three injections at 0, 2 and 6 months)	Routine vaccinations
13–18 yrs	Td/IPV: Tetanus, diphtheria Polio	Routine vaccinations

The BCG and MMR vaccinations are live vaccinations and therefore cannot be used in immunocompromised children.

Managing the Critically Ill Child, ed. Richard Skone *et al.* Published by Cambridge University Press.

Chapter 39

Common syndromes in the critically ill child

Oliver Bagshaw

Introduction

There are nearly 7000 described syndromes and diseases that are known to occur in children. Syndromes may be caused by:

- chromosome abnormalities
- single gene defects
- familial association
- the environment
- no apparent reason.

It is impossible for even an experienced paediatrician to have knowledge of all possible syndromes. However, every doctor should have an understanding of the common syndromes that have implications in the critically ill child.

A syndrome is defined as a group of symptoms and signs that are characteristic of a particular disorder. Many conditions in children that have implications for the anaesthetist do not have the term 'syndrome' associated with them. However, for the sake of completeness, we will assume that all of the conditions mentioned in this chapter have the characteristics of a syndrome.

In keeping with the fact that most of these children will be encountered in a resuscitation scenario, the information on each condition is presented in an 'ABC' format, so that the treating clinician can quickly refer to the specific, relevant abnormalities in a systematic manner.

Common syndromes

Down syndrome

Trisomy 21 (Down syndrome) is one of the commonest, best-known and most easily recognized chromosome abnormality syndromes in children. It occurs in about 1.5 per 1000 live births, the incidence increasing with increasing maternal age.

Airway

Trisomy 21 causes the following difficulties when managing the airway:

Managing the Critically Ill Child, ed. Richard Skone *et al.* Published by Cambridge University Press.

- a large tongue, which is more likely to protrude from the mouth; this may make attempts at intubation more difficult, as the tongue may have a tendency to herniate over the laryngoscope blade and obscure the view of the larynx
- a narrower than normal larynx, which in some cases may be related to subglottic stenosis; an endotracheal tube 0.5–1 mm ID smaller than predicted should be used, to avoid causing laryngeal oedema and post-extubation stridor.

Breathing

There is an increased incidence of respiratory tract complications due to a number of different factors. These include:

- airway abnormalities
- hypotonia
- relative obesity
- cardiovascular anomalies
- immune deficiency
- gastroesophageal reflux
- obstructive sleep apnoea.

Sedative and narcotic agents are likely to make this worse and should be used with caution in the non-intubated patient.

Circulation

Cardiovascular anomalies occur in up to 50% of children with trisomy 21. The commonest anomalies are (see Chapter 6 for details):

- ventriculoseptal defect (VSD); depending on the size this may cause significant left to right shunting
- endocardial cushion defect, which most often presents with atrioventricular septal defect and left to right shunting of blood
- persistent ductus arteriosus – like endocardial cushion defects, this can lead to increased pulmonary blood flow and heart failure
- tetralogy of Fallot; this leads to reduced pulmonary flow and hypoxia.

Another feature of these children is increased atropine sensitivity. This should be taken into account if administering atropine for vagolytic effects. However, they are also characterized by reduced sympathetic activity, which may counteract this effect.

Disability

Neurological problems include:

- significant learning disabilities, which may compromise understanding of any intended interventions; parental presence may help to calm any fears and anxieties
- atlantoaxial instability, which may be found in up to 20% of children with trisomy 21; it should be assumed to be present unless radiological investigations have proved otherwise; frank atlantoaxial subluxation with spinal cord compression is much rarer (2%) and is nearly always associated with neurological symptoms, including:
  - neck pain
  - decreased mobility

- abnormal gait
- torticollis
- sensory deficits.

The head should be maintained in the neutral position when intubating these patients and when managing them post-intubation.

Other

- Hypothyroidism.
- Potential for haematological malignancies, such as acute lymphoblastic leukaemia, with anaemia, thrombocytopenia and increased infection risk.
- Increased sensitivity to volatile anaesthetic agents.

Cystic fibrosis

Cystic fibrosis (CF) is an inherited disorder of the chloride channels in various epithelial surfaces, resulting in the production of abnormally viscid secretions, which block organ passages. The frequency of occurrence depends on ethnic group, with Caucasian people having the highest incidence (1 in 3000 live births).

Airway

There are no airway abnormalities attributable to this condition. However, patients with CF are prone to gastroesophageal reflux, with an incidence of approximately 20% in children.

Breathing

One of the most prominent features of CF is the pulmonary manifestation of the disease. Mucus plugging and pulmonary infiltrates lead to recurrent chest infections, which may in turn lead to:

- chronic cough
- pulmonary obstructive disease
- bronchiectasis
- haemoptysis
- hypoxia
- cor pulmonale.

Intubation may be straightforward, but ventilation can be problematic, with copious secretions, bronchospasm, atelectasis, hypoxaemia, gas trapping and barotrauma all occurring in anaesthetized patients.

Active infection, particularly in the lungs, should always be considered in these patients – *Pseudomonas aeruginosa* and *Staphylococcus aureus* are the most common infecting organisms.

Circulation

Advanced lung disease may have secondary effects on the CVS, with the development of pulmonary hypertension, right ventricular failure and cor pulmonale. Intubating patients with known pulmonary hypertension is a high-risk procedure. Expert advice should be sought first, where possible.

Disability

Children with CF do not usually suffer from intellectual impairment.

Other

- Patients with CF may be malnourished and underweight, due to impaired pancreatic exocrine function, although this is proving less of a problem with modern enzyme therapy.
- The endocrine function of the pancreas may be affected as well, leading to diabetes mellitus. Hypo- or hyperglycaemia should always be considered in a patient with CF who has a depressed conscious level.
- Hepatic involvement may lead to impaired function, with cholestasis and reduced production of clotting factors.

Muscular dystrophy

Several types of muscular dystrophy (MD) exist; some exhibit X-linked inheritance (Duchenne, Becker) while others demonstrate autosomal dominant inheritance (limb-girdle, facioscapulohumeral). All patients are characterized by an abnormality of the dystrophin proteins in skeletal muscle, which leads to impaired function. The muscle dysfunction varies in both severity and the muscles affected, depending on the type of dystrophy. Weakness is usually progressive and leads to significant disability. Duchenne (DMD) is the commonest and most severe form of the disease.

Airway

There are no specific airway problems for patients with muscular dystrophy, although patients have been reported with a larger than normal tongue. Other problems include:

- swallowing difficulties, which may lead to recurrent aspiration
- gastric hypomotility, which may also increase the aspiration risk.

Breathing

- Progressive respiratory and abdominal muscle weakness is characteristic. Combined with aspiration episodes, this makes recurrent chest infections common.
- Diaphragmatic function is initially preserved, but will eventually deteriorate. Respiratory failure is the main mode of death.
- Scoliosis is often present and may lead to restrictive lung problems.

Circulation

As a muscle, the heart is often affected in patients with muscular dystrophy.

- Patients may develop cardiomyopathy. They may be relatively asymptomatic, due to limited activity. Heart failure often appears in adolescence.
- Arrhythmias are rare, but can occur with fibrosis of the conducting system, and may include heart block. The ECG is usually abnormal, with sinus tachycardia, tall R waves in the right chest leads and deep Q waves in the left chest leads.
- Hyperkalaemia and cardiac arrest may occur following administration of suxamethonium or volatile anaesthetic agents. Suxamethonium is contraindicated in MD and volatile anaesthetic agents should be used with caution.

Disability

- Developmental delay occurs in some, but not all patients.
- Difficulty with verbal communication may be related to respiratory failure.

Other

- Patients may be obese, due to replacement of muscle with fat, and inactivity.
- The association between MD and malignant hyperthermia is unproven and probably does not exist.
- Congenital adrenal hypoplasia may also be present, necessitating steroid-replacement therapy.

CHARGE association

CHARGE is an autosomal dominant disorder characterized by a number of different but characteristic abnormalities. Not all are present in patients, although several of the major and minor features need to be present for the diagnosis to be made. CHARGE is an acronym of several of the common features (Coloboma, Heart defects, Atresia of choanae, Retarded growth, Genital abnormalities, Ear abnormalities).

Airway

- Choanal atresia or stenosis may be present, resulting in complete airway obstruction or respiratory distress. This will usually have been treated in older children, but re-stenosis can occur and the nasal passages may be small for age.
- Cleft lip and/or palate.
- Cranial nerve involvement can lead to swallowing problems.
- Profuse oral secretion production is characteristic of the condition.
- Laryngomalacia may be present, causing stridor.

Breathing

- Recurrent aspiration may occur in relation to profuse secretions, swallowing difficulties or the presence of a trachea-oesophageal fistula.
- Vertebral anomalies such as hemivertebrae and scoliosis may give rise to restrictive lung disease.
- Facial abnormalities may make facemask ventilation difficult.

Circulation

- Congenital heart defects such as septal defects, conotruncal abnormalities and vessel stenosis are very common.

Disability

Common findings in this association are:

- developmental delay
- hearing loss
- cranial nerve anomalies
- seizure disorder.

Other

- Renal abnormalities may occur which can adversely affect renal function.
- Truncal hypotonia.

VATER/VACTERL association

This condition is also a collection of congenital abnormalities, characterized by the main features of Vertebral anomalies, Anal atresia, (Cardiac defects), Tracheo-Esophageal fistula, Renal and Limb abnormalities. Many other abnormal features have been described.

Airway

- Choanal atresia may lead to airway obstruction.
- Micrognathia may cause airway obstruction and difficulties with intubation.
- Tracheo-oesophageal fistula may cause recurrent aspiration and difficulty in bagging as the stomach distends.

Breathing

- Aspiration and pneumonia from trachea-oesophageal fistula.
- Hypoplastic lungs.
- Restrictive lung disease from vertebral anomalies and scoliosis.
- Increased pulmonary blood flow secondary to congenital heart disease.

Circulation

The cardiac defects seen in VACTERL association include:

- VSD
- PDA
- tetralogy of Fallot
- transposition of the great arteries.

Disability

The condition can be associated with hydrocephalus and other CNS abnormalities such as absent corpus callosum.

Other

- Renal anomalies are very common, including urethral atresia, renal agenesis and hydronephrosis.
- Bowel obstruction secondary to imperforate anus or duodenal atresia may occur.
- Limb abnormalities may make IV and arterial access difficult.

Inborn errors of metabolism

The inborn errors of metabolism (IEM) constitute a constellation of conditions characterized by deficiencies of certain enzymes. Under certain conditions this can lead to an accumulation of toxic metabolites (see Chapter 12).

More severe symptoms usually occur in the neonate and infant, when a diagnosis has often not yet been made. Decompensation nearly always occurs as a result of metabolic stress, due to intercurrent illness, change in feed or a period of starvation. An IEM should always be considered in the differential diagnosis of the collapsed infant.

Airway

- Encephalopathy and coma are a common presenting feature and may lead to loss of the airway.
- Seizure may also occur and lead to airway compromise.
- Vomiting may lead to aspiration.

Breathing

- Apnoea is a common presenting feature in encephalopathic infants.
- Respiratory distress and increased work of breathing may be present as a result of LRTI, acidosis or ammonia-induced central hyperventilation.

Circulation

- Cardiomyopathy may develop in older children (see Chapter 12).
- Circulatory collapse may be due to the accumulation of cardiotoxic metabolites.
- Poor feeding and vomiting may have led to significant dehydration.
- Primary or secondary lactic acidosis may be present, with a profound anion gap.

Disability

Neurological signs are often the most significant presenting feature of the infant with IEM. Causes include:

- encephalopathy and coma (usually secondary to hyperammonaemia)
- seizures
- hypoglycaemia
- raised intracranial pressure
- 'shock' and poor cerebral perfusion
- profound metabolic derangement.

Don't forget possible underlying CNS infection as a cause of neurological abnormality Older children may already have developed significant developmental delay

Other

- Hepatic disturbances are common in the acute stages of illness.
- Key management actions include administration of glucose-containing IV solutions, urgent PICU referral if significant hyperammonaemia is present (poor outcome if treatment is delayed), administration of carnitine, benzoate and phenylacetate and urgent consultation with an IMD specialist.

Mucopolysaccharidoses

The name includes several conditions characterized by deficiency of the enzymes responsible for mucopolysaccharide degradation in tissues. Accumulation of mucopolysaccharides in various tissues leads to progressive cellular damage and destruction.

Airway

These children provide a particular challenge for anyone trying to manage their airway. Even hand ventilation may be difficult. This is due to:

- the presence of a large, thick tongue, short neck and immobile cervical spine, which can make these patients very difficult to intubate; the problem tends to get worse as the child gets older
- obstructive sleep apnoea, which is commonly present
- copious secretions necessitating antisialogogue treatment
- MPS deposition in the airway, which may mean that a smaller than anticipated ET Tube needs to be used.

Breathing

- Skeletal deformities and chest wall involvement may lead to restrictive lung disease.
- Thick secretions may increase the risk of respiratory complications, including recurrent chest infections.

Circulation

Cardiac involvement presents as:

- valvular disease such as mitral and aortic valve thickening
- left ventricular hypertrophy
- pulmonary hypertension.

Disability

In addition to developmental delay these children may have physical problems such as:

- odontoid hypoplasia, creating instability of the cervical spine
- progressive narrowing of the spinal canal, which may cause myelopathy, which can be worsened by recurrent flexion and extension of the cervical spine
- hydrocephalus.

Other

- Prolonged bleeding times can occur in some conditions.
- Joint contractures.
- Coarse, dry skin making IV access more difficult.

Specialist paediatric metabolic units dealing with MPS patients are a good source of advice and in the UK are situated in Manchester Children's Hospital, Birmingham Children's Hospital and Great Ormond Street Hospital, London.

Summary

Due to the large and varied number of conditions that may be encountered in critically ill children, it is best for the attending physicians to use their combined knowledge and experience to manage the child appropriately. Table 39.1 is a brief summary of some of the problems that may be encountered in syndromic children and the specific syndromes to which they relate.

Table 39.1. Pathological conditions that may be encountered during critical care management and some of the syndromes in which they are most common.[a]

	Problem	Syndromes
Airway	Obstructed upper airway	Choanal atresia, craniosynostoses, Beckwith syndrome, cystic hygroma
	Difficult intubation	Pierre–Robin syndrome, Goldenhar syndrome, Treacher–Collins syndrome, hemifacial microsomia, MPS, osteopetrosis, epidermolysis bullosa, Klippel–Feil syndrome, cystic hygroma
	Impaired bulbar function	Myasthenia gravis, leukodystrophy
Breathing	Hypoventilation	Spinal muscular atrophy, muscular dystrophy, central hypoventilation syndrome, myasthenia gravis, Leigh disease, Jeune syndrome
	Diaphragmatic weakness	Myasthenia gravis, SMA, muscular dystrophy, mitochondrial disease
	Increased risk of chest infection	Cystic fibrosis, cerebral palsy, myopathies, sickle-cell disease, MPS, pulmonary alveolar proteinosis, prune belly, immune deficiency syndromes
	Restrictive lung disease	Prader–Willi syndrome, achondroplasia, Jeune syndrome, MPS, arthrogryposis, osteopetrosis
Circulation	Congenital cardiac abnormalities	Down syndrome, VACTERL, CHARGE, DiGeorge syndrome, velocardiofacial syndrome, Noonan syndrome, Marfan syndrome, Turner syndrome, Shone complex, Alagille syndrome, Cornelia de Lange syndrome
	Cardiomyopathy	Muscular dystrophy, Pompe disease, IEM, MPS, haemochromatosis, mitochondrial disease, Friedrich ataxia, Kawasaki disease, arthrogryposis, SLE
	Arrhythmias	Wolf–Parkinson–White syndrome, Prader–Willi syndrome, congenital lupus, Lown–Ganong–Levine syndrome, long QT syndrome, Rett syndrome
	Raised lactate	Mitochondrial disease, Leigh disease, pyruvate dehydrogenate deficiency
Disability	Raised ICP	Achondroplasia, craniosynostoses, Dandy–Walker malformation, Arnold–Chiari malformation, spina bifida
	Unstable cervical spine	MPS, achondroplasia, Klippel–Feil, Ehlers–Danlos, arthrogryposis
	Hypoglycaemia	MCADD, Prader-Willi syndrome, glycogen storage disease, Beckwith syndrome, several IEM
	Seizures	Cerebral palsy, several IEM (particularly with hyperammonaemia), leukodystrophy, Lennox–Gastaut syndrome, Dandy–Walker malformation, absent corpus callosum, Cornelia de Lange syndrome, West syndrome, tuberous sclerosis, Sturge–Weber syndrome, Rett syndrome
Other	Hepatic insufficiency	Alagille syndrome, haemochromatosis, glycogen storage disease, mitochondrial disease, galactosamia, Budd–Chiari syndrome, α_1-antitrypsin deficiency, Wilson disease, tyrosinaemia
	Renal insufficiency	Nephrotic syndrome, haemolytic–uraemic syndrome, Goodpasture syndrome, polycystic kidney disease, SLE
	Scoliosis	Muscular dystrophy, achondroplasia, osteogenesis imperfecta, CHARGE, cerebral palsy, spinal muscular atrophy, Prader-Willi syndrome, neurofibromatosis, Marfan syndrome, Klippel–Feil syndrome, arthrogryposis
	Malignant hyperpyrexia risk	Central core disease, multiminicore disease, King–Denborough syndrome, Brody myopathy
	Anaemia	Sickle-cell disease, thalassaemia, haemoglobin C disease, G-6-PD deficiency, haemolytic uraemic syndrome, hereditary spherocytosis, Fanconi anaemia, Diamond–Blackfan anaemia

[a]Muscular dystrophies are not thought to be associated with malignant hyperpyrexia, although triggering agents such as halothane and suxamethonium can precipitate rhabdomyolysis and hyperkalaemia. Suxamethonium should also be avoided in any other myopathic or neuropathic disorder that causes significant muscular weakness, due to the risks of massive potassium release and life-threatening arrhythmias.

IEM, inborn errors of metabolism; MCADD, medium chain acyl-coA dehydrogenase deficiency; MPS, mucopolysaccharidosis; SLE, systemic lupus erythematosus; G-6-PD, glucose-6-phosphate dehydrogenase.

Further reading

Baum VC, O'Flaherty JE. *Anesthesia for Genetic, Metabolic, and Dysmorphic Syndromes of Childhood*, 2nd edn. Lippincott, Williams and Wilkins, 2007.

Bissonnette B, Dalens B. *Syndromes: Rapid Recognition and Perioperative Implications.* McGraw-Hill Professional, 2006.

http://www.orpha.net.

http://www.rarediseases.org.

Index